Nutrition in ICU Patients

Andreas Rümelin · Konstantin Mayer
Thomas W. Felbinger
Editors

Nutrition in ICU Patients

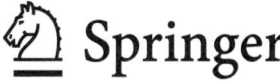

Editors
Andreas Rümelin
Department of Anesthesiology
Hospital "Land Hadeln"
Otterndorf, Germany

Thomas W. Felbinger
Department of Anesthesiology,
Perioperative and Pain Medicine,
Harlaching and Neuperlach Medical Centers
The Munich Municipal Hospitals Group Ltd
München, Germany

Konstantin Mayer
Department of Pneumology
Infectiology, and Sleep Medicine,
ViDia Hospitals
Karlsruhe, Germany

Faculty of Medicine
University of Giessen
Giessen, Germany

ISBN 978-3-032-00817-6   ISBN 978-3-032-00818-3 (eBook)
https://doi.org/10.1007/978-3-032-00818-3

Translation from the German language edition: "Ernährung des Intensivpatienten" by Andreas Rümelin et al., © Springer-Verlag Berlin Heidelberg 2013. Published by Springer. All Rights Reserved.

© The Editor(s) (if applicable) and The Author(s), under exclusive license to Springer Nature Switzerland AG 2025

This work is subject to copyright. All rights are solely and exclusively licensed by the Publisher, whether the whole or part of the material is concerned, specifically the rights of reprinting, reuse of illustrations, recitation, broadcasting, reproduction on microfilms or in any other physical way, and transmission or information storage and retrieval, electronic adaptation, computer software, or by similar or dissimilar methodology now known or hereafter developed.
The use of general descriptive names, registered names, trademarks, service marks, etc. in this publication does not imply, even in the absence of a specific statement, that such names are exempt from the relevant protective laws and regulations and therefore free for general use.
The publisher, the authors and the editors are safe to assume that the advice and information in this book are believed to be true and accurate at the date of publication. Neither the publisher nor the authors or the editors give a warranty, express or implied, with respect to the material contained herein or for any errors or omissions that may have been made.

This Springer imprint is published by the registered company Springer Nature Switzerland AG
The registered company address is: Gewerbestrasse 11, 6330 Cham, Switzerland

If disposing of this product, please recycle the paper.

Foreword

Let food be thy medicine and medicine be thy food.
  —Hippocrates

In 1883, the Russian poet and physician Anton Chekhov (1860–1904) described the medical history of a 61-year-old female patient hospitalized with severe lobar pneumonia, a mostly fatal condition in the pre-antibiotic era. Chekhov prescribed a low-carbohydrate diet, consisting of soups, milk, eggs, and low amounts of meat. The patient recovered after 29 days of critical illness [1]. This case vignette points out the significance of diets as a cornerstone in the treatment of critically ill patients in the nineteenth century.

Times have changed—but isn't high-quality, evidence-based nutritional therapy still one of the cornerstones of therapy for critically ill patients?

Since the evolution of the first modern Critical Care Unit at the University of Pittsburgh in 1959, intensive care medicine revolutionized the treatment of critical illness worldwide from the end of the 1980s onwards [2].

Developments in nutritional therapy initially kept pace with this revolution.

In 1968, Dudrick et al. fed beagle puppies with a solution of dextrose, protein hydrolysate, vitamins, and minerals via a central venous line for up to 256 days. They were the first to show that normal and comparable growth and development could be achieved in animals fed entirely intravenously [3]. In 1974, Jurgens et al. from St. Georg Hospital Hamburg, Germany, designed programmes of parenteral nutrition with emulsified fat for infants and children [4]. In 1980, Gauterer et al. described the first endoscopic placement of a gastrostomy tube [5].

To foster research, the American Society for Parenteral and Enteral Nutrition (ASPEN) was founded in 1975, followed by the establishment of European Society for Parenteral and Enteral Nutrition (ESPEN) in 1980.

Due to major advances in supportive treatment of acute organ failure, more and more patients subsequently survived the initial phase of conditions such as septic or cardiogenic shock, fecal peritonitis, multiple trauma, or extensive burns. About a quarter, however, enter the chronic phase of critical illness, during which they require vital organ support often for weeks, sometimes months. The term protracted critical illness was coined for this condition at the end of the 1990s. Nutrition was increasingly considered a potential intervention to attenuate muscle wasting and improve functional recovery.

Groundbreaking research came from the group of Greet van den Berghe, Leuven, Belgium, who was able to show that protracted critical illness, characterized by feeding-resistant wasting of protein and reesterification of fatty acids, is associated with a low-activity status of the somatotropic and thyrotropic axis [6].

Artificial nutrition is nowadays routinely provided to the majority of patients admitted to the intensive care unit (ICU) with enteral nutrition administered twice as frequently as parenteral nutrition (48% versus 24%) [7].

Despite this, we still have an incomplete understanding about the optimal route, timing, and dose to provide. Clinical practice guidelines are largely based on expert opinion or observational data rather than on evidence. The ASPEN 2016 Critical Care Guidelines provide 95 individual recommendations, of which just 3 are based on high or moderate-to-high quality evidence (i.e., a high-quality randomized controlled trial (RCT)) and 55 are based on "expert opinion" alone [8].

It is therefore not surprising that many established nutritional therapy practices that were based on expert consensus or low-quality studies have been refuted by recent large multicentric randomized trials. A prominent example had been the concept of intensive insulin therapy for the treatment of stress hyperglycaemia, which was enthusiastically recommended in many clinical practice guidelines since 2001, but did not take into account the influence of accompanying high-dose parenteral glucose therapy to avoid severe hypoglycaemia [9].

A recent review article by Arabi et al. highlighted the future intensive care medicine research agenda in nutrition and metabolism [10]. The authors recommend to initiate RCT's on the topics of (1) the optimal protein dose combined with standardized active and passive mobilization during different phases of critical illness, (2) nutritional assessment, (3) nutritional strategies in critically obese patients, and (4) on the effects of continuous versus intermittent enteral nutrition [10].

As a critical care trialist, I strongly agree with the recommendations made regarding phase III (efficacy) RCTs trial design in nutritional support.

First, patient-centred outcomes must include long-term functional outcomes. Surrogate outcomes are misleading in clinical efficacy trials and should not be used. *Second*, phase III RCTs must be adequately powered and power calculations must be performed using realistic event rates and expected effect size. *Third*, the time course of critical illness must be taken into account. It is of utmost importance to distinguish between acute, subacute, and chronic critical illness. *Fourth*, the heterogeneity of the critical care population must be taken into account. The focus should be on patients with organ failure, in which outcomes are likely to be most influenced by nutritional support. Further, specific phenotypes should be identified (e.g., patients with previous poor nutrition, postoperative patients, and those with sepsis).

The importance of nutrition in critical care is increasingly recognized. However, the implementation of randomized clinical trials requires public funding, and additional efforts are required to convince public funding bodies to support these trials in the future.

The textbook *Nutrition in the ICU* makes an important contribution to this.

I would like to thank the editors and authors for their efforts to provide an excellent up-to-date overview about what we know and what we don't in nutritional therapy for the critically ill.

Suggested Readings

1. Steger F, Kosenko O. Diagnosis and treatment of lobar pneumonia in the pre-antibiotic era Anton Chekhov's medical report (1883). Microbes Infect. 2022;24(2):104889. https://doi.org/10.1016/j.micinf.2021.104889.
2. Weil MH, Tang W. From intensive care to critical care medicine: a historical perspective. Am J Respir Crit Care Med. 2011;183(11):1451–3. https://doi.org/10.1164/rccm.201008-1341OE. Epub 2011 Jan 21. PMID: 21257788.
3. Dudrick SJ, Wilmore DW, Vars HM, Rhoads JE. Long-term total parenteral nutrition with growth, development, and positive nitrogen balance. Surgery. 1968;64(1):134–42. PMID: 4968812.
4. Jürgens P, Dolif D, Panteliadis C, Hofert C. Controlled parenteral nutrition of premature infants. In: Parenteral nutrition in infancy and childhood. vol. 46. 1974. ISBN: 978-1-4684-3251-0.
5. Gauderer MW, Ponsky JL, Izant RJ Jr. Gastrostomy without laparotomy: a percutaneous endoscopic technique. J Pediatr Surg. 1980;15(6):872–5. https://doi.org/10.1016/s0022-3468(80)80296-x. PMID: 6780678.
6. Van den Berghe G, de Zegher F, Bouillon R. Clinical review 95: acute and prolonged critical illness as different neuroendocrine paradigms. J Clin Endocrinol Metab. 1998;83(6):1827–34. https://doi.org/10.1210/jcem.83.6.4763. PMID: 9626104.
7. Hiesmayr M, Fischer A, Veraar C, Mora B, Tarantino S, Weimann A, Volkert D. Ernährungspraxis auf Intensivstationen: nutritionDay 2007–2021 [Nutrition practices in intensive care units: nutritionDay from 2007–2021]. Med Klin Intensivmed Notfmed. 2023;118(2):89–98. German. https://doi.org/10.1007/s00063-023-00996-y. Epub 2023 Feb 28. PMID: 36853418; PMCID: PMC9992071.
8. Chapple LS, Ridley EJ, Chapman MJ. Trial design in critical care nutrition: the past, present and future. Nutrients. 2020;12(12):3694. https://doi.org/10.3390/nu12123694. PMID: 33265999; PMCID: PMC7760682.

9. Gunst J, Umpierrez GE, Van den Berghe G. Managing blood glucose control in the intensive care unit. Intensive Care Med. 2024;50(12):2171–4. https://doi.org/10.1007/s00134-024-07687-y. Epub 2024 Oct 29. PMID: 39470800; PMCID: PMC11588876.
10. Arabi YM, Casaer MP, Chapman M, et al. The intensive care medicine research agenda in nutrition and metabolism. Intensive Care Med. 2017;43:1239–56. https://doi.org/10.1007/s00134-017-4711-6.

Department of Anaesthesiology and Intensive Care Medicine
Jena University Hospital,
Jena, Germany

Dr. Frank M. Brunkhorst

Preface

Dear reader,

This book is intended to be a helpful guide for you when treating your patients in the intensive care unit, beyond the treatment of cardiovascular and organ functions.

We editors ultimately decided to provide you with this handbook because we see major differences in the nutritional tasks of healthy people and patients requiring intensive care.

The hormonal and consecutive metabolic changes in our patients—together with any regional perfusion and oxidation disorders that have occurred—may lead to a complex medical picture.

Metabolic pathways such as gluconeogenesis, lipolysis, and proteolysis, which are responsible for ensuring sufficient glucose as an energy source for the cell structures that can only obtain energy from glucose, are excessively stimulated. Radicals, which can be generated in the context of oxidative phosphorylation, metal ions, the "respiratory burst" of granulocytes, or the activation of xanthine oxidase, endanger cell integrity. The immune system of our patients is also impaired, resulting in an increase or impairment of the immune function.

Individual organ functions of the lungs, liver, or kidneys can be temporarily impaired, but above all the gastrointestinal tract, which together with the lymphatic system has the greatest cellular immune competence.

We are increasingly treating the combination of an excessive catabolic metabolic state, increased radical generation, and altered immune function by using selected nutrient components.

The selection of fatty acids in the lipid emulsions may be able to influence the duration and severity of the disease.

Last but not least, the targeted use of insulin to prevent hyperglycaemia is also important.

We are aware that we can only present you with a snapshot. We are eagerly awaiting the opportunity to develop our concepts further, for example through bedside monitoring of immune function.

We are also eagerly awaiting the question of whether we will ever be able to make clinical use of the finding that individual nutrients influence hormone secretion in the hypothalamic-pituitary axis.

What we would like to give you for your everyday clinical practice is that nutrient intake in our patients requiring intensive care has a therapeutic approach.

We would like to thank all the contributors for their tireless efforts in making this book project a success and hope that the reader will derive the greatest possible benefit from our book.

Langen, Germany Andreas Rümelin
Gießen, Germany Konstantin Mayer
München, Germany Thomas W. Felbinger

Contents

Part I Basics

1. **Physiology and Pathophysiology of the Gastrointestinal Tract** 3
   Elke Roeb

2. **Nutritional Status** 13
   Wolfgang H. Hartl

3. **Nutrition in ICU Proteins and Amino Acids** 27
   Ellen Dresen

4. **Carbohydrate Metabolism and Insulin Resistance in Critically Ill Patients: Implications for the Management of Insulin and Medical Nutrition Therapy** 45
   Christian von Loeffelholz and Gunnar Elke

5. **Lipids in Nutritional Therapy** 63
   Andreas Edel and Kathrin Scholtz

Part II Clinical Application

6. **Nutritional Adjustment** 95
   Thomas W. Felbinger, Konstantin Mayer, and Andreas Rümelin

7. **Enteral and Parenteral Nutrition in the ICU** 99
   Arved Weimann and Geraldine de Heer

8. **Immunonutrition and Pharmaconutrition** 123
   Aileen Hill and Christian Stoppe

9. **Excel Worksheet for Calculating an Adapted Nutrition Plan** 137
   Ulrich Fauth

10. **Children and Adolescents** 141
    Frank Jochum, Antonia Nomayo, Harry Nomayo, and Hanna Petersen

11	**Obesity and Cachexia** .... Matthias Pirlich	159
12	**Gastrointestinal Sonography in Nutritional Management: A Clinical Perspective** .... Nick Weidner	169

Part III Organ Dysfunction and Specific Conditions

13	**Nutrition in Patients with Kidney Disease** .... Wilfred Druml	185
14	**Nutrition in Liver Disease** .... Jule K. Adams and Alexander Koch	195
15	**Nutrition in Lung Disease** .... Matthias Hecker	209
16	**Pancreatic Disease in ICU** .... Johann Ockenga	213
17	**Nutritional Management in Patients with Severe Traumatic Brain Injury** .... Maximilian Fichtl and Thomas W. Felbinger	223
18	**Sepsis** .... Benjamin Tan and Markus A. Weigand	231
19	**Nutrition Therapy in Major Burns** .... Mette M. Berger	241
20	**Special Enteral Diets: Synbiotics** .... Arved Weimann and Geraldine de Heer	253

Part IV Special Aspects

21	**Early Mobilisation in ICU** .... Laura Homann and Stefan J. Schaller	261
22	**Ethical Challenges of Artificial Nutrition in Intensive Care: Navigating the Borders Between Self-Determination, Authenticity, and Best Interest** .... Norbert W. Paul	275

Part I
Basics

Physiology and Pathophysiology of the Gastrointestinal Tract

Elke Roeb

Trailer
In the chapter pathophysiology, the major nutrition-relevant organ structures and their primary disturbances in ICU patients are discussed. First, a functional description of the esophagus and stomach, and the gastrointestinal motility are presented. The pharmacological modulation of motility and characteristics of postoperative motility (disturbances) are discussed in detail. Constipation and intestinal translocation are among the most common pathophysiological disorders of intensive care patients, yet the therapeutic options appear limited. Stress bleeding after peptic lesions, however, can be prevented by careful prophylaxis or at least might be significantly reduced. The disturbed intestinal perfusion could be influenced by the diet of intensive care patients. Still unclear, however, are dietary recommendations in case of shock liver, as enteral nutrition often is disturbed and parenteral nutrition is associated with hepatic and cholestatic side effects.

1.1 Pathophysiology of the Intestinal Tract

Esophagus
Hormonal and neural mechanisms control esophageal motility and function of the lower esophageal sphincter. The proximal esophagus is controlled by the vagus nerve via nicotinic receptors and the distal esophagus via muscarinic receptors. Relaxation of smooth circular muscles in the esophagus occurs via nitric oxide (NO) and vasoactive intestinal peptide (VIP). Reflux is promoted by influences reducing the pressure of the lower esophageal sphincter. These include β-adrenergic

E. Roeb (✉)
Department of Gastroenterology, Justus Liebig University Giessen,
University Hospital Giessen, Giessen, Germany
e-mail: elke.roeb@innere.med.uni-giessen.de

© The Author(s), under exclusive license to Springer Nature
Switzerland AG 2025
A. Rümelin et al. (eds.), *Nutrition in ICU Patients*,
https://doi.org/10.1007/978-3-032-00818-3_1

agonists, sildenafil, secretin, progesterone, paracrine influences but also pregnancy, obesity, and high-fat foods (e.g., western diet).

Stomach
The exocrine secretion of the stomach is affected by hydrochloric acid, pepsinogen, mucosal, and intrinsic factors. Furthermore, gastrin (produced by G-cells) and histamine (mast cells, enterochromaffin cells) as well as somatostatin are secreted (from D-cells). Any disorder of gastric emptying is reflected by an increased gastric reflux (can be observed easily by a gastric tube). A reflux of more than 1 L indicates that the physiological knee-jerk relaxation of the pylorus is disturbed.

Intestinal Motility
The gastrointestinal motor and secretion are regulated by the autonomic and enteric nervous system, hormones, cytokines, and other transmitters. Every day about 9 L of fluid pass through the gastrointestinal tract. Two liters come from supplied food and 7 L from the endogenous gastrointestinal secretion. In jejunum, the reabsorption of electrolytes occurs along with a large part of the aqueous liquid. In the proximal small intestine (due to increased mucosal permeability), the exchange of osmolarity between chyme and blood works faster than in the rest of the intestine. In the ileum, the reabsorption of water slowly decreases and the intestinal content is pooled. Water- and fat-soluble dietary components are primarily reabsorbed in the proximal small intestine, with the exception of vitamin B12, which is absorbed in the terminal ileum only. A vitamin B12 deficiency can lead to Addison's anemia and even to funicular myelosis. A connection with dementia and neuropathy was discussed. A recently published study demonstrated a high prevalence of subclinical vitamin B12 deficiency, which represents a possible risk factor for disease burden among apparently healthy urban adults [23].

Various mucosal diseases, that affect the proximal intestine, therefore lead to different deficiencies. In extensive disease of the distal intestine, any bacterial overgrowth of the small intestine in addition to chronic cholestasis might interfere with adequate intraluminal bile acid concentration and thus interfere with a proper absorption of fat and liposoluble vitamins (ADEK). Early stages of vitamin deficiency symptoms are not clinically detectable until they lead to tremendous diseases, e.g., the usually irreversible spinocerebellar degeneration in case of vitamin E deficiency.

Suggestibility of Pharmacological Motility
A consensus is emerging that the gastric symptoms of functional dyspepsia are caused mainly by gastric motility abnormalities and gastric hypersensitivity [14, 17]. The commonly used dopamine antagonists metoclopramide (MCP) and domperidone are both able to stimulate esophageal, gastric, as well as duodenal motility. MCP is a pure dopamine antagonist. In addition to its peripheral action, the acceleration of gastric peristalsis and increasing frequency of opening the pylorus, MCP leads to central, sometimes neuroleptic, side effects, since it partially overcomes the blood-brain barrier. The effect of MCP in postoperative nausea seems to be

controversial [30]. Domperidone prevents the binding of dopamine toward the D2 dopamine receptor. Thus, dopamine reduces nausea, retching, and vomiting through this central effect. The positive impact of that piperidine derivative on motility is not yet understood. In addition to an increase in prolactin levels, the extension of QT intervals, especially with risk of ventricular arrhythmia, is a relevant side effect of domperidone in ICU patients. The numerous hormones that change their concentrations in critically ill patients and affect gastrointestinal motility include ghrelin, motilin, cholecystokinin, peptide YY, ACTH, and incretins [6, 28]. Figure 1.1 gives an overview.

Effective substance groups for the symptomatic treatment of diarrhea are still opiates and opioids (for example, loperamide). Their operation modus takes place exclusively locally in the gut by inhibiting the peristalsis. By concomitant administration of verapamil, ketoconazole, or HIV protease inhibitors, the blood-brain barrier can be overcome and central side effects such as respiratory depression may occur [3].

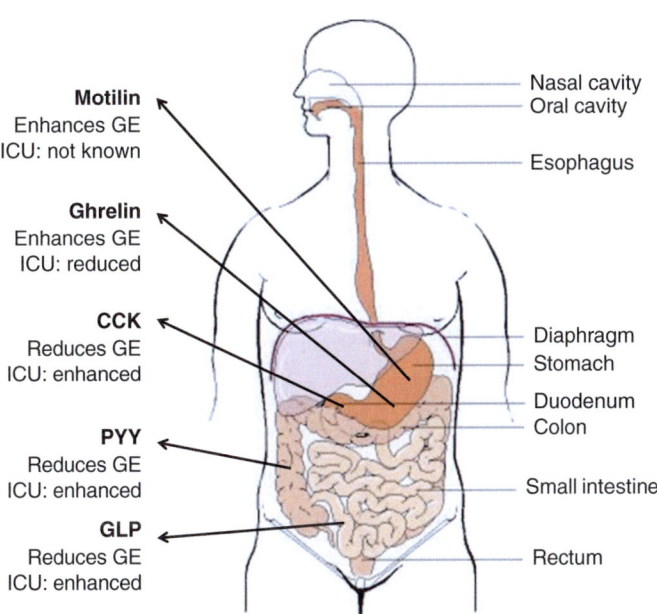

Fig. 1.1 Hormones influencing gastric and intestinal motility in healthy subjects and intensive care (ICU) patients. Hormonal effects in healthy individuals and in critically ill patients are shown. Cholecystokinin (CCK) and peptide YY (PYY) are released in response to enteral feeding and play an important role in gastric emptying. Glucagon-like peptide is released in the distal small intestine and colon. It acts as enterogastrone [16]. CCK cholecystokinin, GLP glucagon-like peptide, GE gastric emptying, ICU intensive care unit, PYY peptide YY

> **Note**
> At supratherapeutic doses, loperamide causes both QRS and QT prolongation. Supratherapeutic dosages of loperamide are advertised on several drug use websites and online forums as a treatment for opioid withdrawal and to produce euphoric effects. With regard to the current prescription-based opioid abuse, toxicity of loperamide, an opioid agonist that is readily available without a prescription, is more common [31].

Table 1.1 Substances which act tone-enhancing and tone-reducing

Tone- and motility-enhancing prokinetic drugs	Tone- and motility-reducing
β-adrenergic receptor antagonists	$β_2$-adrenergic receptor agonists
Choline rezeptor agonists	calcium antagonists
Dopamine antagonists Domperidone Metoclopramide Itopride	Cholecystokinin
Erythromycin/Azithromycin	Choline receptor antagonists (tricyclic antidepressants)
Gastrin	Diazepam
Ghrelin agonists Ulimorelin + TZP-102	Dopamine
Others Motilin receptor agonist (Camicinal) Neostigmine Alternative medicine Acupuncture	Glucagon
Prostaglandin $F_{2α}$ ($PGF_{2α}$) Prostaglandin E_2	Nitrates
	Opiate
Serotonin/5-HT_4-agonists TAK-964 Cisapride Mosapride Prucalopride	Serotonin
	Theophylline

According to Arzneimitteltherapie in der Gastroenterologie, Schölmerich, Sewing Hsg. (2003) and Crone [5] with ongoing studies

Table 1.1 gives an overview of substances that act tonus- or motility enhancing or tonus- or motility reducing.

Postoperative Gastrointestinal Motility

After abdominal operations, nausea, bloating of the abdomen, lack of bowel sounds, or obstruction of feces occur. Motoric function of the stomach returns to normal after 6–12 h; of the colon, on average, not before 3 days. Some of the motility disorders are due to impaired coordination and not to absent gastrointestinal activity. Also, imbalance of electrolytes, hypoxemia, and hyperglycemia have negative effects on the gastrointestinal motility. Erythromycin, intravenously applied, might speed up gastric emptying but, however, it has no influence on the postoperative ileus [6].

Metoclopramide seems to be the most studied prokinetic agent (49% of studies) followed by erythromycin (31%). But data provided no firm evidence on the balance between the desirable and undesirable effects of prokinetic agents. Studies addressing prokinetic agents in hospitalized adults had considerable variations in indications, drugs, and outcomes assessed, and the certainty of evidence was judged to be low to very low in a recent review [5].

1.2　Constipation

Constipation is among the most common disorders of the colon. Chronic constipation of ICU patients is often induced by medication. Important roles herein are played by, e.g., psychotropics, sedatives, aluminum-containing antacids (aluminum sulfate), opiates (morphine), iron preparations, diuretics, antihypertensives, Parkinson disease treatments, and antiepileptics. Other causes include lack of oral nutrition, lack of hydration, metabolic diseases or disorders of the electrolyte balance (often a potassium deficiency), and lack of physical exercise acts favoring as well. The therapeutically applicable substances include osmotic laxatives, hydragogue substances, and motility enhancing laxatives such as agonists of the serotonin 5-HT4 receptor. The subcutaneously administration of methylnaltrexone rapidly leads to defecation in patients with advanced intensive care abidance or those with opioid-induced constipation. This substance is approved, however, for the treatment of opioid-induced constipation in adults only, in a palliative setting that does not respond adequately to conventional laxatives. Methylnaltrexone does not seem to affect a central analgesia and does not lead to opioid withdrawal. In 2008, methylnaltrexone bromide came into the German market as a peripherally acting antagonist of the μ-opioid receptor. The recommended dose of methylnaltrexone bromide is, depending on body weight, 8 mg or 12 mg every other day. The rate of fecal evacuation of 48% (placebo 15%) after a single injection according to a study by Thomas et al. [26] corresponds approximately to our experience. Opioid-induced constipation is a burdensome clinical problem independent of opioid subtype. Timely intensification of prophylactic laxative treatment, especially when opioid doses increase, may help to prevent opioid-induced constipation.

In summary, clinically overt opioid-induced constipation requires a more intensive laxative regimen with, for example, methylnaltrexone [18].

1.3 Bacterial Translocation

- The concept of bacterial translocation (introduced by Berg & Garlington [1]) defines the passage of living enteral bacteria from the intestinal lumen through the mucosa into mesenteric lymph nodes and other organs: Of the more than 500 enterally detectable bacteria, very few translocate, particularly aerobic and facultative anaerobic gram-negative bacteria such as *E. coli, Enterobacteriaceae, Pseudomonas aeruginosa*, enterococci and streptococci. Three main mechanisms are made responsible for the occurrence of systemic spread of translocated bacteria following bacterial translocation:

    (a) Luminal factors with bacterial overgrowth, collection of non-commensal bacteria with different virulence and colonization factors;
    (b) Disorders of physical and secretory mucosal barrier, changes in bacterial adherence by different concentrations of IgA, bile acids, mucins, and chloride: The increase in penetration is facilitated by oxidative stress, mucosal acidosis, and ATP depletion. Especially, the villi of enteral mucosa are affected by threatening or overt hypoxia. Here, the oxygen saturation is lower than in the arterial blood. In the villus region, a decrease in blood circulation quickly results in acidosis with ATP depletion. This affects especially intensive care patients with hemorrhagic, septic, or cardiogenic shock;
    (c) Defects in the immune system: Here locally T-cell activation and the release of chemokines and cytokines play an important role. The so-called *gut associated lymphatic tissue* (GALT) is one of the most important defense mechanisms of bacterial translocation and represents the largest immune organ in humans. Systemically, the activation of the reticuloendothelial system in liver and spleen is of importance.

According to a very recent review article, the microbiota is recognized as one of the important factors that can worsen the clinical conditions of patients who are already very frail in the intensive care unit. At the same time, the microbiota also plays a crucial role in the prevention of ICU-associated complications. By using probiotics, synbiotics, or fecal microbiota transplantation (FMT), the integrity of the microbiota and the gut might be preserved, which will later help maintain homeostasis in ICU patients [32].

As a marker for the integrity of intestinal enterocytes, the biomarker citrulline, a non-proteinogenic, α-amino acid can be used. Citrulline is synthesized almost exclusively in enterocytes [20, 21]. The microbiological detection of bacteria in peripheral blood corresponds to advanced stages of disease. In spontaneous bacterial peritonitis in patients with liver cirrhosis and necrotizing pancreatitis, bacterial translocation is considered as a proven pathomechanism. In patients with liver cirrhosis after spontaneous bacterial peritonitis or acute variceal bleeding, a selective intestinal decontamination should be done for prophylaxis according to appropriate guidelines [2, 9].

1.4 Bleeding Out of Peptic Stress Lesions

The protective mechanisms of a healthy stomach are based on a functional balance between aggressive (acid, pepsin, free oxygen radicals, endogenous mediators) and protective factors (mucus, bicarbonate, cell regeneration, mucosal blood circulation, radical scavengers). Nowadays, stress bleeding rarely arises by increasing aggressive factors during intensive care therapy, but rather due to the loss of protective capabilities of the gastric mucosa. Here, patients are at risk with a ventilation time of more than 5 days and coagulation disorders. Shock and hypotension represent significant risk factors of stress bleeding. Stress lesions mostly consist of multiple erosions in the gastric fundus and corpus. Often, you can find the lesions in hypoacid patients. An active acid producing stomach is—according to our current understanding of general intensive care patients—no pathological condition, but rather an indication of an adequate blood supply and power supply [27]. The key to prevention of ICU complications in stress bleeding is not the use of specific drugs but an optimized intensive medical treatment program (early fluid resuscitation, ensuring oxygenation, prevention of infection, optimization of circulatory regulation, sufficient analgesia) [27]. For an overview of drugs that lead to inhibition of acid secretion in the stomach, see Table 1.2 below.

Among ICU patients requiring mechanical ventilation, stress ulcer prophylaxis with use of proton pump inhibitors vs. histamine-2 receptor blockers resulted in hospital mortality rates of 18.3% vs. 17.5%, respectively, a difference that did not reach any significance [19]. There were also no different rates of *Clostridioides difficile* infection and ICU and hospital lengths of stay. However, the interpretation of data may be limited by crossover in the use of the assigned medication [19].

Table 1.2 Medications for inhibition of gastric acid secretion

Pharmacological group	Mechanism of action
Antacids	Acid neutralization, absorbents for pepsin, and bile acids
Histamin-H_2-antagonists	Competitive and reversible inhibition of histamine to H_2 receptors of parietal cells
Pirenzepine	Parasympatholytics, inhibiting M1—receptors of enterochromaffin like cells (inhibition of histamine release)
Prostaglandins (Misoprostol)	E1 prostaglandin, stimulates prostaglandin receptors of parietal cells, promotes bicarbonate and mucus production
Proton pump inhibitors (PPIs)	Prodrug, irreversible inhibition of H+/K+-ATPase in parietal cells, neutralization of gastric acid
Alginate-containing formulations	Alginate taken on demand is an effective and safe option for the treatment of breakthrough symptoms in GERD patients on PPI

According and updated with regard to Arzneimitteltherapie in der Gastroenterologie, Schölmerich, Sewing Hsg. (2003)

1.5 Disturbed Intestinal Perfusion

A disturbed perfusion of the digestive tract occurs early in the context of critical diseases [4] and may also exist during normal systemic blood pressure, normal oxygen saturation, and unimpaired cardiac output. The determination of the perfusion of gastrointestinal mucosa in principle is clinically measurable by tonometry of the stomach [10, 12], contrast-enhanced or duplex sonography [8], and multislice computed tomography [13, 22]. All of these methods are technically complex, error-prone, and clinically neither sufficiently validated nor established outside scientific questions. It remains unclear also whether or which specific therapeutic implications should draw a disturbed gastrointestinal perfusion. Therefore, in general, supportive measures to improve oxygenation and blood flow are recommended at the same time as far as waiver of vasopressors—as clinically possible [29]. A rapid onset of fluid resuscitation is necessary. Supplementation of dobutamine (in septic patients with norepinephrine) in addition to the early enteral nutrition is the most important step to improve oxygenation in the splanchnic [8]. In a very recent Chinese study, high respiratory efforts might decrease perfusion of peripheral tissues and splanchnic organs. This status should therefore be avoided to protect splanchnic and peripheral organs in mechanically ventilated patients [33]. The so-called nonocclusive mesenteric ischemia is a detrimental disease associated with progressive organ failure and a high mortality. Whether local intra-arterial prostaglandin application might hold promise as a rescue treatment strategy has to be evaluated in the future [24].

1.6 Shock Liver and Cholestasis

In more than half of the critically ill patients in the ICU, liver dysfunction is detected [7]. Presumably, pathogenetically, the complex arterial and venous supply plays an important role. Both changes in the splanchnic area, right ventricular disorders, and hypoxia affect the liver cells structurally and functionally. Hepatocyte damage lead to impaired glucose metabolism with reduced gluconeogenesis and systemic energy deficiency. The hepatic detoxification function is reduced in addition to further deterioration by resultant cholestasis. Sludge formation in the gallbladder occurs in critically ill patients typically 5–10 days following the initiation of intensive therapeutic interventions. After 6 weeks, 100% of parenterally fed patients reveal biliary sludge. Stone-free cholecystitis, which can be secured by means of sonography in up to 90%, is a common cause of fever, leukocytosis, and sepsis [25].

Cholestasis is more common in patients with diarrhea and vice versa. Diarrhea and cholestasis both occur in approximately one quarter of ICU patients, with significant proportion manifesting beyond the first week in the ICU [15]. In addition, the incidence of cholestasis is higher than that of hypoxic hepatitis but does not increase the 28-day case fatality rate of ICU patients, suggesting that cholestatic liver dysfunction may be an early adaptation of the liver to critical diseases [11].

References

1. Berg RD, Garlington AW. Translocation of certain indigenous bacteria from the gastrointestinal tract to the mesenteric lymph nodes and other organs in a gnotobiotic mouse model. Infect Immun. 1979;23(2):403–11.
2. Bernard B, Grangé JD, Khac EN, Amiot X, Opolon P, Poynard T. Antibiotic prophylaxis for the prevention of bacterial infections in cirrhotic patients with gastrointestinal bleeding: a meta-analysis. Hepatology. 1999;29(6):1655–61.
3. Cheng Z, Zhang J, Liu H, Li Y, Zhao Y, Yang E. Central nervous system penetration for small molecule therapeutic agents does not increase in multiple sclerosis- and Alzheimer's disease-related animal models despite reported blood-brain barrier disruption. Drug Metab Dispos. 2010;38(8):1355–61.
4. Creteur J. Gastric and sublingual capnometry. Curr Opin Crit Care. 2006;12(3):272–7.
5. Crone V, Møller MH, Baekgaard ES, Perner A, Bytzer P, Alhazzani W, Krag M. Use of prokinetic agents in hospitalised adult patients: a scoping review. Acta Anaesthesiol Scand. 2023;67(5):588–98.
6. Deane A, Chapman MJ, Fraser RJ, Horowitz M. Bench-to-bedside review: the gut as an endocrine organ in the critically ill. Crit Care. 2010;14(5):228.
7. Drolz A, Horvatits T, Roedl K, Fuhrmann V. Shock liver and cholestatic liver in critically ill patients. Med Klin Intensivmed Notfmed. 2014;109(4):228–34.
8. Gatt M, MacFie J, Anderson AD, Howell G, Reddy BS, Suppiah A, Renwick I, Mitchell CJ. Changes in superior mesenteric artery blood flow after oral, enteral, and parenteral feeding in humans. Crit Care Med. 2009;37(1):171–6.
9. Gerbes AL, Labenz J, Appenrodt B, Dollinger M, Gundling F, Gülberg V, Holstege A, Lynen-Jansen P, Steib CJ, Trebicka J, Wiest R, Zipprich A. Aktualisierte S2k-Leitlinie der Deutschen Gesellschaft für Gastroenterologie, Verdauungs- und Stoffwechselkrankheiten (DGVS) Komplikationen der Leberzirrhose [Updated S2k-Guideline "Complications of liver cirrhosis". German Society of Gastroenterology (DGVS)]. Z Gastroenterol. 2019;57(5):e168.
10. Graf J, Königs B, Mottaghy K, Janssens U. In vitro validation of gastric air tonometry using perfluorocarbon FC 43 and 0.9% sodium chloride. Br J Anaesth. 2000;84(4):497–9.
11. Huimin S, Jing W, Chang HU, Chang L, Jianguo LI. Effects of cholestasis and hypoxic hepatitis on prognosis of ICU patients: a retrospective study based on MIMIC III database. Nan Fang Yi Ke Da Xue Xue Bao. 2020;40(6):771–7.
12. Janssens U, Graf J, Koch KC, Hanrath P. Gastric tonometry: in vivo comparison of saline and air tonometry in patients with cardiogenic shock. Br J Anaesth. 1998;81(5):676–80.
13. Kamimura K, Oosaki A, Sugahara S, Mori S. Survival of three nonocclusive mesenteric ischemia patients following early diagnosis by multidetector row computed tomography and prostaglandin E1 treatment. Intern Med. 2008;47(22):2001–6.
14. Keller J, Wedel T, Seidl H, Kreis ME, van der Voort I, Gebhard M, Langhorst J, Lynen Jansen P, Schwandner O, Storr M, van Leeuwen P, Andresen V, Preiß JC, Layer P, Allescher H, Andus T, Bischoff SC, Buderus S, Claßen M, Ehlert U, Elsenbruch S, Engel M, Enninger A, Fischbach W, Freitag M, Frieling T, Gillessen A, Goebel-Stengel M, Gschossmann J, Gundling F, Haag S, Häuser W, Helwig U, Hollerbach S, Holtmann G, Karaus M, Katschinski M, Krammer H, Kruis W, Kuhlbusch-Zicklam R, Lynen Jansen P, Madisch A, Matthes H, Miehlke S, Mönnikes H, Müller-Lissner S, Niesler B, Pehl C, Pohl D, Posovszky C, Raithel M, Röhrig-Herzog G, Schäfert R, Schemann M, Schmidt-Choudhury A, Schmiedel S, Schweinlin A, Schwille-Kiuntke J, Stengel A, Tesarz J, Voderholzer W, von Boyen G, von Schönfeld J. Update S3-Leitlinie Intestinale Motilitätsstörungen: definition, Pathophysiologie, Diagnostik und Therapie. Gemeinsame Leitlinie der Deutschen Gesellschaft für Gastroenterologie, Verdauungs- und Stoffwechselkrankheiten (DGVS) und der Deutschen Gesellschaft für Neurogastroenterologie und Motilität (DGNM). Z Gastroenterol. 2022;60(2):192–218. German
15. Kiss O, Maizik J, Tamme K, Orav A, van de Poll MCG, Blaser AR. Diarrhea and elevation of plasma markers of cholestasis are common and often occur concomitantly in critically ill patients. J Crit Care. 2020;60:120–6.

16. Marathe CS, Rayner CK, Jones KL, Horowitz M. Effects of GLP-1 and incretin-based therapies on gastrointestinal motor function. Exp Diabetes Res. 2011;2011:279530.
17. Miwa H, Oshima T, Tomita T, Fukui H, Kondo T, Yamasaki T, Watari J. Recent understanding of the pathophysiology of functional dyspepsia: role of the duodenum as the pathogenic center. J Gastroenterol. 2019;54(4):305–11.
18. Neefjes ECW, van der Wijngaart H, van der Vorst MJDL, Ten Oever D, van der Vliet HJ, Beeker A, Rhodius CA, van den Berg HP, Berkhof J, Verheul HMW. Optimal treatment of opioid induced constipation in daily clinical practice – an observational study. BMC Palliat Care. 2019;18(1):31.
19. PEPTIC Investigators for the Australian and New Zealand Intensive Care Society Clinical Trials Group, Alberta Health Services Critical Care Strategic Clinical Network, and the Irish Critical Care Trials Group, Young PJ, Bagshaw SM, Forbes AB, Nichol AD, Wright SE, Bailey M, Bellomo R, Beasley R, Brickell K, Eastwood GM, Gattas DJ, van Haren F, Litton E, Mackle DM, McArthur CJ, McGuinness SP, Mouncey PR, Navarra L, Opgenorth D, Pilcher D, Saxena MK, Webb SA, Wiley D, Rowan KM. Effect of stress ulcer prophylaxis with proton pump inhibitors vs histamine-2 receptor blockers on in-hospital mortality among ICU patients receiving invasive mechanical ventilation: the PEPTIC randomized clinical trial. JAMA. 2020;323(7):616–26.
20. Peters JH, Beishuizen A, Keur MB, Dobrowolski L, Wierdsma NJ, van Bodegraven AA. Assessment of small bowel function in critical illness: potential role of citrulline metabolism. J Intensive Care Med. 2011;26(2):105–10.
21. Peters JH, Wierdsma NJ, Beishuizen A, Teerlink T, van Bodegraven AA. Intravenous citrulline generation test to assess intestinal function in intensive care unit patients. Clin Exp Gastroenterol. 2017;28(10):75–81.
22. Saber AA, Azar N, Dekal M, Abdelbaki TN. Computed tomographic scan mapping of gastric wall perfusion and clinical implications. Am J Surg. 2015;209(6):999–1006.
23. Sivaprasad M, Shalini T, Reddy PY, Seshacharyulu M, Madhavi G, Kumar BN, Reddy GB. Prevalence of vitamin deficiencies in an apparently healthy urban adult population: assessed by subclinical status and dietary intakes. Nutrition. 2019;63–64:106–13.
24. Stahl K, Busch M, Maschke SK, Schneider A, Manns MP, Fuge J, Wiesner O, Meyer BC, Hoeper MM, Hinrichs JB, David S. A retrospective analysis of nonocclusive mesenteric ischemia in medical and surgical ICU patients: clinical data on demography, clinical signs, and survival. J Intensive Care Med. 2020;35(11):1162–72.
25. Theodorou P, Maurer CA, Spanholtz TA, Phan TQ, Amini P, Perbix W, Maegele M, Lefering R, Spilker G. Acalculous cholecystitis in severely burned patients: incidence and predisposing factors. Burns. 2009;35(3):405–11.
26. Thomas J, Karver S, Cooney GA, Chamberlain BH, Watt CK, Slatkin NE, Stambler N, Kremer AB, Israel RJ. Methylnaltrexone for opioid-induced constipation in advanced illness. N Engl J Med. 2008;358(22):2332–43.
27. Tryba M. Stressblutungsprophylaxe. In: Eckard J, Forst H, Burchardi H, editors. Intensivmedizin. Bd. 5, X-6; 2006, S. 1–19.
28. Van den Berghe G. Adrenal function/dysfunction in critically ill patients: a concise narrative review of recent novel insights. J Anesth. 2021;35(6):903–10.
29. van Haren FM, Sleigh JW, Pickkers P, Van der Hoeven JG. Gastrointestinal perfusion in septic shock. Anaesth Intensive Care. 2007;35(5):679–94.
30. Wallenborn J, Eberhart L, Kranke P. Postoperative Übelkeit und Erbrechen—Alles beim Alten in der Pharmakotherapie von PONV? Anästhesiol Intensivmed Notfallmed Schmerzther. 2009;44:296–305.
31. Wightman RS, Hoffman RS, Howland MA, Rice B, Biary R, Lugassy D. Not your regular high: cardiac dysrhythmias caused by loperamide. Clin Toxicol (Phila). 2016;54(5):454–8.
32. Zanza C, Romenskaya T, Thangathurai D, Ojetti V, Saviano A, Abenavoli L, Robba C, Cammarota G, Franceschi F, Piccioni A, Longhitano Y. Microbiome in Critical Care: An Unconventional and Unknown Ally. Curr Med Chem. 2022;29(18):3179–88.
33. Zhou Y, Chi Y, He H, Cui N, Wang X, Long Y. High respiratory effort decreases splanchnic and peripheral perfusion in patients with respiratory failure during mechanical ventilation. J Crit Care. 2023;75:154361.

Nutritional Status

Wolfgang H. Hartl

2.1 Assessment of Nutritional Status—General Aspects

Traditional intensive care unit (ICU) scores do not take into account the nutritional status of patients. Malnutrition is present in up to 80% of critically ill patients on admission or can develop during their stay in the ICU [1]. As a surrogate of malnutrition, international guidelines recommend the assessment of lean body mass (LBM), especially in underweight, obese and overweight patients. Predictive formulae can provide estimates of LBM, but may differ significantly from actual LBM. LBM or muscle mass can be better estimated using dual-energy X-ray absorptiometry or CT (computed tomography)/MRI (magnetic resonance imaging) scans [2]. ICU research has used various indices or scores, anthropometry, muscle ultrasound, CT scan and/or bioelectrical impedance analysis (BIA) monitoring to assess nutritional risk and to identify malnourished patients [3].

The primary diagnostic aim is to identify malnutrition on admission to the ICU; a secondary aim is to monitor nutritional status during the ICU stay and, if necessary, to adjust nutritional therapy to changes in nutritional status.

2.2 Malnutrition as a Risk Factor for Critical Illness

A retrospective analysis of more than 6000 critically ill patients showed that protein-energy malnutrition on admission to intensive care—defined as disease-related weight loss, underweight, loss of muscle mass and reduced energy or protein

---

W. H. Hartl (✉)
Surgical Critical Care, Department of General, Visceral, and Transplantation Surgery,
University Medical Center, Campus Großhadern, Ludwig-Maximilians-Universität Munich,
Munich, Bavaria, Germany
e-mail: whartl@med.uni-muenchen.de

© The Author(s), under exclusive license to Springer Nature
Switzerland AG 2025
A. Rümelin et al. (eds.), *Nutrition in ICU Patients*,
https://doi.org/10.1007/978-3-032-00818-3_2

intake—was associated with twice the risk of death compared with non-malnourished patients [1]. In principle, pre-existing malnutrition associated with acute organ failure is an independent, significant predictor of poorer prognosis (increased ICU length of stay, ICU readmission rate, incidence of infection) [4].

2.3 Definition of Malnutrition

The Global Leadership Initiative on Malnutrition (GLIM) definition of malnutrition, agreed by international professional societies in 2019, includes phenotypic and aetiological criteria that can be applied to critically ill patients. Phenotypic criteria are as follows: involuntary weight loss, low BMI, reduced muscle mass and a history of reduced food intake or absorption and severity of underlying disease/inflammation. In each case, one aetiological or phenotypic criterion must be met for a clinical diagnosis of malnutrition to be made. Biochemically, this corresponds to an abnormal ratio of total body protein mass (lean body mass, predominantly muscle mass) to total body weight [5]. The following causes of malnutrition are distinguished:

- A specific acute illness: acute severe inflammation/infection (sepsis, burns, trauma).
- Reduced caloric intake, e.g. chronic starvation without inflammation or due to fasting (e.g. socio-economic or prolonged peri-interventional fasting).
- A specific chronic disease: chronic inflammation of mild or moderate severity (e.g. malabsorption in chronic pancreatitis, chronic inflammatory bowel disease, pancreatic cancer, rheumatoid arthritis, sarcopenic obesity).

2.4 Nutritional Status and Medical Nutrition Therapy (MNT)

The purpose of determining nutritional status at ICU admission is to improve prognostic confidence and to identify those patients who will benefit from close monitoring and guideline-directed nutrition. However, simple control of calorie/protein intake (especially in the acute phase of critical illness) based on nutritional status ("the worse, the more") has now been abandoned. Poorly controlled "aggressive" caloric intake in the acute phase may actually increase morbidity and mortality. Individualised MNT based on metabolic and gastrointestinal tolerance is particularly important in this phase [6].

The aim of MNT must be to prevent calorie, protein and micronutrient deficiencies or to avoid worsening of pre-existing malnutrition, but not to worsen the prognosis by inappropriate, overly aggressive substrate feeding. These objectives are particularly relevant for

- Patients at risk who are already primarily malnourished on admission.

- Patients who, because of their underlying condition, are at high risk of developing malnutrition as an additional risk during their stay in the ICU.

Malnourished patients require particularly careful consideration of the indications/contraindications and individual metabolic tolerance of MNT. In particular, MNT also requires appropriate monitoring, which should include follow-up of nutritional status [1].

2.5 Laboratory and Physical Methods for Determining Nutritional Status in Critically Ill Patients

2.5.1 Concentrations of Visceral Proteins (Albumin, Prealbumin)

There is an association between inflammation and malnutrition, but not between malnutrition and concentrations of visceral proteins. In critically ill patients, concentrations of these proteins correlate well with patients' risk of adverse outcomes rather than with protein-energy malnutrition. Therefore, serum albumin and prealbumin should not be used as surrogates for total body protein, total muscle mass or nutritional status in critically ill patients [7].

2.5.2 Anthropometry

In critically ill patients, accurate clinical assessment of nutritional status using conventional parameters (especially weight and BMI) at admission (and during the course of the disease) may be complicated by significant interstitial fluid retention ("capillary leakage"). The hyperhydration that can be observed depending on the stage of the disease makes current body weight and BMI calculated from height unreliable parameters for assessing nutritional status [1].

Another simple anthropometric parameter is mean arm circumference, which has been shown to predict the risk of major complications and increased mortality in hospitalised patients with a body weight < 15th percentile. However, in critically ill patients, fluid retention and capillary leakage also limit the use of this diagnostic tool.

2.5.3 Creatinine/Cystatin C ratio (CCR)

CCR can be calculated as the ratio between creatinine and cystatin-C (serum creatinine × 100/serum cystatin-C). This index offers a more objective alternative for predicting and possibly monitoring the degree of catabolism or muscle mass, also in conjunction with the imaging techniques discussed below. A low sarcopenia index is associated with lower muscle mass. However, it is necessary to measure the concentration of cystatin C in serum [8].

According to a recent meta-analysis, CCR in hospitalised adults correlates significantly with skeletal muscle mass and handgrip strength as assessed by computed tomography. CCR is also a reliable predictor of mortality and morbidity. In critically ill patients, lower CCR is associated with shorter duration of mechanical ventilation and ICU stay. However, there are no cut-off values yet to define an individually increased risk of mortality or to guide specific nutritional interventions [9].

2.5.4 Handgrip Strength

In cooperative patients without pre-existing or acquired neurological comorbidity (critical illness polyneuropathy or myopathy), dynamometry with measurement of hand grip strength is a simple and quantifiable method for functional (progression) monitoring of muscle strength. Handgrip strength correlates with the length of ICU stay and with the rate of reintubation after mechanical ventilation. An association with the sonographic cross-sectional area of the rectus femoris muscle has been shown in patients with sepsis [1].

A significant increase in handgrip strength was observed in cancer patients treated with different nutritional strategies, suggesting that this tool could be also used to guide MNT in these patients [10]. However, according to a recent meta-analysis in unselected hospitalised patients, intensified nutritional therapy neither increased handgrip strength nor improved mortality [11]. In contrast, a post hoc analysis of the EFFORT trial in non-critically ill hospitalised patients at nutritional risk showed that individualised nutritional support was most effective in reducing mortality in patients in the ≤10th percentile compared with those in the >10th percentile [12]. It is not currently known whether similar effects would be seen in appropriate subgroups of critically ill patients.

A prerequisite for reliable measurement is a standardised examination technique without patient restrictions. As validated cut-off values for critically ill patients are still lacking, the value of dynamometry lies primarily in intra-individual monitoring (serial dynamometry) [1].

2.6 Screening Tools for Determining Nutritional Status in Critically Ill Patients

For screening malnutrition in adults (including critically ill patients), there are no tools with high validity, reliability and strong supporting evidence. Most tools achieve only moderate validity, agreement and reliability, and have large variations in individual results [13]. Nevertheless, their use continues to be recommended by international guidelines (albeit with low evidence), and their specifics are discussed below (Table 2.1).

2 Nutritional Status

Table 2.1 Screening tools to assess the prevalence of malnutrition in critically ill patients

Screening tool	Parameter
NUTRIC (Nutrition Risk in Critically Ill)	Age
	APACHE (Acute Physiology and Chronic Health Evaluation) II-Score
	SOFA (Sepsis-related Organ Failure Assessment)-Score
	Number of comorbidities
	Hospital length-of-stay before ICU admission
	IL 6 (interleukin-6) (optional)
NRS-2002 (Nutritional Risk Screening)	BMI ≤ 20.5 kg/m²
	Weight loss of >5% of the body weight within the last 3 months
	Reduced food intake
	Severity of the disease
MNA (Mini Nutritional Assessment)	Reduced food intake
	Extent of weight loss
	Mobility
	BMI
	Psychological stress/problems
SGA (Subjective Global Assessment)	Weight
	Food intake
	Gastrointestinal symptoms
	Functional status
mGLIM (modified Global Leadership Initiative on Malnutrition)	Nutrition Risk Score 2002 ≥ 3 points
	Reduced handgrip strength (cut-off for females 8 kg, for males 16 kg)
	Weight loss of >5% of the body weight within the last 6 months
	Reduced food intake (<50% of energy requirements during the last week)

2.6.1 NRS, MNA, SGA

To identify malnutrition in non-intensive care patients, the European Society for Clinical Nutrition and Metabolism (ESPEN) recommends a two-step approach using the well-validated Nutritional Risk Score (NRS). If one of the pre-screening questions listed in Table 2.1 is answered with "yes", the main screening is performed, in which the nutritional status and disease severity are quantified more precisely using a graduated score. Scores >3 indicate a high-risk patient, and scores ≥5 indicate a high-risk patient with signs of manifest malnutrition [1].

The Mini Nutritional Assessment (MNA) is a screening tool for assessing the nutritional status of people aged >65 years in home care, hospital or nursing home settings and also has a two-stage structure: a preliminary medical history of 6 items (A-F) with a maximum of 14 points (MNA short form) and a medical history of 12 items (G-R)—including two anthropometric measurements (upper arm circumference and calf circumference)—with a maximum of 16 points (MNA long form) [1].

The Subjective Global Assessment (SGA) is a simple, reproducible bedside method that quantifies a patient's nutritional status based on history (weight change, food intake, gastrointestinal symptoms, exercise capacity, underlying medical condition) and clinical examination findings (subcutaneous adipose tissue, muscle mass, oedema). In critically ill patients, malnutrition diagnosed by SGA is associated with a higher rate of ICU readmission, longer hospital stay and higher in-hospital mortality [1].

Compared with the MNA, the NRS has a higher sensitivity in assessing prognosis, whereas the NRS specificity is lower compared with the SGA and the MNA short form. A large meta-analysis found a prevalence of malnutrition in hospitalised patients of 38–78% using the NRS, SGA and MNA. The SGA was clearly superior to the MNA in predicting malnutrition. However, the association between screening and the risk of malnutrition was not very consistent. For all tools, there was an independent association between the presence of malnutrition and a worse prognosis. However, the SGA and MNA were better than the NRS at estimating the prognosis associated with nutritional status [4].

Limitations

All these scores have limitations for use in critically ill patients because they require a history that can only be reliably obtained from patients who are awake and able to provide information. External history is often difficult to obtain or unreliable in routine clinical practice. A further limiting factor is that the NRS always assigns a score of three to critical illness, which means that all critically ill patients are at risk of malnutrition on admission and no further differentiation is possible. In addition to the medical history, the SGA requires trained assessors. The usefulness of the MNA is limited by the fact that it was originally developed to assess the nutritional status of elderly, non-critically ill patients >65 years of age [1].

2.6.2 NUTRIC-Score

The Nutrition Risk in Critically Ill (NUTRIC) score was developed specifically for intensive care patients to estimate the likelihood of a complicated course of intensive care ("prolonged ICU length-of-stay") and the associated nutritional risk. The score is based on the APACHE II and SOFA scores, among others. The starting point is a predominantly non-malnourished patient, so typical nutritional status parameters are not included. In addition to the APACHE II and SOFA scores, other parameters include age, number of comorbidities and length of hospital stay prior to ICU admission. The variable interleukin (IL)-6 concentration is optional, depending on availability. A score < 6 points (if IL-6 concentration is not available: <5) indicates a low risk of developing malnutrition; a score of six points or more (if IL-6 concentration is not available: five points or more) indicates an increased risk of a complicated course with a prolonged stay in the ICU [1].

Only the 2016 American Society for Parenteral and Enteral Nutrition (A.S.P.E.N.) guideline recommends the NUTRIC score on admission to the ICU, based on expert opinion. In principle, the NUTRIC score is not suitable for assessing nutritional status but only reflects the overall risk influenced by inflammation/infection and multi-organ dysfunction. Therefore, it is recommended that this score be used in conjunction with an additional nutritional assessment, such as body composition. Another limitation is that controlling the intensity of nutritional therapy according to the level of the NUTRIC score is not associated with specific effects on morbidity/mortality [14–16].

2.6.3 mGLIM (Modified Global Leadership Initiative on Malnutrition)

The use of mGLIM was evaluated in a post hoc analysis of a multicentre randomised trial of nutritionally vulnerable hospitalised patients. Of 1917 eligible participants at nutritional risk, 1181 (61.6%) were diagnosed with malnutrition based on mGLIM criteria. The incidence of adverse clinical outcomes was significantly higher in mGLIM-positive participants compared with mGLIM-negative individuals. The ability of intensified MNT to reduce adverse clinical outcomes was greater in mGLIM-positive than in mGLIM-negative participants [17]. However, in critically ill patients, the use of mGLIM criteria to predict adverse clinical outcomes and responsiveness to a specific type of MNT is still unknown.

2.7 Technical Procedures for Determining Nutritional Status in Critically Ill Patients

In a systematic review of six studies of muscle loss in intensive care patients, a loss of muscle mass of up to approximately 20% was observed in the first 14 days after admission. These studies used γ-neutron activation, computed tomography (CT) or ultrasound to quantify muscle mass [1]. However, a definitive evaluation of the usefulness and reliability of CT morphological and sonographic methods or bioimpedance analysis for assessing body muscle mass in critically ill patients remains to be performed [18]. Nevertheless, a brief overview of the characteristics of these diagnostic techniques is given below.

2.7.1 Muscle Sonography

Muscle sonography is a non-invasive, bedside procedure that can be used to diagnose muscle wasting as a sign of malnutrition and to estimate fat-free mass. It also allows repeated measurements to be made, providing a quantitative assessment of muscle mass changes. When used correctly, it has high reliability in the study of muscle thickness and muscle cross-sectional area [19].

However, there is no single standardised measurement specification, although the quadriceps femoris or rectus femoris muscles are usually measured in cross section. The measuring point for the rectus femoris muscle is usually on the line from the anterior superior iliac spine to the proximal edge of the patella (at a distance of 60% of the total length from the anterior superior iliac spine). The cross-sectional area of the rectus femoris muscle or, technically simpler, the thickness (diameter) of the quadriceps consisting of the rectus femoris and vastus intermedius muscles is measured. To date, the reliability of the cross-sectional area measurement has been best analysed. In healthy people, quadriceps cross-sectional area correlates very well with total muscle mass on MRI ($r = 0.88$ for men, $r = 0.89$ for women) [1]. Serial measurements in critically ill patients showed a high correlation between the thickness of the quadriceps muscle measured by ultrasound and by computed tomography (CT) [20]. Serial measurements may also help to track loss of muscle mass and possibly muscle function, and may be used as a marker of disease severity and potential adverse outcomes [21].

Several reviews have analysed the value of skeletal muscle ultrasound in critically ill patients. About 75% of the studies found that skeletal muscle ultrasound (cross-sectional area, muscle thickness and echo intensity) showed significant associations with functional capacity, length of stay, readmission and survival. However, there was significant heterogeneity in ultrasound technique and outcome measures among the included studies, which prevented consistency and comparison between studies. Reporting of ultrasound methodology was not comprehensive and often did not provide a full understanding of the specific methods used [22–24].

Limitations

The limiting factor for all sonographic methods is that changes in hydration status can significantly affect the measurement results and that it is not the quadriceps muscle mass but the lumbar muscle mass that best correlates with total body protein mass. Furthermore, in critically ill patients, only the sum of muscle thickness at the mid-upper arm and bilateral thighs (or one thigh if both thighs cannot be imaged) may be the ultrasound protocol that best relates to CT muscle area at L3 [25].

The muscle US technique is not easy to perform as it has a long learning curve due to the many errors that can occur in its execution. It provides qualitative rather than quantitative results and the main difficulty is in interpreting or distinguishing the contours of the muscle and its adjacent structures. Therefore, this technique is highly dependent on the skill of the operator [19]. In addition, there is no consensus on cut-off values to define sarcopenia or an increased risk of mortality, and the relationship between muscle ultrasound and dietary or physical intervention has yet to be demonstrated [21].

In 2020, the American Society for Parenteral and Enteral Nutrition Clinical Guidelines concluded that no recommendations could be made at this time to support the use of US in clinical practice because of the limited data supporting its validity in any specific patient population [26]. The use of advanced techniques such as shear wave elastography (SWE), super microvascular imaging (SMI) and contrast-enhanced quadriceps anterior rectus ultrasound (CEUS) remains to be established.

2.7.2 Computer Tomography (CT)

For clinical reasons, critically ill patients undergo abdominal CT scans not only before admission to intensive care, but often several times during their hospital stay. CT morphological findings can therefore be used not only to analyse body composition but also to monitor changes in skeletal muscle mass. A cadaver validation study showed that quantitative analysis of the musculature in the lumbar spine area (usually at L3) in the computed tomographic abdominal cross-section (CSA) correlates well with the muscle mass of the whole body [27]. CT-derived muscle area has been validated for the assessment of total skeletal muscle mass in healthy volunteers [28], and in critically ill patients there is a strong correlation between CT-morphological muscle mass and patient prognosis (mortality, duration of mechanical ventilation and intensive care unit/hospital length-of-stay) [29, 30, 31]. The incidence of skeletal muscle mass loss diagnosed by serial computed tomographies in intensive care patients is estimated to be 60–70% [1].

Several software programs are available for mathematical analysis, such as ImageJ, which is freely available from the National Institute of Health (Bethesda, MD, USA) and Sliceomatic by TomoVision, Montreal, Quebec, Canada. To calculate total body muscle mass, the software extrapolates findings at a single L3 level to total skeletal muscle mass using the Shen equation and tissue density [28].

Limitations
There are no internationally accepted cut-off values for the diagnosis of sarcopenia based on CT scan measurements. More recently, sarcopenia has been defined using the skeletal muscle index (SMI), which estimates the area of total skeletal muscle (cm^2) in relation to height squared (m^2). Sarcopenia was assumed if a patient's SMI was in the lowest sex-specific SMI quartile. However, in hospitalised medical patients at nutritional risk, low SMI was not a significant predictor of clinical response to intensified MNT [32, 33].

CT scans are also affected by hydration status, as muscles can become oedematous. Furthermore, CT scans assess muscle mass indirectly using equations based on algorithms that are not validated in the critically ill population with altered hydration, altered membrane capacitance and unreliable body weight. Disproportionate muscle distribution cannot be assessed by CT analysis at a single L3 level [28].

For reasons of radiation safety and cost, CT scans should only be used when there is a clinical indication for such a scan and when appropriate expertise in body composition assessment is available locally.

2.7.3 Bioelectrical Impedance Analysis (BIA)

Non-invasive BIA focuses on the electrical conductivity of the body, which is determined by measuring the total body resistance (impedance) when an alternating current (50 kHz at 0.8 mA) is applied through electrodes placed on the back of the hand and foot. The body impedance is inversely proportional to the body water content (ohmic resistance) and depends on the body proportions (i.e. the cross-sectional area of the conductor). When an alternating current is applied, the cell membranes act like a capacitor and determine the capacitive resistance. This capacitor-like effect of the cell membranes leads to a shift in the phase angle [1].

Body weight, which is entered into the software along with height as the basis for calculating the variables, should ideally be measured at the time of the BIA examination. In addition, when using the extracellular water (ECW) parameter, a reduction in the albumin level should also be taken into account. Fat-free mass, body cell mass and fat mass can then be calculated using different algorithms [1].

Limitations

The measurement of fat-free mass and body cell mass by BIA must be considered very unreliable, especially in the case of extreme shifts in hydration status. Comparative studies in critically ill patients with an abdominal CT scan have shown poor agreement between BIA and CT-derived muscle mass [28].

Another methodological limitation is that the BIA devices on the market use different equations to calculate body composition based on the measured resistance (R) and/or reactance (Xc). Equations for muscle mass have been developed by Talluri, Janssen and Kyle. In critically ill patients, the Talluri equations may be superior to other equations [28].

Phase Angle

In intensive care patients, calculations of fat-free mass are much less informative than phase angle, which is independent of weight but dependent on age and sex. However, because phase angle must be considered as a sum parameter of tissue quality, which in turn depends on hydration status, the extent of capillary leakage and lean body mass, its correlation with nutritional status is limited.

The decrease in phase angle measured by BIA or bioelectrical impedance vector analysis (BIVA) is probably associated with increased morbidity and mortality, although many studies have a high risk of bias and consequently the quality of evidence is low or very low [34]. The benefits of controlling MNT based on phase angle have not been demonstrated.

There are currently too many uncertainties (including standardisation and cut-off values) and discrepancies in the interpretation of BIA measurements in critical illness to justify major therapeutic consequences [35]. No recommendations can be made at this time to support the use of BIA in the clinical setting, as data to support its validity in any specific patient population is limited by the proprietary nature of the manufacturer-specific BIA regression models used to generate body composition data [26].

2.8 Current Guideline Recommendations for Assessing the Nutritional Status of Critically Ill Patients

Due to the generally weak evidence base, current international guidelines do not provide clear recommendations on the precise methodology or level of human resources that should be available to assess nutritional status. A recent survey analysed 18 national clinical practice guidelines. All mention heterogeneous criteria for assessing nutritional status. The most commonly mentioned criteria are reduced food intake, loss of muscle mass, weight loss and low BMI. The most frequently mentioned tool was the SGA. None of the guidelines provided a clear rationale for the use of specific criteria or tools for nutritional assessment [36]. To establish a standardised process for assessing nutritional status in critically ill patients, there is a need for validation studies of bedside methods and the development of globally standardised assessment protocols [37].

Table 2.2 shows recommendation by German, North American and European guidelines for assessing the nutritional status of critically ill patients.

Table 2.2 Guideline recommendations for assessing the nutritional status of critically ill patients (according to [1])

Society	Parameter
DGEM Guideline "Intensive Care Medicine"	Subjective Global Assessment (SGA) or
	BMI < 18.5 kg/m^2 or
	Involuntary weight loss of >10% of the body weight within the last 3–6 months or
	BMI < 20 kg/m^2 and involuntary weight loss of >5% of the body weight within the last 3–6 months or
	Fasting > 7 days
	Non-invasive serial measurements of skeletal muscle mass using sonography/MRI/CT on admission and during intensive care unit stay
A.S.P.E.N. Guideline "Intensive Care Medicine"	Risk assessment by validated scores, Nutritional Risk Score (NRS), Nutrition Risk in the Critically Ill (NUTRIC)
	Inappropriate energy intake
	Loss of body weight
	Loss of muscle mass and subcutaneous fat tissue
	Oedema
	Reduced functional status
ESPEN Guideline "Intensive Care Medicine"	History and clinical examination
	Reduced BMI
	Involuntary weight loss
	If possible: Determination of body composition including muscle mass and strength

A.S.P.E.N. American Society for Parenteral and Enteral Nutrition, *BMI* body mass index, *CT* computerised tomography, *DGEM* German Society for Medical Nutrition Therapy, *ESPEN* European Society for Clinical Nutrition and Metabolism, *MRI* magnetic resonance imaging

References

1. Weimann A, Hartl WH, Adolph M, Angstwurm M, Brunkhorst FM, Edel A, de Heer G, Felbinger TW, Goeters C, Hill A, Kreymann KG, Mayer K, Ockenga J, Petros S, Rümelin A, Schaller SJ, Schneider A, Stoppe C, Elke G. Assessment and technical monitoring of nutritional status of patients in intensive and intermediate care units: position paper of the Section Metabolism and Nutrition of the German Interdisciplinary Association for Intensive and Emergency Medicine (DIVI). Med Klin Intensivmed Notfmed. 2022;117(Suppl 2):37–50.
2. Hermans AJH, Laarhuis BI, Kouw IWK, van Zanten ARH. Current insights in ICU nutrition: tailored nutrition. Curr Opin Crit Care. 2023;29(2):101–7.
3. Wischmeyer PE, Bear DE, Berger MM, De Waele E, Gunst J, McClave SA, Prado CM, Puthucheary Z, Ridley EJ, Van den Berghe G, van Zanten ARH. Personalized nutrition therapy in critical care: 10 expert recommendations. Crit Care. 2023;27(1):261.
4. Lew CCH, Yandell R, Fraser RJL, Chua AP, Chong MFF, Miller M. Association between malnutrition and clinical outcomes in the intensive care unit: a systematic review. JPEN J Parenter Enteral Nutr. 2017;41(5):744–58.
5. Jensen GL, Cederholm T, Correia MITD, Gonzalez MC, Fukushima R, Higashiguchi T, de Baptista GA, Barazzoni R, Blaauw R, Coats AJS, Crivelli A, Evans DC, Gramlich L, Fuchs-Tarlovsky V, Keller H, Llido L, Malone A, Mogensen KM, Morley JE, Muscaritoli M, Nyulasi I, Pirlich M, Pisprasert V, de van der Schueren M, Siltharm S, Singer P, Tappenden KA, Velasco N, Waitzberg DL, Yamwong P, Yu J, Compher C, Van Gossum A. GLIM criteria for the diagnosis of malnutrition: a consensus report from the Global Clinical Nutrition Community. JPEN J Parenter Enteral Nutr. 2019;43(1):32–40.
6. Hartl WH, Elke G. Nutrition during the acute phase of critical illness: discussions on NUTRIREA-3. Lancet Respir Med. 2023;11(7):e61.
7. Evans DC, Corkins MR, Malone A, Miller S, Mogensen KM, Guenter P, Jensen GL, ASPEN Malnutrition Committee. The use of visceral proteins as nutrition markers: an ASPEN position paper. Nutr Clin Pract. 2021;36(1):22–8.
8. Elke G, Hartl WH, Adolph M, Angstwurm M, Brunkhorst FM, Edel A, Heer G, Felbinger TW, Goeters C, Hill A, Kreymann KG, Mayer K, Ockenga J, Petros S, Rümelin A, Schaller SJ, Schneider A, Stoppe C, Weimann A. Laboratory and calorimetric monitoring of medical nutrition therapy in intensive and intermediate care units: second position paper of the Section Metabolism and Nutrition of the German Interdisciplinary Association for Intensive Care and Emergency Medicine (DIVI). Med Klin Intensivmed Notfmed. 2023;118(Suppl 1):1–13.
9. Zheng WH, Zhu YB, Yao Y, Huang HB. Serum creatinine/cystatin C ratio as a muscle mass evaluating tool and prognostic indicator for hospitalized patients: a meta-analysis. Front Med (Lausanne). 2023;9:1058464.
10. Victoria-Montesinos D, García-Muñoz AM, Navarro-Marroco J, Lucas-Abellán C, Mercader-Ros MT, Serrano-Martínez A, Abellán-Aynés O, Barcina-Pérez P, Hernández-Sánchez P. Phase angle, handgrip strength, and other indicators of nutritional status in cancer patients undergoing different nutritional strategies: a systematic review and meta-analysis. Nutrients. 2023;15(7):1790.
11. van Zwienen-Pot JI, Reinders I, de Groot LCPGM, Beck AM, Feldblum I, Jobse I, Neelemaat F, de van der Schueren MAE, Shahar DR, Smeets ETHC, Tieland M, Wijnhoven HAH, Volkert D, Visser M. Effects of nutritional interventions in older adults with malnutrition or at risk of malnutrition on muscle strength and mortality: results of pooled analyses of individual participant data from nine RCTs. Nutrients. 2023;15(9):2025.
12. Kaegi-Braun N, Tribolet P, Baumgartner A, Fehr R, Baechli V, Geiser M, Deiss M, Gomes F, Kutz A, Hoess C, Pavlicek V, Schmid S, Bilz S, Sigrist S, Brändle M, Benz C, Henzen C, Thomann R, Rutishauser J, Aujesky D, Rodondi N, Donzé J, Stanga Z, Mueller B, Schuetz P. Value of handgrip strength to predict clinical outcomes and therapeutic response in malnourished medical inpatients: secondary analysis of a randomized controlled trial. Am J Clin

Nutr. 2021;114(2):731–40. https://doi.org/10.1093/ajcn/nqab042. Erratum in: Am J Clin Nutr. 2021;114(2):826–7.
13. Skipper A, Coltman A, Tomesko J, Charney P, Porcari J, Piemonte TA, Handu D, Cheng FW. Adult malnutrition (undernutrition) screening: an evidence analysis center systematic review. J Acad Nutr Diet. 2020;120(4):669–708.
14. Arabi YM, Aldawood AS, Al-Dorzi HM, Tamim HM, Haddad SH, Jones G, McIntyre L, Solaiman O, Sakkijha MH, Sadat M, Mundekkadan S, Kumar A, Bagshaw SM, Mehta S, PermiT Trial Group. Permissive underfeeding or standard enteral feeding in high- and low-nutritional-risk critically ill adults. Post Hoc analysis of the PermiT trial. Am J Respir Crit Care Med. 2017;195(5):652–62.
15. Wang CY, Fu PK, Chao WC, Wang WN, Chen CH, Huang YC. Full versus trophic feeds in critically ill adults with high and low nutritional risk scores: a randomized controlled trial. Nutrients. 2020;12(11):3518.
16. Hung KY, Chen TH, Lee YF, Fang WF. Using body composition analysis for improved nutritional intervention in septic patients: a prospective interventional study. Nutrients. 2023;15(17):3814.
17. Kaegi-Braun N, Boesiger F, Tribolet P, Gomes F, Kutz A, Hoess C, Pavlicek V, Bilz S, Sigrist S, Brändle M, Henzen C, Thomann R, Rutishauser J, Aujesky D, Rodondi N, Donzé J, Stanga Z, Lobo DN, Cederholm T, Mueller B, Schuetz P. Validation of modified GLIM criteria to predict adverse clinical outcome and response to nutritional treatment: a secondary analysis of a randomized clinical trial. Clin Nutr. 2022;41(4):795–804.
18. Mundi MS, Patel JJ, Martindale R. Body composition technology: implications for the ICU. Nutr Clin Pract. 2019;34(1):48–58.
19. Ruiz-Santana S, Hernández-Socorro CR. Novel tools to assess muscle sarcopenic process in ICU patients: are they worthwhile? J Clin Med. 2023;12(10):3473.
20. Peres LM, Luis-Silva F, Menegueti MG, Lovato WJ, do Espirito Santo DA, Donadel MD, Sato L, Malek-Zadeh CH, Basile-Filho A, Martins-Filho OA, Auxiliadora-Martins M. Validation study of ultrasonography versus computed tomography for measuring muscle mass loss in critically ill patients: CT mUS study. Crit Care. 2023;27(1):310.
21. De Rosa S, Umbrello M, Pelosi P, Battaglini D. Update on lean body mass diagnostic assessment in critical illness. Diagnostics (Basel). 2023;13(5):888.
22. Casey P, Alasmar M, McLaughlin J, Ang Y, McPhee J, Heire P, Sultan J. The current use of ultrasound to measure skeletal muscle and its ability to predict clinical outcomes: a systematic review. J Cachexia Sarcopenia Muscle. 2022;13(5):2298–309.
23. Weinel LM, Summers MJ, Chapple LA. Ultrasonography to measure quadriceps muscle in critically ill patients: a literature review of reported methodologies. Anaesth Intensive Care. 2019;47(5):423–34.
24. Nascimento TS, de Queiroz RS, Ramos ACC, Martinez BP, Da Silva E, Silva CM, Gomes-Neto M. Ultrasound protocols to assess skeletal and diaphragmatic muscle in people who are critically ill: a systematic review. Ultrasound Med Biol. 2021;47(11):3041–67.
25. Lambell KJ, Tierney AC, Wang JC, Nanjayya V, Forsyth A, Goh GS, Vicendese D, Ridley EJ, Parry SM, Mourtzakis M, King SJ. Comparison of ultrasound-derived muscle thickness with computed tomography muscle cross-sectional area on admission to the intensive care unit: a pilot cross-sectional study. JPEN J Parenter Enteral Nutr. 2021;45(1):136–45.
26. Sheean P, Gonzalez MC, Prado CM, McKeever L, Hall AM, Braunschweig CA. American society for parenteral and enteral nutrition clinical guidelines: the validity of body composition assessment in clinical populations. JPEN J Parenter Enteral Nutr. 2020;44(1):12–43.
27. Mitsiopoulos N, Baumgartner RN, Heymsfield SB, Lyons W, Gallagher D, Ross R. Cadaver validation of skeletal muscle measurement by magnetic resonance imaging and computerized tomography. J Appl Physiol (1985). 1998;85(1):115–22.
28. Looijaard WGPM, Stapel SN, Dekker IM, Rusticus H, Remmelzwaal S, Girbes ARJ, Weijs PJM, Oudemans-van Straaten HM. Identifying critically ill patients with low muscle mass: agreement between bioelectrical impedance analysis and computed tomography. Clin Nutr. 2020;39(6):1809–17.

29. Yang H, Wan XX, Ma H, Li Z, Weng L, Xia Y, Zhang XM. Prevalence and mortality risk of low skeletal muscle mass in critically ill patients: an updated systematic review and meta-analysis. Front Nutr. 2023;10:1117558.
30. Jiang T, Lin T, Shu X, Song Q, Dai M, Zhao Y, Huang L, Tu X, Yue J. Prevalence and prognostic value of preexisting sarcopenia in patients with mechanical ventilation: a systematic review and meta-analysis. Crit Care. 2022;26(1):140.
31. Meyer HJ, Wienke A, Surov A. Computed tomography-defined low skeletal muscle mass as a prognostic marker for short-term mortality in critically ill patients: a systematic review and meta-analysis. Nutrition. 2021;91–92:111417.
32. Mueller L, Mentil N, Staub N, Griot S, Olpe T, Burn F, Schindera S, Mueller B, Schuetz P, Stanga Z, Baumgartner A. Association of thoracic skeletal muscle index with clinical outcome and response to nutritional interventions in patients at risk of malnutrition-secondary analysis of a randomized trial. Nutrients. 2023;15(4):817.
33. Baumgartner A, Olpe T, Griot S, Mentil N, Staub N, Burn F, Schindera S, Kaegi-Braun N, Tribolet P, Hoess C, Pavlicek V, Bilz S, Sigrist S, Brändle M, Henzen C, Thomann R, Rutishauser J, Aujesky D, Rodondi N, Donzé J, Stanga Z, Mueller B, Schuetz P. Association of CT-based diagnosis of sarcopenia with prognosis and treatment response in patients at risk of malnutrition – a secondary analysis of the effect of early nutritional support on frailty, functional outcomes, and recovery of malnourished medical inpatients trial (EFFORT) trial. Clin Nutr. 2023;42(2):199–207.
34. Lima J, Eckert I, Gonzalez MC, Silva FM. Prognostic value of phase angle and bioelectrical impedance vector in critically ill patients: a systematic review and meta-analysis of observational studies. Clin Nutr. 2022;41(12):2801–16.
35. Moonen HPFX, Van Zanten ARH. Bioelectric impedance analysis for body composition measurement and other potential clinical applications in critical illness. Curr Opin Crit Care. 2021;27(4):344–53.
36. Soriano-Moreno DR, Dolores-Maldonado G, Benites-Bullón A, Ccami-Bernal F, Fernandez-Guzman D, Esparza-Varas AL, Caira-Chuquineyra B, Taype-Rondan A. Recommendations for nutritional assessment across clinical practice guidelines: a scoping review. Clin Nutr ESPEN. 2022;49:201–7.
37. Smith LO, Olieman JF, Berk KA, Ligthart-Melis GC, Earthman CP. Clinical applications of body composition and functional status tools for nutrition assessment of hospitalized adults: a systematic review. JPEN J Parenter Enteral Nutr. 2023;47(1):11–29.

Nutrition in ICU Proteins and Amino Acids

Ellen Dresen

3.1 Biochemical Structure and Classification of Amino Acids and Proteins

Amino acids are organic compounds characterized by four key elements: amino group ($-NH_2$), carboxylic acid group ($-COOH$), hydrogen atom (H), and variable amino acid chain (Fig. 3.1).

Amino acids represent the building blocks of proteins, which are each characterized by an individual sequence of single amino acids linked together via peptide bonds. A total of 20 amino acids are needed to build up all the proteins present in the human body, which are required to preserve its structure and function.

Based on the human body's capacity to endogenously synthesize the amino acids needed to build up body proteins by using carbon and nitrogen precursors and specific enzymatic pathways, the amino acids are differentiated into dispensable amino acids (endogenous synthesis) and indispensable amino acids (no endogenous synthesis). Besides, under certain conditions (e.g., critical illness), specific amino acids cannot be synthesized by endogenous mechanisms in adequate amounts—e.g., due to increased requirements and/or impaired enzymatic synthesis—and, thus, become conditionally indispensable [25, 49]. Table 3.1 shows the classification of all 20 amino acids required to build up body proteins.

Proteins can be divided into:

- Fibrous proteins in supporting and protective tissues, e.g., keratin (hair), collagen (connective tissue), fibrin (blood), myosin (muscle)

E. Dresen (✉)
University Hospital Würzburg, Department of Anaesthesiology, Intensive Care, Emergency and Pain Medicine, Würzburg, Germany
e-mail: Dresen_E@ukw.de

Fig. 3.1 Basic structure of amino acids. COOH carboxylic acid group, H hydrogen atom, H₂N amino group, R variable amino acid chain

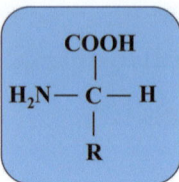

Table 3.1 Classification of indispensable, dispensable, and conditionally indispensable amino acids, according to [25, 49]

Indispensable amino acids	Dispensable amino acids	Conditionally indispensable amino acids
Isoleucine	Alanine	Arginine
Leucine	Asparagine	Cysteine
Lysine	Aspartic acid	Glutamine
Methionine	Glutamic acid	Histidine
Phenylalanine	Glycine	Tyrosine
Threonine	Proline	
Tryptophan	Serine	
Valine		

- Globular proteins in tissue fluids and secretions, e.g., albumins and globulins (blood), caseinogen (milk)
- Plant proteins such as glutelins (e.g., glutenin in wheat, hordenin in barley) and prolamines (e.g., gliadin in wheat, zein in maize)

Further, based on their chemical structure, proteins are divided into enzymes, receptor proteins, immunoglobulins, structural proteins, contractile proteins, and carrier proteins [12].

3.2 Physiological Functions of Amino Acids and Proteins

In general, central functions of amino acids and proteins include provision of nitrogen and (conditionally) indispensable substrates (amino acids), synthesis of endogenous proteins (e.g., enzymes, carrier proteins, hormones, immune proteins), synthesis of body tissues (e.g., muscle, organ, and connective tissues), and synthesis of signaling substances (e.g., adrenaline, noradrenaline, serotonin), and biogenic amins (e.g., dopamine, histamine). By providing 4 kcal/g protein, the contribution as energy source is of minor significance during nutrition in physiological conditions. However, in fasting/starvation and stress metabolism, proteins may deliver glucoplastic amino acids (e.g., alanine, glycine, serin, glutamine) for the synthesis of glucose via gluconeogenesis [12, 57]. Specific functions of single amino acids further comprise protection from free radicals, synthesis of deoxyribonucleic acid (DNA) and ribonucleic acid (RNA), transportation of oxygen, and involvement in diverse processes in carbohydrate and fat metabolism [48].

3.3 Protein and Amino Acid Metabolism in Health and Critical Illness

In healthy people, there exists balance between protein degradation (catabolism) and synthesis (anabolism), which is called protein turnover. Protein intake by nutrition, de novo synthesis of amino acids, and amino acids becoming available through degradation of body protein (e.g., from muscle, intestine, liver, kidney, and skin) contribute to a pool of free amino acids. These free amino acids are used for further metabolism of precursors of diverse metabolic mechanisms, degraded and excreted as nitrogen components via urine and skin, or used as energy substrates. Further, there is a loss of indigestible components via faeces (Fig. 3.2).

However, in critical illness there occur extensive alterations—among others—in protein metabolism leading to imbalances. In detail, critical conditions such as acute/chronic inflammation, tumors, sepsis, trauma, and burn injuries are accompanied by a disease-induced release of hormones (e.g., cortisol, glucagon, adrenalin, noradrenalin) and cytokines (e.g., tumor necrosis factor-alpha [TNF-α], interleukine-1 [IL-1] and IL-6). These factors trigger an increase in protein catabolism, which is characterized by the following:

- Decreased protein synthesis due to inhibition of activated protein kinase B (Akt)/mechanistic target of rapamycin in complex 1 (mTORC1) pathway [2, 13]
- Increased protein degradation due to enhancement in proteolytic cascades of ubiquitin-proteasome pathway [1]
- Increased synthesis of acute phase proteins [44]
- Use of glucoplastic amino acids as energy sources [4]

Furthermore, protein catabolism is additionally boosted by bed rest/immobility and the patients´ individual nutrition status. In consequence, intensified protein

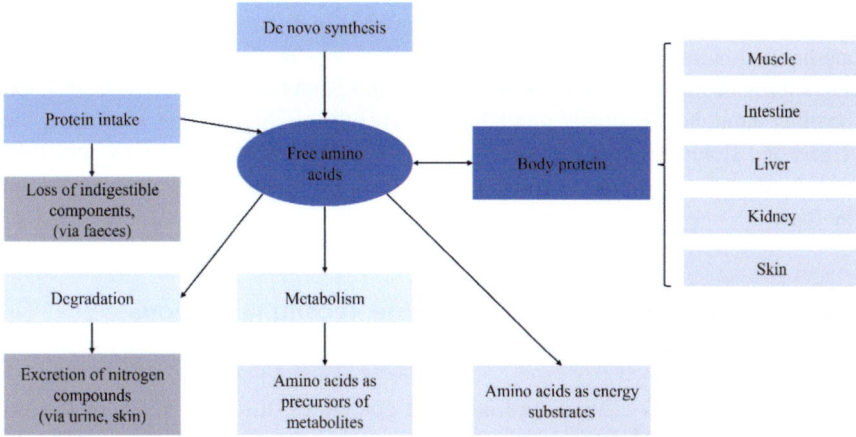

Fig. 3.2 Protein and amino acid metabolism in health, modified according to [12]

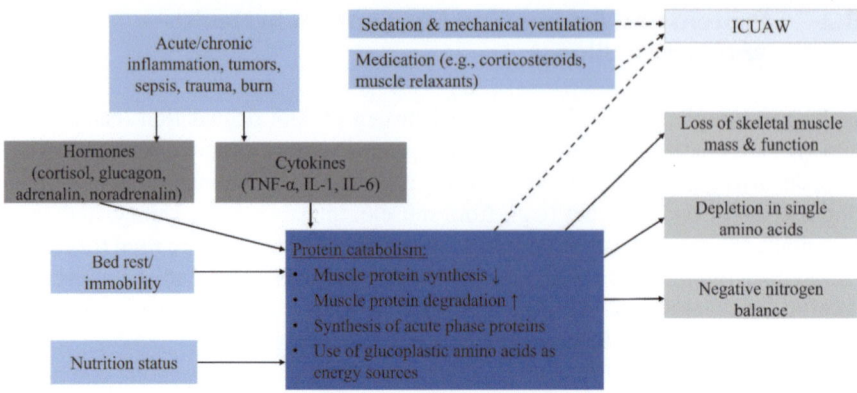

Fig. 3.3 Alterations in protein metabolism during critical illness. TNF-α tumor necrosis factor-alpha, ICUAW intensive care unit acquired weakness, IL-1 interleukine-1, IL-6 interleukine-6

catabolism during critical illness may lead to loss of skeletal muscle mass and function, depletion in single amino acids, and negative nitrogen balance. In addition, critical illness-associated medical treatments such as sedation, medication (i.e., administration of corticosteroids and muscle relaxants), and (prolonged) mechanical ventilation may further increase the risk for the development of iatrogenic muscle weakness, so-called intensive care unit acquired weakness (ICUAW) [29, 42, 43, 54]. Figure 3.3 summarizes the alterations in protein metabolism during critical illness.

3.4 Protein/Amino Acid Supply in Critically Ill ICU Patients

In routine clinical practice, appropriate provision of proteins/amino acids within a balanced medical nutrition therapy approach is an essential element of medical care. However, the optimal dosing and timing of protein supply in critically ill patients in general and in specific sub-cohorts is controversially discussed since years. On the one hand, this fact is also reflected by current recommendations on protein/amino acid supply of international critical care nutrition guidelines [3, 10, 31, 46, 47]. On the other hand, heterogeneity in methods and results of clinical trials evaluating the effects of different protein dosages on diverse clinical outcome measures published over time and also very recently, further fuel the controversial discussions on the topic.

3.4.1 Current International Guideline Recommendations on Protein/Amino Acid Supply

Current international critical care nutrition guidelines differ markedly in recommendations on protein dosage and intake timing in critically ill patients (Table 3.2).

Table 3.2 Current international critical care nutrition guideline recommendations on protein/amino acid supply in critically ill patients

Guideline	Recommendation	Grade of recommendation/quality of evidence/consensus
ASPEN 2016 [31]	1.2–2.0 g protein/kg BW/d (higher dosage may be indicated in burn or multi-trauma patients)	QoE: Very low
	High risk/severely malnourished patients: ≥1.2 g protein/kg BW/d when requiring PN (over first week of ICU admission)	QoE: Very low
	Obese patients: 2.0 g/kg iBW/d (BMI 30–40 kg/m²) up to 2.5 g/kg iBW/d (BMI ≥40 kg/m²)	QoE: N/A
	Patients with acute renal failure/acute kidney injury: 1.2–2.0 g protein/kg BW/d	QoE: N/A
	Patients receiving hemodialysis or CRRT: 2.5 g protein/kg BW/d	QoE: Very low
	Patients with open abdomen: Additional 15.0–30.0 g protein/L of exudate loss	QoE: N/A
	Patients with burn injury: 1.5–2.0 g protein/kg BW/d	QoE: N/A
	Septic patients: 1.2–2.0 g/protein/kg BW/d	QoE: N/A
	Immune-modulating enteral formulations containing arginine and glutamine: Should not be used routinely	QoE: Very low
	Immune-modulating formulas containing arginine: To be considered in patients with severe trauma, traumatic brain injury, and major surgery (postoperatively)	QoE: Very low
	Supplemental enteral glutamine: Not to be added to EN routinely	QoE: Moderate
	Supplemental parenteral glutamine: Not to be used routinely	QoE: Moderate
ESPEN 2019 [46]	1.3 g/kg protein equivalents/d (to be increased progressively)	GoR: 0 strong consensus (91%)
	Obese patients: Protein delivery to be guided by urinary nitrogen losses or lean body mass determination (e.g., via CT); if not available, 1.3 g protein/kg aBW/d	GoR: GPP—consensus (89%)
	Additional EN doses of glutamine:	
	Patients with burns >20% body surface area: 0.3–0.5 g/kg BW/d for 10–15 days	GoR: B—strong consensus (95%)
	Patients with trauma: 0.2–0.3 g/kg BW/d for the first 5 days	GoR: 0—strong consensus (91%)
	Patients with complicated wound healing: 0.2–0.3 g/kg BW/d up to 15 days	GoR: 0—strong consensus (91%)
	No indication in patients except those with burn injury and trauma	GoR: B—strong consensus (92.31%)
	Parenteral glutamine-dipeptide: Not to be given in unstable and complex ICU patients (especially not in those suffering from liver/renal failure)	GoR: A—strong consensus (92.31%)

(continued)

Table 3.2 (continued)

Guideline	Recommendation	Grade of recommendation/ quality of evidence/ consensus
DGEM 2019 [10]	*Acute phase of critical illness:*	
	1.0 g protein/kg BW/d and 1.2 g amino acids/kg BW/d respectively as target	Consensus (87.5%)
	To be initiated with 75% of target and progressively increased according to individual metabolic tolerance to reach 100% of target until the end of acute phase (approx. 4–7 days after onset of critical illness)	Consensus (82%)
	Post-acute/convalescence/rehabilitation phase of critical illness: 1.0 g protein/kg BW/d and 1.2 g amino acids/kg BW/d to be covered by 100% or higher	Consensus (88%)
	Chronic phase of critical illness: 1.0 g protein/kg BW/d and 1.2 g amino acids/kg BW/d to be covered by 100%	Strong consensus (91%)
	Protein loss via drainages/bandages: Shall be balanced in case of open abdomen	Strong consensus (91%)
	Immune-modulating enteral nutrition (e.g., containing arginine and glutamine) Shall not be used in critically ill patients	Consensus (83%)
	Enteral glutamine pharmacotherapy: Shall not be used in critically ill patients	Strong consensus (94%)
	Enteral arginine pharmacotherapy: Shall not to be used in critically ill patients	Strong consensus (100%)
	Parenteral glutamine pharmacotherapy: Can be used in patients receiving parenteral nutrition, who do not suffer from severe liver, kidney, or multiorgan dysfunction	Consensus (87%)
	Amino acid solutions enriched with branched-chain amino acids: Shall not be used routinely in critically ill patients	Consensus (84%)
	Obese patients (BMI $\geq$ 30 kg/m^2): 1.5 g protein/kg iBW/d and 1.8 g amino acids/kg iBW/d, respectively	Strong consensus (94%)
ASPEN 2022 [3]	No modification compared to the 2016 guideline recommendation of 1.2–2.0 g protein/kg BW/d	EG: low SoR: weak

(continued)

Table 3.2 (continued)

Guideline	Recommendation	Grade of recommendation/ quality of evidence/ consensus
ESPEN 2023 [47]	1.3 g protein equivalents/kg BW/d can be delivered progressively	GoR: 0—strong consensus (92%)
	Obese patients (no modification compared to 2019 guideline recommendation): Protein delivery to be guided by urinary nitrogen losses or lean body mass determination (e.g., via CT); if not available, 1.3 g protein/kg aBW/d	GoR: GPP—consensus (89%)
	Additional enteral doses of glutamine (no modifications compared to 2019 guideline recommendations):	
	Patients with burns >20% body surface area: 0.3–0.5 g/kg BW/d for 10–15 days	GoR: B—strong consensus (95%)
	Patients with trauma: 0.2–0.3 g/kg BW/d for the first 5 days	GoR: 0—strong consensus (91%)
	Patients with complicated wound healing: 0.2–0.3 g/kg BW/d up to 15 days	GoR: 0—strong consensus (91%)
	No indication in patients except those with burn injury and trauma	GoR: B—strong consensus (92%)
	Parenteral glutamine-dipeptide (no modification compared to 2019 guideline recommendation): Not to be given in unstable and complex ICU patients (especially not in those suffering from liver/renal failure)	GoR: A—strong consensus (92%)

aBW adjusted body weight, *ASPEN* American Society for Parenteral and Enteral Nutrition, *BW* body weight, *CRRT* continuous renal replacement therapy, *CT* computed tomography, *DGEM* German Society for Clinical Nutrition and Metabolism, *EG* evidence grade, *EN* enteral nutrition, *ESPEN* European Society for Clinical Nutrition and Metabolism, *GoR* grade of recommendation, *GPP* good practice point, *iBW* ideal body weight, *N/A* not applicable, *PN* parenteral nutrition, *QoE* quality of evidence, *SoG* strength of GRADE

3.4.2 Current Evidence on Protein/Amino Acid Supply from Clinical Trials

3.4.2.1 Total Protein/Amino Acid Supply

Determining protein/amino acid requirements in critically ill patients and defining optimal dosing and timing of supply strategies are ongoing subject of debate [9]. However, due to great methodological differences (e.g., target population/inclusion criteria, intervention/protein targets, concomitant nutrition therapy, study duration, outcome measures) resulting in conflicting results, overall evidence from clinical trials is low.

A large international, observational data-base study (n = 16,489 critically ill patients) showed an association of late (day 5–11) standard protein diet (median, 0.99 g/kg BW/d; interquartile range [IQR], 0.89–1.09 g/kg BW/d) and reduced in-hospital mortality and increased discharges alive from hospital [17]. However, both early (day 1–4) standard (median, 0.99 g/kg BW/d; IQR, 0.27–0.66 g/kg BW/d) and high protein intake (median, 1.41 g/kg BW/d; IQR, 1.29–1.6 g/kg BW/d) had no effect on the patient outcomes in the acute phase of critical illness [17].

In addition, observational data from the EuroPN study (n = 1,172 ICU patients) emphasized an association of daily moderate protein intake of 0.8–1.2 g/kg BW/day (median, 1.0 g/kg BW/d; confidence interval [CI], 0.9, 1.11 g/kg BW/d) initiated early within 48 h after ICU admission and fewer days of mechanical ventilation compared with higher (>1.2 g/kg BW/d; median, 1.51 g/kg BW/d; CI, 1.36, 1.76) or lower intakes (<0.8 g/kg BW/d; median, 0.28 g/kg BW/d; CI, 0.0, 0.55 g/kg BW/d) [30].

Data from a retrospective cohort study (n = 2,618 ICU patients) indicated that early high protein supply of ≥1.2 g/kg BW/d at day 4 was associated with lower rates of ICU and hospital mortality compared to early low protein supply of <1.2 g/kg BW/d at day 4 [56].

In recent years, few randomized controlled trials (RCT) evaluating the effects of various dosages of protein supply on diverse clinical and functional outcome parameters have been published.

In a prospective, monocentric RCT (n = 42 adult ICU patients), higher protein intake of 1.5 ± 0.5 g/kg BW/day (mean ± standard deviation) compared to lower protein intake (1.0 ± 0.5 g/kg BW/day) within a balanced medical nutrition approach initiated on day ≥10 after ICU admission did not show a statistically significant effect on skeletal muscle mass changes (Δ quadriceps muscle layer thickness [QMLT]) [7]. Moreover, the different dosages of protein supply did not result in any differences regarding severity of illness, biochemical markers of clinical routine, duration of mechanical ventilation, ICU LOS, and episodes of pneumonia, sepsis, and infected wounds [7].

A prospective single-center RCT (n = 41 ICU patients) showed improved diaphragm atrophy and muscle mass after high protein intake (1.70 ± 0.2 g/kg BW/d) compared to standard protein intake (1.06 ± 0.1 g/kg BW/d), both started within 24–48 h after ICU admission [64]. However, dosage of protein intake had no effect on the duration of mechanical ventilation and ICU LOS, weaning from mechanical ventilation, and ICU mortality [64].

The results of the EFFORT Protein trial, an international, multicenter, pragmatic, registry-based randomized trial ($n = 1,301$ ICU patients) indicated that high protein (≥ 2.2 g/kg BW/day) compared to usual protein (≤ 1.2 g/kg BW/day) supply initiated within 96 h of ICU admission and continued for up to 28 days did not result in shorter time to discharge alive from hospital [21]. But, a subgroup analysis revealed that in patients with acute kidney injury and high organ failure scores, high protein intake was associated with prolonged time to discharge alive and increased 60-day mortality [21].

Findings from the pragmatic, multicenter, open-label RCT NUTRIREA-3, which evaluated the effects of low protein supply (0.2–0.4 g/kg BW/d) compared to standard protein supply (1.0–1.3 g/kg BW/d) both initiated within 24 h after intubation in patients with shock indicated an association of initial lower protein supply and faster recovery and fewer complications, while no effects on mortality could be observed [41].

A systematic review and meta analyses (SRMA) including 19 RCTs confirmed that higher protein supply (1.31 ± 0.48 g/kg BW/d) compared to lower protein supply (0.90 ± 0.30 g/kg BW/d) did not improve clinical and functional outcome measures (e.g., mortality, infectious complications, ICU and hospital LOS, duration of mechanical ventilation, muscle mass changes, hand grip strength, quality of life) [26]. But, achieving a protein supply of ≥ 1 g/kg BW/d within 4–10 days after ICU admission may preserve skeletal muscle mass and improve activities of daily living, as shown in an SRMA including 14 RCTs [36]. However, a recent updated SRMA with trial sequential analysis (TSA) reveals the previously observed finding of preservation of skeletal muscle mass by higher protein supply as type-1 error. Furthermore, especially in patients with acute kidney injury, high protein intake (1.49 ± 0.48 g/kg BW/d) compared to lower protein intake (0.92 ± 0.30 g/kg BW/d) may be harmful [27].

> In summary, based on current evidence from recent clinical trials, a medical nutrition therapy approach following early initiation of protein/amino acid supply at moderate dosages being progressively increased to reach individual targets (e.g., 1.3 g protein equivalents/kg BW/d as recommended by the European Society for Clinical Nutrition and Metabolism [ESPEN]) until the end of the acute phase of critical illness should be implemented in routine clinical practice.

3.4.2.2 Supply of Single/Specific Amino Acids and Combinations

Besides quantitative dosage of protein and amino acids provided via EN and PN, respectively, the protein quality (amino acid pattern) within balanced nutrition approaches as well as targeted supply of single amino acids and specific combinations are subject of research since years.

In this context, a secondary analysis of an RCT ($n = 42$ ICU patients) could not show any associations between protein quality as represented by the amino acid pattern provided via EN + PN and skeletal muscle mass changes in long-term immobilized ICU patients [8].

Results of a single-center, double-blind RCT ($n = 35$ critically ill patients with sepsis or acute respiratory distress syndrome) evaluating the effects of a specific combination of five amino acids (threonine, proline, serine, cysteine and leucine) or placebo within an EN feeding regimen for 21 days indicated that amino acid supplementation increased plasma citrulline levels, reduced alanine aminotransferase and alkaline phosphatase levels, and improved twitch airway pressure and anterior quadriceps volume [18].

With regard to glutamine supplementation in critically ill patients in general, evidence from large scale clinical trials (e.g., [19, 60]) and SRMAs (e.g., [32, 37, 50, 51]) is still controversial. This is reflected in current international critical care nutrition guidelines by the fact that, at present, glutamine supplementation cannot be recommended for critically ill patients in general—only few recommendations are defined for specific sub-populations of critically ill patients such as patients with burn injuries. However, in this context, the results of an international, multicenter RCT—the RE-ENERGIZE trial—indicated that enteral glutamine supplementation (0.5 g/kg BW/d) compared to placebo provided to patients with second- or third-degree burn injury ($n = 1,209$) did not reduce time to discharge alive from hospital and mortality [20]. In addition, a SRMA further strengthened the evidence that enteral or parenteral glutamine supplementation (monosubstrates) does not improve patient outcomes (e.g., mortality, infectious complications) [37]. Based on these most recent data, revision of the guideline recommendation regarding glutamine supplementation in patients with burn injuries may be indicated.

Furthermore, with regard to muscle protein metabolism and preservation of skeletal muscle mass, the branched-chain amino acids valine, leucine, and isoleucine provided in a ratio of 1: 2: 1, beta-hydroxy-beta-methylbutyrate (HMB), taurine, and creatine are of special interest in clinical research, but overall evidence is still limited [28, 33, 34, 40, 45, 58, 59, 63].

> Irrespective of the current evidence on (high-dose) supplementation of specific amino acids (e.g., glutamine), all indispensable, conditionally indispensable, and dispensable amino acids are an essential element of adequate medical nutrition therapy in the critical care setting. Thus, until more valid data regarding specific requirements for single amino acids in this specific patient cohort are available, the quality of protein supply should comprise all these amino acids in physiological dosages.

3.4.3 The Role of Amino Acid/Protein Supply and Exercise in the Critical Care Setting

Besides individualized, phase- and disease-specific medical nutrition therapy providing adequate amounts of protein, physical rehabilitation by targeted mobilization and exercise training during the ICU stay is an essential element of medical care to preserve muscle mass and, thereby, to improve the patients' functional recovery and overall outcome. Therefore, combined interventions (targeted protein/amino acid supply and physical rehabilitation) are increasingly subject of research in the field of critical care nutrition [14, 24, 39, 52].

In this context, a RCT evaluating the effects of a 6-week intervention of enhanced physiotherapy and structured exercise and provision of a supplement drink containing glutamine and essential amino acids (2 × 2 factorial design) showed improved 6-minute walk distance test in patients receiving the combined nutrition and rehabilitation intervention [22].

A monocenter RCT ($n = 117$ ICU patients) evaluating the effects of different protein dosages with and without targeted rehabilitation showed that high protein intake of around 1.5 g/kg BW/day compared to medium protein intake of 0.8 g/kg BW/day by day 10 of ICU admission resulted in decreased femoral muscle volume loss, but only when combined with active early exercise (belt-type electrical muscle stimulation) [35]. Results of another monocenter RCT ($n = 181$ ICU patients) emphasized that higher amounts of protein (median, 1.48 g/kg BW/d; IQR, 1.25–1.64 g/kg BW/d) compared to lower protein intake (median, 1.19 g/kg BW/d; IQR, 0.96–1.26 g/kg BW/d) in combination with early exercise (cycle ergometry) improved quality of life (physical component sum score) and mortality [5].

A single-center, open-label pilot trial ($n = 62$ ICU patients) comparing EN (16.7% protein calories) with conventional physiotherapy (control, group 1), EN (16.7% protein calories) with cycle ergometry (group 2), and protein-enriched EN (25% protein calories) with cycle ergometry (group 3) showed no differences in clinical endpoints such as length of mechanical ventilation, ICU mortality, ICU and hospital length of stay, and re-intubation rate [23]. However, it must be mentioned that no functional measures have been evaluated in this trial and that no data on actual protein intake are provided.

Further, a recent SRMA with TSA confirms that higher protein supply combined with early physical rehabilitation may improve quality of life and functional outcome measures, but requires further investigations [27].

The promising effects of combined targeted protein/amino acid and rehabilitation interventions demonstrated by recent clinical trials may further be supported by the results of currently running RCTs (e.g., NEXIS: NCT03021902; EFFORT-X: NCT04261543).

3.5 Methods to Evaluate Amino Acid/Protein/Muscle Metabolism

In the context of determining protein/amino requirements, defining targets for adequate protein/amino acid supply, and assessing the efficiency of actual protein/amino acid intake, appropriate methods for use in research and clinical practice must be implemented. However, due to certain difficulties in performance in ICU patients and inaccuracies in clinical practice, the methods should be selected carefully according to the technical and personnel availability and feasibility at individual institutions, performed in line with standardized protocols, and obtained results should be interpreted under consideration of the individual patients´ whole clinical picture [61]. The implementation of a mixture of different methods to assess protein/amino acid metabolism might be advantageous.

Table 3.3 provides an overview of various methods to evaluate protein/amino acid metabolism for use in clinical practice.

Table 3.3 Methods to evaluate protein/amino acid metabolism in clinical practice [6, 11, 15, 16, 38, 45, 53, 55, 61, 62]

Methods	Practical guidance
Nitrogen balance	Traditional parameter to evaluate protein metabolism Measurement of nutritional nitrogen intake and nitrogen excretion via 24-h urine samples → Aim: Nitrogen balance defined as +/−4 g/d Indicator of protein catabolism and anabolism Influenced by, e.g., energy intake, growth, injuries, postoperative stress, microbiota Limitations: only expression of net nitrogen exchange, losses via drains and wounds not considered, risk of overestimation especially in case of (critical) illness, imprecise in kidney diseases, high effort in routine clinical practice
Urea-to-creatinine ratio	(Muscle) protein catabolism goes along with increased urea production and a decrease in creatinine resulting from loss of muscle mass Increased urea-to-creatinine ratio as marker of (muscle) protein catabolism Easy to conduct in routine clinical practice → promising parameter for catabolic signature and potential interventional target Influenced by, e.g., medication, protein intake, gastrointestinal bleeding, hypovolemia, acute kidney injury Limitations: values might be invalid in critically ill patients
3-methylhistidine	Measure of (muscle) protein degradation Component of muscle cells (actin and myosin), released during muscle protein catabolism Adjustment with regard to muscle mass → 3-methylhistidin/creatinine ratio Influenced by, e.g., meat consumption in case of normal oral nutrition Limitations: High individual variance, only applicable in case of artificial nutrition (enteral and/or parenteral nutrition), measurement in serum/urine not part of routine diagnostics

(continued)

Table 3.3 (continued)

Methods	Practical guidance
Ultrasound	Evaluation of skeletal muscle mass: quadriceps muscle layer thickness or cross-sectional area Easy and quick to conduct in routine clinical practice → ensure consistence in measurement point, compression, and position of patient during measurement Influenced by, e.g., water retention Limitations: no cut-offs defined yet
Computed tomography	Analysis of body composition Evaluation of skeletal muscle mass at third lumbar spine vertebra (L3) via abdominal computed tomography scan → strong correlation with whole body muscle mass Influenced by, e.g., water retention Limitations: high costs, exposure to radiation → only applicable if computed tomography scans obtained for medical reasons
Bioelectrical impedance analysis	Traditionally used for evaluation of nutrition status via phase angle → valuable tool to predict mortality In stable patients without large water retention/fluid shifts, evaluation of fat mass and fat free mass possible Influenced by, e.g., water retention, feeding state, body weight Limitations: different equations to calculate body composition used in available devices

References

1. Bodine SC, Baehr LM. Skeletal muscle atrophy and the E3 ubiquitin ligases MuRF1 and MAFbx/atrogin-1. Am J Physiol Endocrinol Metab. 2014;307:E469–84. https://doi.org/10.1152/ajpendo.00204.2014.
2. Bodine SC, Stitt TN, Gonzalez M, Kline WO, Stover GL, Bauerlein R, Zlotchenko E, Scrimgeour A, Lawrence JC, Glass DJ, Yancopoulos GD. Akt/mTOR pathway is a crucial regulator of skeletal muscle hypertrophy and can prevent muscle atrophy in vivo. Nat Cell Biol. 2001;3:1014–9. https://doi.org/10.1038/ncb1101-1014.
3. Compher C, Bingham AL, McCall M, Patel J, Rice TW, Braunschweig C, McKeever L. Guidelines for the provision of nutrition support therapy in the adult critically ill patient: American society for parenteral and enteral nutrition. J Parenter Enter Nutr. 2022;46:12–41. https://doi.org/10.1002/jpen.2267.
4. Cuthbertson DP, Zagreb HC. The metabolic response to injury and its nutritional implications. JPEN J Parenter Enteral Nutr. 1979;3:108–29. https://doi.org/10.1177/014860717900300302.
5. de Azevedo JRA, Lima HCM, Frota PHDB, Nogueira IROM, de Souza SC, Fernandes EAA, Cruz AM. High-protein intake and early exercise in adult intensive care patients: a prospective, randomized controlled trial to evaluate the impact on functional outcomes. BMC Anesthesiol. 2021;21:283. https://doi.org/10.1186/s12871-021-01492-6.
6. Dickerson RN. Using nitrogen balance in clinical practice. Hosp Pharm. 2005;40:1081–7. https://doi.org/10.1177/001857870504001210.
7. Dresen E, Weißbrich C, Fimmers R, Putensen C, Stehle P. Medical high-protein nutrition therapy and loss of muscle mass in adult ICU patients: a randomized controlled trial. Clin Nutr. 2021;40:1562–70. https://doi.org/10.1016/j.clnu.2021.02.021.
8. Dresen E, Siepmann L, Weißbrich C, Weinhold L, Putensen C, Stehle P. Is the amino acid pattern in medical nutrition therapy crucial for successfully attenuating muscle mass loss in adult

ICU patients? Secondary analysis of a RCT. Clin Nutr ESPEN. 2022;47:36–44. https://doi.org/10.1016/j.clnesp.2021.12.021.
9. Dresen E, Notz Q, Menger J, Homayr AL, Lindner M, Radke DI, Stoppe C, Elke G. What the clinician needs to know about medical nutrition therapy in critically ill patients in 2023: a narrative review. Nutr Clin Pract. 2023;38:479–98. https://doi.org/10.1002/ncp.10984.
10. Elke G, Hartl W, Kreymann K, Adolph M, Felbinger T, Graf T, de Heer G, Heller A, Kampa U, Mayer K, Muhl E, Niemann B, Rümelin A, Steiner S, Stoppe C, Weimann A, Bischoff S. Clinical nutrition in critical care medicine – guideline of the German Society for Nutritional Medicine (DGEM). Aktuel Ernahrungsmed. 2019;43:341–408. https://doi.org/10.1055/a-0713-8179.
11. Elke G, Hartl WH, Adolph M, Angstwurm M, Brunkhorst FM, Edel A, de Heer G, Felbinger TW, Goeters C, Hill A, Kreymann KG, Mayer K, Ockenga J, Petros S, Rümelin A, Schaller SJ, Schneider A, Stoppe C, Weimann A. Laborchemisches und kalorimetrisches Monitoring der medizinischen Ernährungstherapie auf der Intensiv- und Intermediate Care Station. Med Klin Intensivmed Notfmed. 2023;118(Suppl 1):1–13. https://doi.org/10.1007/s00063-023-01001-2.
12. Fürst P, Stehle P. Proteine und Aminosäuren. In: Hartig W, Druml W, Fürst P, Biesalski H-K, Weimann A, editors. Ernährungs- und Infusionstherapie: Standards für Klinik, Intensivstation und Ambulanz; 232 Tabellen. 8th ed. Thieme, s.l.; 2004. p. 9–20.
13. Gordon BS, Kelleher AR, Kimball SR. Regulation of muscle protein synthesis and the effects of catabolic states. Int J Biochem Cell Biol. 2013;45:2147–57. https://doi.org/10.1016/j.biocel.2013.05.039.
14. Gropper S, Hunt D, Chapa DW. Sarcopenia and psychosocial variables in patients in intensive care units: the role of nutrition and rehabilitation in prevention and treatment. Crit Care Nurs Clin North Am. 2019;31:489–99. https://doi.org/10.1016/j.cnc.2019.07.004.
15. Gunst J, Kashani KB, Hermans G. The urea-creatinine ratio as a novel biomarker of critical illness-associated catabolism. Intensive Care Med. 2019;45:1813–5. https://doi.org/10.1007/s00134-019-05810-y.
16. Haines RW, Zolfaghari P, Wan Y, Pearse RM, Puthucheary Z, Prowle JR. Elevated urea-to-creatinine ratio provides a biochemical signature of muscle catabolism and persistent critical illness after major trauma. Intensive Care Med. 2019;45:1718–31. https://doi.org/10.1007/s00134-019-05760-5.
17. Hartl WH, Kopper P, Bender A, Scheipl F, Day AG, Elke G, Küchenhoff H. Protein intake and outcome of critically ill patients: analysis of a large international database using piecewise exponential additive mixed models. Crit Care. 2022;26:7. https://doi.org/10.1186/s13054-021-03870-5.
18. Heming N, Carlier R, Prigent H, Mekki A, Jousset C, Lofaso F, Ambrosi X, Bounab R, Maxime V, Mansart A, Crenn P, Moine P, Foltzer F, Cuenoud B, Konz T, Corthesy J, Beaumont M, Hartweg M, Roessle C, Preiser J-C, Breuillé D, Annane D. Effect of an enteral amino acid blend on muscle and gut functionality in critically ill patients: a proof-of-concept randomized controlled trial. Crit Care. 2022;26:358. https://doi.org/10.1186/s13054-022-04232-5.
19. Heyland D, Muscedere J, Wischmeyer PE, Cook D, Jones G, Albert M, Elke G, Berger MM, Day AG. A randomized trial of glutamine and antioxidants in critically ill patients. N Engl J Med. 2013;368:1489–97. https://doi.org/10.1056/NEJMoa1212722.
20. Heyland DK, Wibbenmeyer L, Pollack JA, Friedman B, Turgeon AF, Eshraghi N, Jeschke MG, Bélisle S, Grau D, Mandell S, Velamuri SR, Hundeshagen G, Moiemen N, Shokrollahi K, Foster K, Huss F, Collins D, Savetamal A, Gurney JM, Depetris N, Stoppe C, Ortiz-Reyes L, Garrel D, Day AG. A randomized trial of enteral glutamine for treatment of burn injuries. N Engl J Med. 2022;387(11):1001–10. https://doi.org/10.1056/NEJMoa2203364.
21. Heyland DK, Patel J, Compher C, Rice TW, Bear DE, Lee Z-Y, González VC, O'Reilly K, Regala R, Wedemire C, Ibarra-Estrada M, Stoppe C, Ortiz-Reyes L, Jiang X, Day AG. The effect of higher protein dosing in critically ill patients with high nutritional risk (EFFORT Protein): an international, multicentre, pragmatic, registry-based randomised trial. Lancet. 2023;401(10376):568–76. https://doi.org/10.1016/S0140-6736(22)02469-2.
22. Jones C, Eddleston J, McCairn A, Dowling S, McWilliams D, Coughlan E, Griffiths RD. Improving rehabilitation after critical illness through outpatient physiotherapy classes and

essential amino acid supplement: a randomized controlled trial. J Crit Care. 2015;30:901–7. https://doi.org/10.1016/j.jcrc.2015.05.002.
23. Kagan I, Cohen J, Bendavid I, Kramer S, Mesilati-Stahy R, Glass Y, Theilla M, Singer P. Effect of combined protein-enriched enteral nutrition and early cycle ergometry in mechanically ventilated critically ill patients-a pilot study. Nutrients. 2022;14(8):1589. https://doi.org/10.3390/nu14081589.
24. Kou K, Momosaki R, Miyazaki S, Wakabayashi H, Shamoto H. Impact of nutrition therapy and rehabilitation on acute and critical illness: a systematic review. J UOEH. 2019;41:303–15. https://doi.org/10.7888/juoeh.41.303.
25. Laidlaw SA, Kopple JD. Newer concepts of the indispensable amino acids. Am J Clin Nutr. 1987;46:593–605. https://doi.org/10.1093/ajcn/46.4.593.
26. Lee Z-Y, Yap CSL, Hasan MS, Engkasan JP, Barakatun-Nisak MY, Day AG, Patel JJ, Heyland DK. The effect of higher versus lower protein delivery in critically ill patients: a systematic review and meta-analysis of randomized controlled trials. Crit Care. 2021;25:260. https://doi.org/10.1186/s13054-021-03693-4.
27. Lee Z-Y, Dresen E, Lew CCH, Bels J, Hill A, Hasan MS, Ke L, van Zanten A, van de Poll MCG, Heyland DK, Stoppe C. The effects of higher versus lower protein delivery in critically ill patients: an updated systematic review and meta-analysis of randomized controlled trials with trial sequential analysis. Crit Care. 2024;28:15. https://doi.org/10.1186/s13054-023-04783-1.
28. Liu J, Klebach M, Visser M, Hofman Z. Amino acid availability of a dairy and vegetable protein blend compared to single casein, whey, soy, and pea proteins: a double-blind, cross-over trial. Nutrients. 2019;11:2613. https://doi.org/10.3390/nu11112613.
29. Martindale RG, Heyland DK, Rugeles SJ, Wernerman J, Weijs PJM, Patel JJ, McClave SA. Protein kinetics and metabolic effects related to disease states in the intensive care unit. Nutr Clin Pract. 2017;32:21S–9S. https://doi.org/10.1177/0884533617694612.
30. Matejovic M, Huet O, Dams K, Elke G, Vaquerizo Alonso C, Csomos A, Krzych ŁJ, Tetamo R, Puthucheary Z, Rooyackers O, Tjäder I, Kuechenhoff H, Hartl WH, Hiesmayr M. Medical nutrition therapy and clinical outcomes in critically ill adults: a European multinational, prospective observational cohort study (EuroPN). Crit Care. 2022;26:143. https://doi.org/10.1186/s13054-022-03997-z.
31. McClave SA, Taylor BE, Martindale RG, Warren MM, Johnson DR, Braunschweig C, McCarthy MS, Davanos E, Rice TW, Cresci GA, Gervasio JM, Sacks GS, Roberts PR, Compher C. Guidelines for the provision and assessment of nutrition support therapy in the adult critically ill patient: Society of Critical Care Medicine (SCCM) and American Society for Parenteral and Enteral Nutrition (A.S.P.E.N.). JPEN J Parenter Enter Nutr. 2016;40:159–211. https://doi.org/10.1177/0148607115621863.
32. McRae MP. Therapeutic benefits of glutamine: an umbrella review of meta-analyses. Biomed Rep. 2017;6:576–84. https://doi.org/10.3892/br.2017.885.
33. Mitchell WK, Wilkinson DJ, Phillips BE, Lund JN, Smith K, Atherton PJ. Human skeletal muscle protein metabolism responses to amino acid nutrition. Adv Nutr. 2016;7:828S–38S. https://doi.org/10.3945/an.115.011650.
34. Nakamura K, Kihata A, Naraba H, Kanda N, Takahashi Y, Sonoo T, Hashimoto H, Morimura N. β-Hydroxy-β-methylbutyrate, arginine, and glutamine complex on muscle volume loss in critically ill patients: a randomized control trial. JPEN J Parenter Enter Nutr. 2020;44:205–12. https://doi.org/10.1002/jpen.1607.
35. Nakamura K, Nakano H, Naraba H, Mochizuki M, Takahashi Y, Sonoo T, Hashimoto H, Morimura N. High protein versus medium protein delivery under equal total energy delivery in critical care: a randomized controlled trial. Clin Nutr. 2021;40:796–803. https://doi.org/10.1016/j.clnu.2020.07.036.
36. Nakanishi N, Matsushima S, Tatsuno J, Liu K, Tamura T, Yonekura H, Yamamoto N, Unoki T, Kondo Y, Nakamura K. Impact of energy and protein delivery to critically ill patients: a systematic review and meta-analysis of randomized controlled trials. Nutrients. 2022;14:4849. https://doi.org/10.3390/nu14224849.

37. Ortiz-Reyes L, Lee Z-Y, Chin Han Lew C, Hill A, Jeschke MG, Turgeon AF, Cancio L, Stoppe C, Patel JJ, Day AG, Heyland DK. The efficacy of glutamine supplementation in severe adult burn patients: a systematic review with trial sequential meta-analysis. Crit Care Med. 2023;51:1086–95. https://doi.org/10.1097/CCM.0000000000005887.
38. Page A, Flower L, Prowle J, Puthucheary Z. Novel methods to identify and measure catabolism. Curr Opin Crit Care. 2021;27:361–6. https://doi.org/10.1097/MCC.0000000000000842.
39. Parry SM, Chapple L-AS, Mourtzakis M. Exploring the potential effectiveness of combining optimal nutrition with electrical stimulation to maintain muscle health in critical illness: a narrative review. Nutr Clin Pract. 2018;33:772–89. https://doi.org/10.1002/ncp.10213.
40. Phillips SM, Lau KJ, D'Souza AC, Nunes EA. An umbrella review of systematic reviews of β-hydroxy-β-methyl butyrate supplementation in ageing and clinical practice. J Cachexia Sarcopenia Muscle. 2022;13:2265–75. https://doi.org/10.1002/jcsm.13030.
41. Reignier J, Plantefeve G, Mira J-P, Argaud L, Asfar P, Aissaoui N, Badie J, Botoc N-V, Brisard L, Bui H-N, Chatellier D, Chauvelot L, Combes A, Cracco C, Darmon M, Das V, Debarre M, Delbove A, Devaquet J, Dumont L-M, Gontier O, Groyer S, Guérin L, Guidet B, Hourmant Y, Jaber S, Lambiotte F, Leroy C, Letocart P, Madeux B, Maizel J, Martinet O, Martino F, Maxime V, Mercier E, Nay M-A, Nseir S, Oziel J, Picard W, Piton G, Quenot J-P, Reizine F, Renault A, Richecoeur J, Rigaud J-P, Schneider F, Silva D, Sirodot M, Souweine B, Tamion F, Terzi N, Thévenin D, Thiery G, Thieulot-Rolin N, Timsit J-F, Tinturier F, Tirot P, Vanderlinden T, Vinatier I, Vinsonneau C, Voicu S, Lascarrou J-B, Le Gouge A, Contou D, Pajot O, Jaubert P, Marin N, Simon M, Cour M, Mortaza S, Souday V, Lemerle M, Malfroy S, Berdaguer Ferrari F, Rozec B, Gruson D, Sazio C, Champion S, Boissier F, Veinstein A, Baboi L, Richard J-C, Yonis H, Le Guennec L, Lefevre L, Chommeloux J, Hékimian G, Lemiale V, Mariotte E, Valade S, Tirolien J, Fedun Y, Cerf C, Tachon G, Roustan J, Vimeux S, Bonnivard M, Anguel N, Osman D, Asehnoune K, Roquilly A, Belafia F, Conseil M, Cisse M, Chaouki B, Espenel R, Brasse C, Ena S, Delahaye A, Castanera J, Dulac T, Petua P, Zerbib Y, Brault C, Annane D, Bounab R, Heming N, Boulain T, Jacquier S, Muller G, Favory R, Préau S, Poissy J, Massri A, Lissonde F, Winiszewski H, Vieille T, Jacquier M, Labruyère M, Andreu P, Tadié J-M, Bodenes L, Combaux D, Luis D, Marchalot A, Herbrecht J-E, Clere-Jehl R, Schnell D, Aboad J, Bougon D, Escudier E, Coupez E, Dupuis C, Demailly Z, Galerneau L-M, Chelly J, Pourcine F, van Vong L, Abid S, de Montmollin E, Sonneville R, Guitton C, Chudeau N, Landais M, Pages V, Séjourné C, Rahmani I, Sbouj G, Megarbane B, Deye N, Malissin I. Low versus standard calorie and protein feeding in ventilated adults with shock: a randomised, controlled, multicentre, open-label, parallel-group trial (NUTRIREA-3). Lancet Respir Med. 2023;11(7):602–12. https://doi.org/10.1016/S2213-2600(23)00092-9.
42. Schefold JC, Bierbrauer J, Weber-Carstens S. Intensive care unit-acquired weakness (ICUAW) and muscle wasting in critically ill patients with severe sepsis and septic shock. J Cachexia Sarcopenia Muscle. 2010;1:147–57. https://doi.org/10.1007/s13539-010-0010-6.
43. Schefold JC, Wollersheim T, Grunow JJ, Luedi MM, Z'Graggen WJ, Weber-Carstens S. Muscular weakness and muscle wasting in the critically ill. J Cachexia Sarcopenia Muscle. 2020;11:1399–412. https://doi.org/10.1002/jcsm.12620.
44. Sharma K, Mogensen KM, Robinson MK. Pathophysiology of critical illness and role of nutrition. Nutr Clin Pract. 2019;34:12–22. https://doi.org/10.1002/ncp.10232.
45. Singer P. Protein metabolism and requirements in the ICU. Clin Nutr ESPEN. 2020;38:3–8. https://doi.org/10.1016/j.clnesp.2020.03.026.
46. Singer P, Blaser AR, Berger MM, Alhazzani W, Calder PC, Casaer MP, Hiesmayr M, Mayer K, Montejo JC, Pichard C, Preiser J-C, van Zanten ARH, Oczkowski S, Szczeklik W, Bischoff SC. ESPEN guideline on clinical nutrition in the intensive care unit. Clin Nutr. 2019;38:48–79. https://doi.org/10.1016/j.clnu.2018.08.037.
47. Singer P, Blaser AR, Berger MM, Calder PC, Casaer M, Hiesmayr M, Mayer K, Montejo-Gonzalez JC, Pichard C, Preiser J-C, Szczeklik W, van Zanten AR, Bischoff SC. ESPEN practical and partially revised guideline: clinical nutrition in the intensive care unit. Clin Nutr. 2023;42:1671–89. https://doi.org/10.1016/j.clnu.2023.07.011.

48. Sobotka L, Allison SP, Forbes A, Meier RF, Schneider SM, Soeters PB, Stanga Z, van Gossum A, editors. Basics in clinical nutrition. Prague: Galén; 2019.
49. Stehle P, Kuhn KS, Fürst P. From structure to function: what should be known about building blocks of protein. In: Pichard C, Kudsk KA, editors. From nutrition support to pharmacologic nutrition in the ICU. Berlin, Heidelberg: Springer; 2000. p. 26–37.
50. Stehle P, Ellger B, Kojic D, Feuersenger A, Schneid C, Stover J, Scheiner D, Westphal M. Glutamine dipeptide-supplemented parenteral nutrition improves the clinical outcomes of critically ill patients: a systematic evaluation of randomised controlled trials. Clin Nutr ESPEN. 2017;17:75–85. https://doi.org/10.1016/j.clnesp.2016.09.007.
51. Sun Y, Zhu S, Li S, Liu H. Glutamine on critical-ill patients: a systematic review and meta-analysis. Ann Palliat Med. 2021;10:1503–20. https://doi.org/10.21037/apm-20-702.
52. Sundström-Rehal M, Tardif N, Rooyackers O. Can exercise and nutrition stimulate muscle protein gain in the ICU patient? Curr Opin Clin Nutr Metab Care. 2019;22:146–51. https://doi.org/10.1097/MCO.0000000000000548.
53. Tashiro T. Contribution by skeletal muscle to whole-body protein catabolism in critical illness: usefulness of urinary 3-methylhisitidine excretion. Nutrition. 1998;14:708–10. https://doi.org/10.1016/s0899-9007(98)00070-7.
54. van Gassel RJJ, Baggerman MR, van de Poll MCG. Metabolic aspects of muscle wasting during critical illness. Curr Opin Clin Nutr Metab Care. 2020;23:96–101. https://doi.org/10.1097/MCO.0000000000000628.
55. van Ruijven IM, Stapel SN, Molinger J, Weijs PJM. Monitoring muscle mass using ultrasound: a key role in critical care. Curr Opin Crit Care. 2021;27:354–60. https://doi.org/10.1097/MCC.0000000000000846.
56. van Ruijven IM, Stapel SN, Girbes ARJ, Weijs PJM. Early high protein provision and mortality in ICU patients including those receiving continuous renal replacement therapy. Eur J Clin Nutr. 2022;76(9):1303–8. https://doi.org/10.1038/s41430-022-01103-8.
57. Vaupel P, Biesalski H-K. Proteine. In: Biesalski H-K, Bischoff SC, Pirlich M, Weimann A, editors. Ernährungsmedizin: Nach dem Curriculum Ernährungsmedizin der Bundesärztekammer. 5th ed. Stuttgart, New York: Georg Thieme Verlag; 2018. p. 145–63.
58. Wandrag L, Brett SJ, Frost G, Hickson M. Impact of supplementation with amino acids or their metabolites on muscle wasting in patients with critical illness or other muscle wasting illness: a systematic review. J Hum Nutr Diet. 2015;28:313–30. https://doi.org/10.1111/jhn.12238.
59. Wandrag L, Brett SJ, Frost GS, To M, Loubo EA, Jackson NC, Umpleby AM, Bountziouka V, Hickson M. Leucine-enriched essential amino acid supplementation in mechanically ventilated trauma patients: a feasibility study. Trials. 2019;20:561. https://doi.org/10.1186/s13063-019-3639-2.
60. Wernerman J, Kirketeig T, Andersson B, Berthelson H, Ersson A, Friberg H, Guttormsen AB, Hendrikx S, Pettilä V, Rossi P, Sjöberg F, Winsö O. Scandinavian glutamine trial: a pragmatic multi-centre randomised clinical trial of intensive care unit patients. Acta Anaesthesiol Scand. 2011;55:812–8. https://doi.org/10.1111/j.1399-6576.2011.02453.x.
61. Wernerman J, Morris CR, Paddon-Jones D, Sarav M. Assessment of protein turnover in health and disease. Nutr Clin Pract. 2017;32:15S–20S. https://doi.org/10.1177/0884533617694611.
62. Wischmeyer PE, Puthucheary Z, San Millán I, Butz D, Grocott MPW. Muscle mass and physical recovery in ICU: innovations for targeting of nutrition and exercise. Curr Opin Crit Care. 2017;23:269–78. https://doi.org/10.1097/MCC.0000000000000431.
63. Wittholz K, Fetterplace K, Ali Abdelhamid Y, Presneill JJ, Beach L, Thomson B, Read D, Koopman R, Deane AM. β-Hydroxy-β-methylbutyrate (HMB) supplementation and functional outcomes in multi-trauma patients: a study protocol for a pilot randomised clinical trial (BOOST trial). Pilot Feasibility Stud. 2022;8:21. https://doi.org/10.1186/s40814-022-00990-9.
64. Zhang Q, Zhou J, Zhu D, Zhou S. Evaluation of the effect of high protein supply on diaphragm atrophy in critically ill patients receiving prolonged mechanical ventilation. Nutr Clin Pract. 2022;37:402–12. https://doi.org/10.1002/ncp.10672.

Carbohydrate Metabolism and Insulin Resistance in Critically Ill Patients: Implications for the Management of Insulin and Medical Nutrition Therapy

Christian von Loeffelholz and Gunnar Elke

4.1 Glucose as Standard Carbohydrate in Clinical Nutrition of Critically Ill Patients

Carbohydrates in general are important precursor molecules for glycation of endogenously synthesized lipids, mucopolysaccharides, and protein derivates, while specifically, glucose is the central energy source for maintenance of cellular metabolism [1]. In fact, several cell systems in the human body are more or less completely reliant on this substance, such as erythrocytes, some immunocompetent cells, or cells of the central nervous system. Probably because of this fundamental role, glucose is not an essential metabolite for the human body, since it can be sufficiently synthesized under physiologic conditions. By maintaining a dynamic equilibrium between glucose utilization and endogenous glucose production (EGP), glucose homeostasis is constantly kept at concentrations of ~3.9–5.6 mmol/l [2]. These processes are mainly regulated by insulin and glucagon, and by intermediate metabolites such as glucose, free fatty acids, and carbon-3 compounds (e.g., glycerol, lactate, alanine). Within the human body under in vivo conditions, the liver, and, to a minor extent, the kidney contribute to EGP. Therefore, the liver remains the organ, which is considered mainly responsible for glucose homeostasis, ensuring EGP rates of ~1.8–2.0 mg/kg/min. (7–10 g/h) [2]. However, reciprocally one important exception from the principal nonessential role of glucose in human metabolism

---

C. von Loeffelholz (✉)
Department of Anesthesiology and Intensive Care, Jena University Hospital, Friedrich Schiller University, Jena, Germany
e-mail: christian.von_loeffelholz@med.uni-jena.de

G. Elke
Department of Anaesthesiology and Intensive Care Medicine, University Medical Center Schleswig-Holstein, Kiel, Germany
e-mail: gunnar.elke@uksh.de

© The Author(s), under exclusive license to Springer Nature Switzerland AG 2025
A. Rümelin et al. (eds.), *Nutrition in ICU Patients*,
https://doi.org/10.1007/978-3-032-00818-3_4

needs to be considered by intensivists, which is critically ill patients suffering from functional liver failure [3]. In this specific group, glucose needs to be constantly supplied, which is routinely realized by the parenteral route.

In the past, attempts have been made to introduce several glucose substitutes (e.g., xylitol, fructose, sorbitol) in clinical nutrition. However, in particular, xylitol could exert significant side effects as it is not reabsorbed in the kidney at higher intakes and may thereby cause osmotic diuresis, and oxalate crystals could originate in individual organs [4]. Therefore, sugar substitutes are no longer recommended. Otherwise, glucose can be easily monitored and is nowadays considered the carbohydrate of choice, particularly for parenteral nutrition [4].

Due to its non-essential role under physiologic conditions, it is not trivial to recommend a minimum or maximum intake for glucose. Regarding the abovementioned EGP of ~1.8–2.0 mg/kg/min (7–10 g/h), an 80 kg patient would synthesize 144–160 mg/min. Under fasted conditions, corresponding to ~2.6–2.9 g/kg/24 h. This could be interpreted as a physiological minimum for maintaining basic cell metabolism. However, a large percentage of critically ill patients suffer from stress hyperglycemia. Stress hyperglycemia is reported "to generally refer to transient hyperglycemia during illness" [5]. The American Diabetes Association (ADA) and the American Association of Clinical Endocrinologists consensus on inpatient hyperglycemia define stress hyperglycemia or hospital related hyperglycemia as any blood glucose concentration exceeding 7.8 mmol/l [6–9]. Stress hyperglycemia does not only impact the prognosis of critically ill patients (see subsequent sections), but primarily reflects a condition of severely impaired carbohydrate metabolism during critical illness, which needs to be regarded, when discussing glucose requirements of patients.

> Except for critically ill patients suffering from functional liver failure, glucose is basically not an essential macronutrient, as endogenous glucose production ensures a glucose supply of ~3 g/kg/24 h under physiological conditions.

4.2 The Pathophysiology of Stress Hyperglycemia

In nonobese healthy subjects, ~65% of insulin stimulated systemic glucose uptake are utilized by the skeletal muscle, while adipose tissue accounts for only ~4% of peripheral glucose uptake [10]. On a molecular level, insulin-stimulated glucose transporter (GLUT) 4 translocation is the main responsible mechanism for this phenomenon [11]. Considering that glucose uptake of the central nervous system (CNS) via GLUT1 (insulin independent) lays in a range of ~1 mg/kg/min, the CNS accounts for the majority of the remaining fraction of systemic glucose uptake [10, 12]. Importantly, postprandial insulin concentrations needed for sufficient stimulation of peripheral glucose uptake at the same time effectively suppress EGP and thereby help to keep blood glucose in a physiological range. However, this homeostasis of carbohydrate metabolism becomes severely disturbed by the onset or during critical illness, respectively, resulting in acute stress hyperglycemia.

The pathophysiology of stress hyperglycemia is complex [13, 14]. From a clinician's viewpoint, it remains essential to recognize that stress induced hyperglycemia during the acute phase of critical illness is mainly elicited by inflammation-related insulin resistance (see Fig. 4.1).

Insulin-dependent peripheral glucose uptake is significantly impaired during critical illness, which, due to the central role of skeletal muscle mass, markedly contributes to the phenomenon of stress hyperglycemia. Likewise, insulin-dependent suppression of lipolysis and ketogenesis is affected by insulin resistance, and compromised insulin signaling and secretion capacity are also pertinent in terms of skeletal muscle catabolism, inducing a net release of amino acids along with compromised anticatabolic insulin effects under conditions of systemic inflammation [16–22].

Insulin resistance induces whole body catabolism via stimulation of endogenous energy substrate mobilization. By using in vivo techniques, it was shown in human septic patients that gluconeogenesis can be elevated by more than 90% and appears to be largely non-suppressible, at least with physiological insulin concentrations [18, 20, 22–24]. Thereby, the liver plays a key role and acts as a linchpin mediating metabolic signals between the gut (diet/nutritional intake, microbiota and complex endocrine and autonomic signaling) and the rest of the body [25].

Thus, critically ill patients can generate more than 50% of their energy substrate requirements during the acute phase endogenously, and hyperglycemia, in alliance with insulin requirements, can therefore be viewed as routinely monitored clinical surrogate measures of insulin resistance [4, 15, 26]. The latter has not only

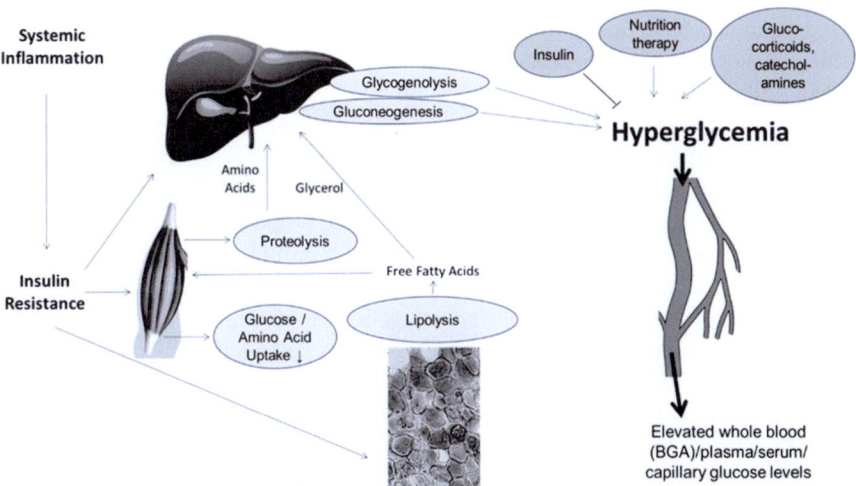

Fig. 4.1 Main pathophysiological traits of stress hyperglycemia. (Adapted according to [15, 16])

consequences in terms of insulin therapy, but also in terms of medical nutrition management during critical illness.

> The main pathophysiologic features of stress hyperglycemia are hepatic (central) and peripheral insulin resistance, eliciting substantial endogenous energy substrate mobilization. During the acute phase of critical illness, patients with stress hyperglycemia can meet a major percentage of their substrate requirements by endogenous sources, which has impact on nutrition management.

4.3 Exogenous Glucose Supply Under Conditions of Stress Hyperglycemia

As for the estimated minimum demand, there are currently no reliable clinical data suggesting a maximum for carbohydrate supply in critically ill subjects [4]. In vivo studies in septic patients indicate that, during systemic inflammation, basal glucose oxidation rates are ~30% lower when compared to healthy controls [27]. Otherwise, under conditions of hyperinsulinemic clamping, maximum glucose oxidation rates of 4.1 mg/kg/min fat free mass were observed in septic collectives, which is almost +100% as compared to control conditions [2, 27]. However, glucose storage capacity remains severely impaired in patients suffering from systemic inflammation, even with hyperinsulinemia. Thus, providing glucose to critically ill patients in excess of 4 mg/kg/min fat free mass is very likely to result in substantial hyperglycemia, even under conditions of high dose continuous insulin infusion for maintenance of blood glucose targets.

Of note, in septic patients without catecholamine support and in absence of septic shock, gluconeogenesis can be suppressed by continuous infusion of supraphysiological insulin doses [20]. By contrast, exclusive infusion of glucose at a rate of 4 mg/kg/min, which, due to related endogenous insulin release, is capable of abolishing gluconeogenesis in healthy volunteers, suppresses EGP in sepsis by only ~50% [21]. Gluconeogenesis from protein sources is unproportionally induced under such conditions, contributing to the well-known catabolic consequences, resulting in a substantial loss of skeletal muscle mass [21–23]. Therefore, the guideline of the German Society for Nutritional Medicine (DGEM) suggests an upper level of 4 g glucose supply/kg/24 h. Moreover, they propose that it is reasonable to interrupt glucose supply completely in patients with insulin requirements of >4 U/h, indicating pronounced insulin resistance with non-suppressible EGP and exclusive provision of substrate requirements by endogenous sources [4].

Intensivists should further regard that glucose is a potentially lipogenic substrate, which can exert unfavorable effects when being excessively consumed. This phenomenon either depends on macronutrient composition or acute dyslipidemia can even be observed in healthy volunteers as a consequence of very low-fat diets enriched in carbohydrates [28]. Therefore, except for the treatment of hypoglycemia, substantial amounts of glucose should not be administered as an exclusive energy substrate over longer periods of time, and particularly not by the parenteral route.

Furthermore, the lipogenic potential of glucose could be predominantly harmful in subjects with a history of disturbed glucose metabolism [29]. Prevalences and incidences of diabetes mellitus are continuously on the rise and a large number of patients admitting to the ICU can be expected to suffer from unknown glucose metabolism disorders [9, 29–31]. Metabolic-associated fatty liver disease (MAFLD) affects >50% of diabetic patients and > 30% of the common population in industrialized countries [32, 33]. MAFLD meanwhile became an indication for liver transplantation, and patients are at increased risk of septic and cardiovascular complications [34, 35]. Moreover, a small postmortem study suggests high prevalences of fatty liver in critically ill patients, and hepatic lipogenesis is known to be significantly upregulated in insulin resistant perioperative fatty liver subjects [36, 37]. Overfeeding with glucose can not only contribute to the onset of MAFLD, but also to a proinflammatory microenvironment [38]. Finally, overnutrition during the acute phase of critical illness and in particular high macronutrient loads by the parenteral route are associated with fatty liver disease and liver dysfunction not only in adults but also in infants [39, 40].

Therefore, it appears reasonable to propose an upper limit of glucose intake of ~4 g/kg/24 h. Furthermore, caloric and macronutrient intake should be strictly managed according to the patient's individual metabolic tolerance, as reflected by blood glucose level and insulin demand, in order to avoid relative overfeeding, particularly in the acute phase of illness, and unfavorable impact on clinical endpoints (see following sections).

> A glucose supply of ~4 g/kg/24 h is considered as upper limit. Glucose should not be administered as an exclusive caloric source over longer periods of time. Caloric and macronutrient supply should be strictly aligned in relation to insulin requirements and blood glucose levels.

4.4 Prevalence of Stress Hyperglycemia and Evidence on Intensive Insulin Therapy in Nondiabetic ICU Patients

Stress hyperglycemia is common in critically ill populations. In a large prospective monocentric observational study, Plummer et al. in 1000 consecutive ICU patients detected dysglycemia to be present in almost 50% of admissions [41]. This is in alliance with findings in, e.g., severe sepsis and perioperative trauma, while in cardiac surgery stress, hyperglycemia can be observed in up to 80% of patients [42–44]. Furthermore, data from pro- and retrospective observational studies indicate a strong association of various measures of stress hyperglycemia with clinical outcomes [42–47]. Not to forget, stress hyperglycemia is associated with an increased risk of incident diabetes after ICU stay [48]. Thus, from a practical viewpoint, stress hyperglycemia is frequently observed in critically ill subjects and related to outcomes in medical and surgical ICU collectives.

The era of targeted blood glucose control in critically ill patients started in the field of cardiovascular surgery, suggesting a reduction in mortality and the number of infections under circumstances of perioperative insulin therapy (reviewed in [47]). Consequently, several large intervention trials on intensive insulin therapy (IIT) were initiated in the following decade. In 2001, the first large randomized controlled trial (RCT) on IIT was published, the LEUVEN I study including mainly cardiac surgery patients. LEUVEN I provided evidence for reduced morbidity and mortality as a consequence of IIT [49]. The results were confirmed in a subgroup of LEUVEN II, particularly in patients receiving critical care for three or more days, but the study failed to prove benefit in the total cohort [50]. Two subsequent multicenter randomized controlled studies on IIT, however, were then prematurely terminated without showing benefit, and the NICE sugar-trial finally provided evidence for elevated 90-day mortality under IIT [47, 51]. Numerous reasons for the observed discrepancies between study results were discussed, a lower rate of achievement of targeted blood glucose range and higher percentage of clinically relevant hypoglycemia among them (reviewed in [47]). Just recently, the largest RCT to date, TGC-Fast, was published in 9230 critically ill adults (45.2% after cardiac surgery, 50% with an ICU length-of-stay ≤3 days) [52]. Patients were either assigned to liberal glucose control (insulin initiated only when the blood glucose level was >11.9 mmol/l) or to tight glucose control (blood glucose level targeted with the use of the LOGIC-Insulin algorithm at 4.4–6.1 mmol/l). Parenteral nutrition was withheld in both groups for 1 week. No in-between group differences were found regarding the primary endpoint ICU length of stay. Further, eight prespecified secondary outcomes suggested that the incidence of new infections, the duration of respiratory and hemodynamic support, the time to discharge alive from the hospital, and mortality in the ICU and hospital were comparable in the two groups, whereas severe acute kidney injury and cholestatic liver dysfunction appeared less prevalent with tight glucose control.

In fact, specifically some nondiabetic ICU collectives with longer ICU stay could benefit from IIT, as evidenced by reduced mortality and lower risk of new kidney injury, critical illness polyneuropathy/myopathy, or surgical site infections [49, 50, 52–55]. However, the risk of symptomatic hypoglycemia under IIT appears to equipoise any potential benefits. Therefore, mainly driven by the results of NICE sugar, a change in ICU blood glucose management toward moderate control was the broadly consented therapeutical consequence, targeting a range of ~7.8–10 mmol/l in critically ill patients [47]. This may represent the best compromise for prevention of clinically relevant hypoglycemia and consequences of exaggerating stress hyperglycemia. Many modern ICU treatment guidelines follow this consideration of risk and benefit (e.g., [4, 6, 56–58]), whereby levels of up to 11 mmol/l can be tolerated in most ICU patients.

> Blood glucose targets of 4.4–6.1 mmol/l could provide benefit for some nondiabetic critically ill subjects with longer ICU stay, which are however compensated by the risk of severe hypoglycemia. Therefore, a target range of ~7.8–10 (−11) mmol/l is broadly accepted for the majority of critically ill patients and represents a compromise between the risk of hypoglycemia and the consequences of exaggerating hyperglycemia.

4.5 Stress Hyperglycemia in Subjects with a Prehospital History of Dysglycemia

Results of RCTs indicate that critically ill patients with preexisting diabetes mellitus have no benefit from IIT, but are exposed to a comparable risk of severe hypoglycemia as nondiabetic patients. The NICE sugar-trial included a predefined group of more than 1200 diabetic subjects and it was shown that in the control arm with less intensive glucose care, severe hypoglycemia (defined as blood glucose levels ≤ 2.2 mmol/l) was still recorded in 0.5% of patients, without reported differences between diabetic and nondiabetic subjects [51]. Analogous circumstances were observed in the combined evaluation of the LEUVEN studies, and in a meta-analysis of randomized controlled trials on blood glucose control for the prevention of surgical site infections [54, 55]. In support of the latter, the recent TGC-Fast RCT even reported no benefit regarding the time of discharge alive from the ICU for the tight glucose control protocol in the substantial subgroup of diabetic patients. However, regarding the safety issue, there was a trend toward a better outcome with liberal glucose control in this subgroup [52].

Therefore, it appears reasonable to question, whether critically ill patients with preexisting diabetes mellitus should be managed according to the same criteria as nondiabetic subjects. Early studies on mainly medical patients suggest that diabetic patients with moderate hyperglycemia (9–11 mmol/l) had the lowest mortality, while not alone severe hyperglycemia (≥ 11 mmol/l), but also euglycemia (<7 mmol/l) were related to higher mortality [59]. There is an ongoing debate on this issue and meanwhile first prospective studies evaluated liberal targets of up to 14 mmol/l. They provide early evidence that this could be without major risk of harm, while significantly reducing hypoglycemic episodes [60–63]. The recent LUCID trial was a multicenter RCT including 419 patients with type 2 diabetes. In the intervention group, insulin therapy started at blood glucose levels >14 mmol/l, targeting 10–14 mmol/l. In control subjects, insulin started at >10 mmol/l with a target of 6–10 mmol/l [62]. The primary outcome was incident hypoglycemia (defined as <4 mmol/l). At least one hypoglycemic event was observed in ~5% of the intervention arm, and in 18% of the comparator group ($p < 0.05$). No major adverse effects were observed, although 90-day mortality tended to increase (29.5% intervention, 24.9% comparator, $p = 0.29$). Yet, the LUCID trial was not powered for this endpoint, and future studies need to evaluate a potential risk of harm for liberal blood glucose targets up to 14 mmol/l in diabetic ICU patients. The latter results are largely in accordance with the study of Rau et al., who retrospectively defined stress hyperglycemia in diabetic patients at blood glucose levels >13.9 mmol/l [64], and with data from observational studies [47, 63]. According to these findings, blood glucose levels exceeding 14 mmol/l appear to be harmful for diabetic subjects and should be generally avoided. Otherwise, blood glucose concentrations >13.9 mmol/l can be tolerated in terminally ill patients who are considered to have short life expectancy.

While 14 mmol/l could be defined as upper blood glucose limit for critically ill diabetic patients, there is currently no broadly consented target range regarding liberal blood glucose control. The landmark study of Egi et al. showed rising mortality with more strict glucose control for ICU patients with pathologic glycated hemoglobin A1c (HbA1c) [65]. This observation has been attributed to rising hypoglycemia risk [47]. In the aforementioned meta-analysis on glycemic control for the prevention of surgical site infections, which included 2836 diabetic and nondiabetic patients, the lowest hypoglycemia rate was observed with blood glucose targets <12.2 mmol/l [54]. This is supported by findings of a recent network meta-analysis [66]. However, increased numbers of surgical site infections were detected with such a more liberal blood glucose control strategy.

Currently there is no evidence for an individualized therapy in diabetic critically ill patients, based upon blood glucose targets delineated from admission HbA1c [67]. Nevertheless, potential benefits of glucose control could depend upon metabolic preadmission condition [14, 61, 65]. At least in patients with controlled glycemia (e.g., admission HbA1c ≤ 7%/53 mmol/mol), some data support blood glucose targets of ~7.8–10 mmol/l [54, 67–69]. For patients with less well controlled preadmission glycemia (e.g., admission HbA1c > 7%/53 mmol/mol), an appropriate blood glucose target remains unclear and further studies are needed to clarify this important question [47]. However, keeping this group <12.2 mmol/l could at least help to minimize the risk of (relative) hypoglycemic events [68].

> Except for those with short life expectancy, blood glucose levels ≥14 mmol/l should be generally avoided in diabetic critically ill ICU patients, even under conditions of poor preadmission metabolic control (HbA1c > 7%/53 mmol/mol). Under circumstances of well controlled preadmission glycemia (HbA1c ≤ 7%/53 mmol/mol), a target range of ~7.8–10 mmol/l could positively impact clinical endpoints as, e.g., the risk of surgical site infections.

4.6 Hypoglycemia

Regardless of whether hypoglycemia occurs spontaneously or is associated with insulin treatment, low blood glucose levels are independently related to increased mortality in critically ill patients [47]. Targeting of euglycemia (e.g., 4.4–6.1 mmol/l) has been related to substantial increases in the risk of iatrogenic hypoglycemia, although in the recent TGC-Fast RCT, severe hypoglycemia occurred in 31 patients (0.7%) in the liberal control group and 47 patients (1.0%) in the tight control group [52]. Otherwise, the TGC-Fast RCT supports previous results, indicating that normalization of blood glucose does not alter ICU, hospital, or postdischarge mortality and, therefore, avoidance of hypoglycemia remains critically important in the ICU. To minimize the risk of hypoglycemic complications, guidelines on the clinical management of diabetes mellitus in hospital indeed suggest not to fall <6.1 mmol/l [7, 70].

Due to the phenomenon of relative hypoglycemia, definition of hypoglycemia is not trivial, particularly in patients with a history of diabetes mellitus [68]. Indeed, definitions of hypoglycemia in randomized studies on critically ill patients vary from <2.2 to <4.4 mmol/l. We suggest to follow the current definition of the ADA (Table 4.1).

Level 2 hypoglycemia is considered the threshold where neuroglycopenic symptoms begin to occur and require immediate reaction. Detecting symptomatic level 2 and 3 hypoglycemia, however, is not trivial in sedated and ventilated ICU patients. This requires structured blood glucose surveillance protocols (see below). To strictly minimize hypoglycemia risk, we suggest to immediately treat level 1 hypoglycemia by using i.v. glucose, and to closely monitor blood glucose and adapt nutritional therapy in case of blood glucose levels <6.1 mmol/l. Furthermore, an ADA consensus report suggested that a patient's overall treatment regimen (e.g., insulin, nutrition, etc.) should be reviewed when a blood glucose value of 3.9 mmol/l is identified, because such readings often predict imminent level 3 hypoglycemia [70]. Finally, episodes of hypoglycemia should be documented in medical records.

> Level 2 hypoglycemia (<3.0 mmol/l) is considered as threshold for neuroglycopenic symptoms. Therefore, level 1 hypoglycemia <3.9 mmol/l should be immediately treated using i.v. glucose, and the patient's overall treatment regimen (e.g., insulin, nutrition, etc.) should be reviewed. Blood glucose levels <6.1 mmol/l should be closely monitored and nutrition therapy should be adapted.

4.7 Surveillance Protocols, Insulin Treatment, and Nutrition Therapy: Cornerstones of Glycemic Management in the ICU

In order to treat hyperglycemia and limit hypoglycemic episodes, intensivists need to monitor blood glucose. A consensus recommendation on the measurement of blood glucose in critically ill stated: "All patients whose severity of illness justifies the presence of invasive vascular monitoring (an indwelling arterial and/or central venous catheter) should have all samples for measurement of the blood glucose concentration taken from the arterial catheter as the first option. If blood cannot be sampled from an arterial catheter or an arterial catheter is temporarily or permanently unavailable, blood may be sampled from a venous catheter as a second option" [71]. In fact, arterial blood gas sampling is close to laboratory analytic

Table 4.1 Definition of hypoglycemia [70]

Level of hypoglycemia	Glycemic criteria (mmol/l)/description
Level 1	<3.9 and ≥3.0
Level 2	<3.0
Level 3	A severe event characterized by altered mental and/or physical status requiring assistance from another person for recovery

standards, feasible to perform, with quick reports of critical results, and provides additional information on electrolyte status. This is imperative, since hypokalemia is frequently observed during treatment of hyperglycemic episodes with insulin, and severe hypokalemia is associated with increased mortality [6].

Monitoring via intermittent testing of capillary blood using point of care methodologies is not recommended for critically ill collectives [6]. Continuous blood glucose monitoring meets several of the criteria of ideal blood glucose measurement [72]. Meanwhile, the FDA approved two continuous monitoring systems for the hospital setting. However, concerns regarding the accuracy of continuous glucose monitoring persist, particularly under conditions of acutely disturbed homeostasis (e.g., vasoconstriction, severe dehydration, hypoxemia, rapidly changing glucose concentrations), which are frequently observed in critically ill subjects. Moreover, devices need to be removed for diagnostic procedures like MRI [6]. Therefore, continuous blood glucose monitoring can currently not be recommended for the critical care setting routine.

> Blood glucose monitoring in critically ill subjects should be realized by using blood gas analysis, ideally taken from an arterial line.

Management of blood glucose surveillance and therapy in critically ill subjects requires structured treatment protocols. Figure 4.2 provides an exemplary schedule including an optional treatment path for liberal glucose control of stress hyperglycemia in patients with poorly controlled preadmission diabetes mellitus.

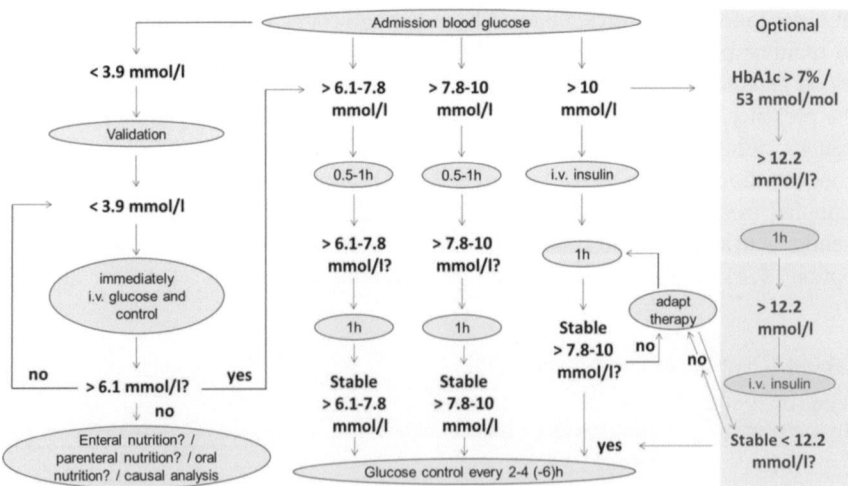

Fig. 4.2 Structured blood glucose management protocol for critically ill subjects. (Modified according to [73])

Prevention and forwarded treatment of hypoglycemic episodes remain a central issue in the ICU. Application with i.v. glucose is the method of choice for level 1 or higher level hypoglycemia. However, blood glucose >3.9 and <6.1 mmol/l are also in need of intervention, preferentially by means of adapted nutrition therapy. Moreover, causal analysis should routinely follow any hypoglycemic episode (e.g., did the patient use high risk hypoglycemic oral antidiabetics shortly before ICU admission?). It is further imperative that if nutritional therapy is interrupted or terminated for any reason, bedside intensivists should pay specific attention to ongoing insulin therapy. In order to minimize the risk of hypoglycemia, insulin therapy should be concomitantly interrupted after nutrition cessation, and blood glucose levels should be closely monitored.

Stress hyperglycemia >10 mmol/l is primarily treated by means of continuous insulin infusion. Bolus applications should not be part of the treatment routine. The rate of insulin infusion needs to be closely adjusted upon the patient's current glucose concentration and the absolute change in blood glucose compared to the last reading. Blood glucose should initially be measured at 1–2 h intervals, depending on the patient's status. During the acute phase, glucose monitoring intervals can then individually be extended to 4–6 h intervals, and after return to homeostasis, even to 8–12 h intervals in order to minimize blood loss.

However, as with hypoglycemia, hyperglycemia treatment is not alone a matter of insulin management, but also of an accurately adapted nutritional therapy including glucose supply. As shown in Fig. 4.1, stress hyperglycemia is closely related to endogenous substrate mobilization during critical illness. Therefore, intensivists should attempt to focus on closely matching nutritional therapy to the patient's situative needs. As stated above, glucose supply can be completely cessated in patients with insulin infusion of >4 U/h for maintenance of blood glucose targets, which indicate that the patient's current substrate requirements are completely met by endogenous sources [4]. However, not only glucose intake, but also application of parenteral lipid emulsions and amino acids should be questioned under such circumstances, as rising free fatty acid levels may further aggravate insulin resistance and EGP [2, 74, 75]. This could result in acceleration of stress hyperglycemia. Data from the first TICACOS trial, where critically ill patients were fully fed by combined enteral and parenteral nutrition during the acute phase of critical illness according to measured resting energy expenditure, showed a longer ICU stay and increased infectious complications [76]. Very recent results of large observational trials and RCTs support the hypothesis that enforced macronutrient intake including glucose during the acute phase of critical illness could negatively impact clinical endpoints [39, 77–81]. In summary, stress hyperglycemia during the acute phase of critical illness should not be accentuated by an excessive nutrition strategy beyond the patient's individual metabolic tolerance.

An empiric clinical protocol for controlling the substrate supply depending on the caloric target was recently published by the German Interdisciplinary Association for Intensive Care and Emergency Medicine (DIVI), which is presented in Fig. 4.3.

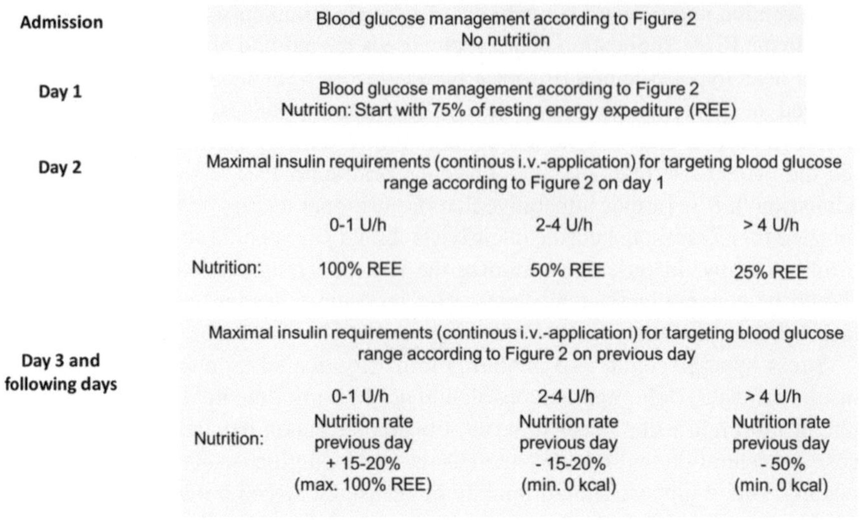

Admission	Blood glucose management according to Figure 2 No nutrition		
Day 1	Blood glucose management according to Figure 2 Nutrition: Start with 75% of resting energy expediture (REE)		
Day 2	Maximal insulin requirements (continous i.v.-application) for targeting blood glucose range according to Figure 2 on day 1		
	0-1 U/h	2-4 U/h	> 4 U/h
Nutrition:	100% REE	50% REE	25% REE
Day 3 and following days	Maximal insulin requirements (continous i.v.-application) for targeting blood glucose range according to Figure 2 on previous day		
	0-1 U/h	2-4 U/h	> 4 U/h
Nutrition:	Nutrition rate previous day + 15-20% (max. 100% REE)	Nutrition rate previous day - 15-20% (min. 0 kcal)	Nutrition rate previous day - 50% (min. 0 kcal)

Fig. 4.3 Protocol of integrated insulin and nutrition therapy in critically ill patients according to the degree of estimated insulin resistance and reciprocal endogenous substrate mobilization. (Adapted according to [26])

Monitoring and therapy of blood glucose in critically ill subjects should follow structured protocols. Management of stress hyperglycemia and hypoglycemia risk are not alone a matter of insulin treatment, but also of management of medical nutrition therapy. Provision of energy substrates should be closely matched to endogenous mobilization as estimated by current insulin demand for reaching blood glucose targets.

References

1. Dashty M. A quick look at biochemistry: carbohydrate metabolism. Clin Biochem. 2013;46:1339–52. https://doi.org/10.1016/j.clinbiochem.2013.04.027.
2. Roden M, Bernroider E. Hepatic glucose metabolism in humans—its role in health and disease. Best Pract Res Clin Endocrinol Metab. 2003;17:365–83. https://doi.org/10.1016/S1521-690X(03)00031-9.
3. Al-Yousif N, Rawal S, Jurczak M, Mahmud H, Shah FA. Endogenous glucose production in critical illness. Nutr Clin Pract. 2021;36:344–59. https://doi.org/10.1002/ncp.10646.
4. Elke G, Hartl WH, Kreymann KG, Adolph M, Felbinger TW, Graf T, de Heer G, Heller AR, Kampa U, Mayer K, et al. DGEM-Leitlinie: Klinische Ernährung in der Intensivmedizin. Aktuel Ernahrungsmed. 2018;43:341–408. https://doi.org/10.1055/a-0713-8179.
5. Dungan KM, Braithwaite SS, Preiser J-C. Stress hyperglycaemia. Lancet. 2009;373:1798–807. https://doi.org/10.1016/S0140-6736(09)60553-5.

6. Pasquel FJ, Lansang MC, Dhatariya K, Umpierrez GE. Management of diabetes and hyperglycaemia in the hospital. Lancet Diabetes Endocrinol. 2021;9:174–88. https://doi.org/10.1016/S2213-8587(20)30381-8.
7. Moghissi ES, Korytkowski MT, DiNardo M, Einhorn D, Hellman R, Hirsch IB, Inzucchi SE, Ismail-Beigi F, Kirkman MS, Umpierrez GE. American Association of Clinical Endocrinologists and American Diabetes Association consensus statement on inpatient glycemic control. Endocr Pract. 2009;15:353–69. https://doi.org/10.4158/EP09102.RA.
8. Farrokhi F, Smiley D, Umpierrez GE. Glycemic control in non-diabetic critically ill patients. Best Pract Res Clin Endocrinol Metab. 2011;25:813–24. https://doi.org/10.1016/j.beem.2011.05.004.
9. American Diabetes Association. (2) Classification and diagnosis of diabetes. Diabetes Care. 2015;38 Suppl:S8–S16. https://doi.org/10.2337/dc15-S005.
10. Ng JM, Azuma K, Kelley C, Pencek R, Radikova Z, Laymon C, Price J, Goodpaster BH, Kelley DE. PET imaging reveals distinctive roles for different regional adipose tissue depots in systemic glucose metabolism in nonobese humans. Am J Physiol Endocrinol Metab. 2012;303:E1134–41. https://doi.org/10.1152/ajpendo.00282.2012.
11. Saltiel AR, Kahn CR. Insulin signalling and the regulation of glucose and lipid metabolism. Nature. 2001;414:799–806. https://doi.org/10.1038/414799a.
12. Wang L, Pavlou S, Du X, Bhuckory M, Xu H, Chen M. Glucose transporter 1 critically controls microglial activation through facilitating glycolysis. Mol Neurodegener. 2019;14:2. https://doi.org/10.1186/s13024-019-0305-9.
13. Umpierrez GE, Pasquel FJ. Management of inpatient hyperglycemia and diabetes in older adults. Diabetes Care. 2017;40:509–17. https://doi.org/10.2337/dc16-0989.
14. Mifsud S, Schembri EL, Gruppetta M. Stress-induced hyperglycaemia. Br J Hosp Med (Lond). 2018;79:634–9. https://doi.org/10.12968/hmed.2018.79.11.634.
15. Wischmeyer PE. Nutrition therapy in sepsis. Crit Care Clin. 2018;34:107–25. https://doi.org/10.1016/j.ccc.2017.08.008.
16. Preiser J-C, Ichai C, Orban J-C, Groeneveld ABJ. Metabolic response to the stress of critical illness. Br J Anaesth. 2014;113:945–54. https://doi.org/10.1093/bja/aeu187.
17. Shaw JH, Wolfe RR. An integrated analysis of glucose, fat, and protein metabolism in severely traumatized patients. Studies in the basal state and the response to total parenteral nutrition. Ann Surg. 1989;209:63–72. https://doi.org/10.1097/00000658-198901000-00010.
18. Donatelli F, Nafi M, Di Nicola M, Macchitelli V, Mirabile C, Lorini L, Carli F. Twenty-four hour hyperinsulinemic-euglycemic clamp improves postoperative nitrogen balance only in low insulin sensitivity patients following cardiac surgery. Acta Anaesthesiol Scand. 2015;59:710–22. https://doi.org/10.1111/aas.12526.
19. Hartl WH, Jauch K-W. Metabolic self-destruction in critically ill patients: origins, mechanisms and therapeutic principles. Nutrition. 2014;30:261–7. https://doi.org/10.1016/j.nut.2013.07.019.
20. Chambrier C, Laville M, Rhzioual BK, Odeon M, Boulétreau P, Beylot M. Insulin sensitivity of glucose and fat metabolism in severe sepsis. Clin Sci (Lond). 2000;99:321–8.
21. Shaw JH, Wolfe RR. Determinations of glucose turnover and oxidation in normal volunteers and septic patients using stable and radio-isotopes: the response to glucose infusion and total parenteral feeding. Aust N Z J Surg. 1986;56:785–91. https://doi.org/10.1111/j.1445-2197.1986.tb02327.x.
22. Dahn MS, Jacobs LA, Smith S, Hans B, Lange MP, Mitchell RA, Kirkpatrick JR. The relationship of insulin production to glucose metabolism in severe sepsis. Arch Surg. 1985;120:166–72. https://doi.org/10.1001/archsurg.1985.01390260036006.
23. Long CL, Kinney JM, Geiger JW. Nonsuppressability of gluconeogenesis by glucose in septic patients. Metabolism. 1976;25:193–201. https://doi.org/10.1016/0026-0495(76)90049-4.
24. Black PR, Brooks DC, Bessey PQ, Wolfe RR, Wilmore DW. Mechanisms of insulin resistance following injury. Ann Surg. 1982;196:420–35. https://doi.org/10.1097/00000658-198210000-00005.

25. Barber TM, Kabisch S, Pfeiffer AFH, Weickert MO. Metabolic-associated fatty liver disease and insulin resistance: a review of complex interlinks. Metabolites. 2023;13:757. https://doi.org/10.3390/metabo13060757.
26. Elke G, Hartl WH, Adolph M, Angstwurm M, Brunkhorst FM, Edel A, de Heer G, Felbinger TW, Goeters C, Hill A, et al. Laborchemisches und kalorimetrisches Monitoring der medizinischen Ernährungstherapie auf der Intensiv- und Intermediate Care Station: Zweites Positionspapier der Sektion Metabolismus und Ernährung der Deutschen Interdisziplinären Vereinigung für Intensiv- und Notfallmedizin (DIVI). Med Klin Intensivmed Notfmed. 2023;118(Suppl 1):1–13. https://doi.org/10.1007/s00063-023-01001-2.
27. Saeed M, Carlson GL, Little RA, Irving MH. Selective impairment of glucose storage in human sepsis. Br J Surg. 1999;86:813–21. https://doi.org/10.1046/j.1365-2168.1999.01140.x.
28. Hudgins LC, Seidman CE, Diakun J, Hirsch J. Human fatty acid synthesis is reduced after the substitution of dietary starch for sugar. Am J Clin Nutr. 1998;67:631–9. https://doi.org/10.1093/ajcn/67.4.631.
29. Chew NWS, Ng CH, Tan DJH, Kong G, Lin C, Chin YH, Lim WH, Huang DQ, Quek J, Fu CE, et al. The global burden of metabolic disease: data from 2000 to 2019. Cell Metab. 2023;35:414–428.e3. https://doi.org/10.1016/j.cmet.2023.02.003.
30. Tönnies T, Hoyer A, Brinks R, Kuss O, Hering R, Schulz M. Spatio-temporal trends in the incidence of type 2 diabetes in Germany. Dtsch Arztebl Int. 2023;120:173–9. https://doi.org/10.3238/arztebl.m2022.0405.
31. Rathmann W, Haastert B, Icks A, Herder C, Kolb H, Holle R, Mielck A, Meisinger C, Wichmann HE, Giani G. The diabetes epidemic in the elderly population in Western Europe: data from population-based studies. Gesundheitswesen. 2005;67(Suppl 1):S110–4. https://doi.org/10.1055/s-2005-858227.
32. Younossi ZM, Golabi P, de Avila L, Paik JM, Srishord M, Fukui N, Qiu Y, Burns L, Afendy A, Nader F. The global epidemiology of NAFLD and NASH in patients with type 2 diabetes: a systematic review and meta-analysis. J Hepatol. 2019;71:793–801. https://doi.org/10.1016/j.jhep.2019.06.021.
33. Younossi Z, Anstee QM, Marietti M, Hardy T, Henry L, Eslam M, George J, Bugianesi E. Global burden of NAFLD and NASH: trends, predictions, risk factors and prevention. Nat Rev Gastroenterol Hepatol. 2018;15:11–20. https://doi.org/10.1038/nrgastro.2017.109.
34. Zhou G-P, Jiang Y-Z, Sun L-Y, Zhu Z-J. Clinical evidence of outcomes following liver transplantation in patients with nonalcoholic steatohepatitis: an updated meta-analysis and systematic review. Int J Surg. 2022;104:106752. https://doi.org/10.1016/j.ijsu.2022.106752.
35. Wang X, Li J, Riaz DR, Shi G, Liu C, Dai Y. Outcomes of liver transplantation for nonalcoholic steatohepatitis: a systematic review and meta-analysis. Clin Gastroenterol Hepatol. 2014;12:394–402.e1. https://doi.org/10.1016/j.cgh.2013.09.023.
36. von Loeffelholz C, Döcke S, Lock JF, Lieske S, Horn P, Kriebel J, Wahl S, Singmann P, de Las Heras Gala T, Grallert H, et al. Increased lipogenesis in spite of upregulated hepatic 5'AMP-activated protein kinase in human non-alcoholic fatty liver. Hepatol Res. 2017;47:890–901. https://doi.org/10.1111/hepr.12825.
37. Koskinas J, Gomatos IP, Tiniakos DG, Memos N, Boutsikou M, Garatzioti A, Archimandritis A, Betrosian A. Liver histology in ICU patients dying from sepsis: a clinico-pathological study. World J Gastroenterol. 2008;14:1389–93. https://doi.org/10.3748/wjg.14.1389.
38. Barazzoni R, Deutz NEP, Biolo G, Bischoff S, Boirie Y, Cederholm T, Cuerda C, Delzenne N, Leon Sanz M, Ljungqvist O, et al. Carbohydrates and insulin resistance in clinical nutrition: recommendations from the ESPEN expert group. Clin Nutr. 2017;36:355–63. https://doi.org/10.1016/j.clnu.2016.09.010.
39. Reignier J, Plantefeve G, Mira J-P, Argaud L, Asfar P, Aissaoui N, Badie J, Botoc N-V, Brisard L, Bui H-N, et al. Low versus standard calorie and protein feeding in ventilated adults with shock: a randomised, controlled, multicentre, open-label, parallel-group trial (NUTRIREA-3). Lancet Respir Med. 2023;11:602–12. https://doi.org/10.1016/S2213-2600(23)00092-9.

40. Gunnar R, Mutanen A, Merras-Salmio L, Pakarinen MP. Histopathological liver steatosis linked with high parenteral glucose and amino acid supply in infants with short bowel syndrome. JPEN J Parenter Enteral Nutr. 2023;47:41–50. https://doi.org/10.1002/jpen.2416.
41. Plummer MP, Bellomo R, Cousins CE, Annink CE, Sundararajan K, Reddi BAJ, Raj JP, Chapman MJ, Horowitz M, Deane AM. Dysglycaemia in the critically ill and the interaction of chronic and acute glycaemia with mortality. Intensive Care Med. 2014;40:973–80. https://doi.org/10.1007/s00134-014-3287-7.
42. Li X, Hou X, Zhang H, Qian X, Feng X, Shi N, Guo R, Sun H, Feng W, Zhao W, et al. Association between stress hyperglycaemia and in-hospital cardiac events after coronary artery bypass grafting in patients without diabetes: a retrospective observational study of 5450 patients. Diabetes Obes Metab. 2023;25(Suppl 1):34–42. https://doi.org/10.1111/dom.15013.
43. Chen Y, Yang X, Meng K, Zeng Z, Ma B, Liu X, Qi B, Cui S, Cao P, Yang Y. Stress-induced hyperglycemia after hip fracture and the increased risk of acute myocardial infarction in non-diabetic patients. Diabetes Care. 2013;36:3328–32. https://doi.org/10.2337/dc13-0119.
44. Leonidou L, Michalaki M, Leonardou A, Polyzogopoulou E, Fouka K, Gerolymos M, Leonardos P, Psirogiannis A, Kyriazopoulou V, Gogos CA. Stress-induced hyperglycemia in patients with severe sepsis: a compromising factor for survival. Am J Med Sci. 2008;336:467–71. https://doi.org/10.1097/MAJ.0b013e318176abb4.
45. Khalfallah M, Abdelmageed R, Elgendy E, Hafez YM. Incidence, predictors and outcomes of stress hyperglycemia in patients with ST elevation myocardial infarction undergoing primary percutaneous coronary intervention. Diab Vasc Dis Res. 2020;17:1479164119883983. https://doi.org/10.1177/1479164119883983.
46. Wernly B, Lichtenauer M, Franz M, Kabisch B, Muessig J, Masyuk M, Kelm M, Hoppe UC, Jung C. Differential impact of hyperglycemia in critically ill patients: significance in acute myocardial infarction but not in sepsis? Int J Mol Sci. 2016;17:1586. https://doi.org/10.3390/ijms17091586.
47. Krinsley JS, Preiser J-C. Is it time to abandon glucose control in critically ill adult patients? Curr Opin Crit Care. 2019;25:299–306. https://doi.org/10.1097/MCC.0000000000000621.
48. Ali Abdelhamid Y, Kar P, Finnis ME, Phillips LK, Plummer MP, Shaw JE, Horowitz M, Deane AM. Stress hyperglycaemia in critically ill patients and the subsequent risk of diabetes: a systematic review and meta-analysis. Crit Care. 2016;20:301. https://doi.org/10.1186/s13054-016-1471-6.
49. van den Berghe G, Wouters P, Weekers F, Verwaest C, Bruyninckx F, Schetz M, Vlasselaers D, Ferdinande P, Lauwers P, Bouillon R. Intensive insulin therapy in critically ill patients. N Engl J Med. 2001;345:1359–67. https://doi.org/10.1056/NEJMoa011300.
50. van den Berghe G, Wilmer A, Hermans G, Meersseman W, Wouters PJ, Milants I, van Wijngaerden E, Bobbaers H, Bouillon R. Intensive insulin therapy in the medical ICU. N Engl J Med. 2006;354:449–61. https://doi.org/10.1056/NEJMoa052521.
51. Finfer S, Chittock DR, Su SY-S, Blair D, Foster D, Dhingra V, Bellomo R, Cook D, Dodek P, Henderson WR, et al. Intensive versus conventional glucose control in critically ill patients. N Engl J Med. 2009;360:1283–97. https://doi.org/10.1056/NEJMoa0810625.
52. Gunst J, Debaveye Y, Güiza F, Dubois J, de Bruyn A, Dauwe D, de Troy E, Casaer MP, de Vlieger G, Haghedooren R, et al. Tight blood-glucose control without early parenteral nutrition in the ICU. N Engl J Med. 2023;389:1180–90. https://doi.org/10.1056/NEJMoa2304855.
53. Hermans G, de Jonghe B, Bruyninckx F, van den Berghe G. Interventions for preventing critical illness polyneuropathy and critical illness myopathy. Cochrane Database Syst Rev. 2014;2014:CD006832. https://doi.org/10.1002/14651858.CD006832.pub3.
54. de Vries FEE, Gans SL, Solomkin JS, Allegranzi B, Egger M, Dellinger EP, Boermeester MA. Meta-analysis of lower perioperative blood glucose target levels for reduction of surgical-site infection. Br J Surg. 2017;104:e95–e105. https://doi.org/10.1002/bjs.10424.
55. van den Berghe G, Wilmer A, Milants I, Wouters PJ, Bouckaert B, Bruyninckx F, Bouillon R, Schetz M. Intensive insulin therapy in mixed medical/surgical intensive care units: benefit versus harm. Diabetes. 2006;55:3151–9. https://doi.org/10.2337/db06-0855.

56. Singer P, Blaser AR, Berger MM, Alhazzani W, Calder PC, Casaer MP, Hiesmayr M, Mayer K, Montejo JC, Pichard C, et al. ESPEN guideline on clinical nutrition in the intensive care unit. Clin Nutr. 2019;38:48–79. https://doi.org/10.1016/j.clnu.2018.08.037.
57. McClave SA, Taylor BE, Martindale RG, Warren MM, Johnson DR, Braunschweig C, McCarthy MS, Davanos E, Rice TW, Cresci GA, et al. Guidelines for the provision and assessment of nutrition support therapy in the adult critically ill patient: Society of Critical Care Medicine (SCCM) and American Society for Parenteral and Enteral Nutrition (A.S.P.E.N.). JPEN J Parenter Enteral Nutr. 2016;40:159–211. https://doi.org/10.1177/0148607115621863.
58. Evans L, Rhodes A, Alhazzani W, Antonelli M, Coopersmith CM, French C, Machado FR, Mcintyre L, Ostermann M, Prescott HC, et al. Surviving sepsis campaign: international guidelines for management of sepsis and septic shock 2021. Intensive Care Med. 2021;47:1181–247. https://doi.org/10.1007/s00134-021-06506-y.
59. Ishihara M. Acute hyperglycemia in patients with acute myocardial infarction. Circ J. 2012;76:563–71. https://doi.org/10.1253/circj.cj-11-1376.
60. Di Muzio F, Presello B, Glassford NJ, Tsuji IY, Eastwood GM, Deane AM, Ekinci EI, Bellomo R, Mårtensson J. Liberal versus conventional glucose targets in critically ill diabetic patients: an exploratory safety cohort assessment. Crit Care Med. 2016;44:1683–91. https://doi.org/10.1097/CCM.0000000000001742.
61. Luethi N, Cioccari L, Biesenbach P, Lucchetta L, Kagaya H, Morgan R, Di Muzio F, Presello B, Gaafar D, Hay A, et al. Liberal glucose control in ICU patients with diabetes: a before-and-after study. Crit Care Med. 2018;46:935–42. https://doi.org/10.1097/CCM.0000000000003087.
62. Poole AP, Finnis ME, Anstey J, Bellomo R, Bihari S, Biradar V, Doherty S, Eastwood G, Finfer S, French CJ, et al. The effect of a liberal approach to glucose control in critically ill patients with type 2 diabetes: a multicenter, parallel-group, open-label randomized clinical trial. Am J Respir Crit Care Med. 2022;206:874–82. https://doi.org/10.1164/rccm.202202-0329OC.
63. Nair BG, Neradilek MB, Newman S-F, Horibe M. Association between acute phase perioperative glucose parameters and postoperative outcomes in diabetic and non-diabetic patients undergoing non-cardiac surgery. Am J Surg. 2019;218:302–10. https://doi.org/10.1016/j.amjsurg.2018.10.024.
64. Rau C-S, Wu S-C, Chen Y-C, Chien P-C, Hsieh H-Y, Kuo P-J, Hsieh C-H. Stress-induced hyperglycemia in diabetes: a cross-sectional analysis to explore the definition based on the trauma registry data. Int J Environ Res Public Health. 2017;14:1527. https://doi.org/10.3390/ijerph14121527.
65. Egi M, Bellomo R, Stachowski E, French CJ, Hart GK, Taori G, Hegarty C, Bailey M. The interaction of chronic and acute glycemia with mortality in critically ill patients with diabetes. Crit Care Med. 2011;39:105–11. https://doi.org/10.1097/CCM.0b013e3181feb5ea.
66. Yamada T, Shojima N, Noma H, Yamauchi T, Kadowaki T. Glycemic control, mortality, and hypoglycemia in critically ill patients: a systematic review and network meta-analysis of randomized controlled trials. Intensive Care Med. 2017;43:1–15. https://doi.org/10.1007/s00134-016-4523-0.
67. Bohé J, Abidi H, Brunot V, Klich A, Klouche K, Sedillot N, Tchenio X, Quenot J-P, Roudaut J-B, Mottard N, et al. Individualised versus conventional glucose control in critically-ill patients: the CONTROLING study-a randomized clinical trial. Intensive Care Med. 2021;47:1271–83. https://doi.org/10.1007/s00134-021-06526-8.
68. Schwartz MW, Krinsley JS, Faber CL, Hirsch IB, Brownlee M. Brain glucose sensing and the problem of relative hypoglycemia. Diabetes Care. 2023;46:237–44. https://doi.org/10.2337/dc22-1445.
69. Umpierrez G, Cardona S, Pasquel F, Jacobs S, Peng L, Unigwe M, Newton CA, Smiley-Byrd D, Vellanki P, Halkos M, et al. Randomized controlled trial of intensive versus conservative glucose control in patients undergoing coronary artery bypass graft surgery: GLUCO-CABG trial. Diabetes Care. 2015;38:1665–72. https://doi.org/10.2337/dc15-0303.
70. American Diabetes Association. 15. Diabetes care in the hospital: standards of medical care in diabetes-2019. Diabetes Care. 2019;42:S173–81. https://doi.org/10.2337/dc19-S015.

71. Finfer S, Wernerman J, Preiser J-C, Cass T, Desaive T, Hovorka R, Joseph JI, Kosiborod M, Krinsley J, Mackenzie I, et al. Clinical review: consensus recommendations on measurement of blood glucose and reporting glycemic control in critically ill adults. Crit Care. 2013;17:229. https://doi.org/10.1186/cc12537.
72. Deane AM, Plummer MP, Ali Abdelhamid Y. Update on glucose control during and after critical illness. Curr Opin Crit Care. 2022;28:389–94. https://doi.org/10.1097/MCC.0000000000000962.
73. Kott M, Elke G. Glukosemanagement in der Intensivmedizin. Aktuel Ernahrungsmed. 2017;42:331–49. https://doi.org/10.1055/s-0043-108683.
74. Weickert MO, Loeffelholz CV, Roden M, Chandramouli V, Brehm A, Nowotny P, Osterhoff MA, Isken F, Spranger J, Landau BR, et al. A Thr94Ala mutation in human liver fatty acid-binding protein contributes to reduced hepatic glycogenolysis and blunted elevation of plasma glucose levels in lipid-exposed subjects. Am J Physiol Endocrinol Metab. 2007;293:E1078–84. https://doi.org/10.1152/ajpendo.00337.2007.
75. Roden M, Stingl H, Chandramouli V, Schumann WC, Hofer A, Landau BR, Nowotny P, Waldhäusl W, Shulman GI. Effects of free fatty acid elevation on postabsorptive endogenous glucose production and gluconeogenesis in humans. Diabetes. 2000;49:701–7. https://doi.org/10.2337/diabetes.49.5.701.
76. Singer P, Anbar R, Cohen J, Shapiro H, Shalita-Chesner M, Lev S, Grozovski E, Theilla M, Frishman S, Madar Z. The tight calorie control study (TICACOS): a prospective, randomized, controlled pilot study of nutritional support in critically ill patients. Intensive Care Med. 2011;37:601–9. https://doi.org/10.1007/s00134-011-2146-z.
77. Heyland DK, Patel J, Compher C, Rice TW, Bear DE, Lee Z-Y, González VC, O'Reilly K, Regala R, Wedemire C, et al. The effect of higher protein dosing in critically ill patients with high nutritional risk (EFFORT Protein): an international, multicentre, pragmatic, registry-based randomised trial. Lancet. 2023;401:568–76. https://doi.org/10.1016/S0140-6736(22)02469-2.
78. Pardo E, Lescot T, Preiser J-C, Massanet P, Pons A, Jaber S, Fraipont V, Levesque E, Ichai C, Petit L, et al. Association between early nutrition support and 28-day mortality in critically ill patients: the FRANS prospective nutrition cohort study. Crit Care. 2023;27:7. https://doi.org/10.1186/s13054-022-04298-1.
79. Matejovic M, Huet O, Dams K, Elke G, Vaquerizo Alonso C, Csomos A, Krzych ŁJ, Tetamo R, Puthucheary Z, Rooyackers O, et al. Medical nutrition therapy and clinical outcomes in critically ill adults: a European multinational, prospective observational cohort study (EuroPN). Crit Care. 2022;26:143. https://doi.org/10.1186/s13054-022-03997-z.
80. Hartl WH, Kopper P, Bender A, Scheipl F, Day AG, Elke G, Küchenhoff H. Protein intake and outcome of critically ill patients: analysis of a large international database using piecewise exponential additive mixed models. Crit Care. 2022;26:7. https://doi.org/10.1186/s13054-021-03870-5.
81. Reignier J, Boisramé-Helms J, Brisard L, Lascarrou J-B, Ait Hssain A, Anguel N, Argaud L, Asehnoune K, Asfar P, Bellec F, et al. Enteral versus parenteral early nutrition in ventilated adults with shock: a randomised, controlled, multicentre, open-label, parallel-group study (NUTRIREA-2). Lancet. 2018;391:133–43. https://doi.org/10.1016/S0140-6736(17)32146-3.

Lipids in Nutritional Therapy

5

Andreas Edel and Kathrin Scholtz

5.1 Basics About Fats

5.1.1 Fats (Triglycerides)

Fats are just one type of lipid, a category of compounds that do not easily mix with water because of their chemical properties. Fats have 9 kcal/g (38 kJ/g), which is the most important energy reserve of the human organism. The majority (90–95%) of fats in a typical Western pattern are triglycerides (TGs) [1], which are esters derived from a single molecule of glycerol and three fatty acids (FAs). Since TGs cannot be absorbed, they must be hydrolyzed. Simple triglycerides are those in which each molecule of glycerol is combined with three molecules of one acid. Only a few glycerides occurring in nature are of the simple type; in most TGs, one molecule of glycerol is combined with two or three different FAs. Depending on the carbon chain length, number and position of double bonds, and linearity (stereospecificity or cis vs. trans), lipids have different physical and chemical properties. FAs in TGs carry between 2 and 24 carbon atoms [2]. Short-chain triglycerides (SCTs) include FAs that range in length from 2 to 4 carbons, medium-chain triglycerides (MCTs) contain FAs ranging from 6 to 12 carbons, and LCTs are composed of FAs with chain length >12 carbons [2, 3]. Fats containing LCTs, which are usually derived from vegetable oils, and MCTs are derived from palm kernel oils, palm oils, and coconut oils [2]. Fibers fermented by bacteria in the colon are the most important source of short-chain fatty acids (SCFAs) [4]. Compared with LCTs, neither SCT nor MCTs require bile salt for absorption or promote chylomicron formation or bile

---

A. Edel (✉) · K. Scholtz
Charité-Universitätsmedizin Berlin, Corporate Member of Freie Universität Berlin and Humboldt-Universität zu Berlin, Department of Anesthesiology and Intensive Care Medicine (CCM I CVK), Berlin, Germany
e-mail: andreas.edel@charite.de; kathrin.scholtz@charite.de

© The Author(s), under exclusive license to Springer Nature Switzerland AG 2025
A. Rümelin et al. (eds.), *Nutrition in ICU Patients*,
https://doi.org/10.1007/978-3-032-00818-3_5

salts for absorption. Given their hydrophilic properties, short- and medium-chain FAs can directly enter the portal venous system [2].

Each lipid class possesses unique biological activity and is therapeutically significant [5]. TG molecules serve as a primary storage form of energy, offer insulation to cells, facilitate the absorption of fat-soluble vitamins [6], and transport FAs within cells and plasma. Lipid metabolism plays a crucial role in maintaining cellular homeostasis by influencing various essential processes such as membrane synthesis and the use of lipids as an energy store. Dietary TG is crucial for lipid metabolism homeostasis [7].

Exogenous TGs originate from food sources, whereas endogenous TGs are generated in the liver. In adipose tissue and the liver, the endogenous pathway predominates, whereas the exogenous pathway is more prominent in the intestine (see Sect. 1.5) [8]. Lipid metabolism encompasses catabolic processes that generate energy and anabolic processes that produce various lipid species. Typically, lipids possess a head group with a distinct chemical composition that binds to hydrophobic tails composed of fatty acyl chains or sphingoid bases [9]. The function and structure of lipids are determined by their uptake, synthesis, storage, and consumption across different cellular organelles.

Daily TGs intake is 60–150 g/day [10]. Dietary fats also include cholesterol, phospholipids (PLs), and many other lipids (e.g., vitamins) [1].

5.1.2 Fatty Acids

Fatty acids (FAs) are carboxylic acids with aliphatic chains. They are the main components of triglycerides (TGs) and are classified as saturated fatty acids (SFAs), monounsaturated fatty acids (MUFAs), and polyunsaturated fatty acids (PUFAs) based on the presence and number of double bonds in their molecular structure [11]. The $n - x$ (n minus x) nomenclature provides names for individual compounds and classifies them according to their likely biosynthetic properties in humans. A double bond is located on the xth carbon-carbon bond, originating from the methyl end of the molecular backbone. For instance, linoleic acid is categorized as an $n - 6$ acid and is expected to follow the same biosynthetic pathway as other members of this family because it holds a similar position in the FAs classification system. If all carbon-to-carbon bonds are singular, the acid is considered saturated. However, if any of the bonds are double or triple, the acid is unsaturated and exhibits increased reactivity. The degree of unsaturation and chain length play vital roles in regulating the metabolic stage of FAs, affecting the functionality of cells, tissues, and lipid mediators produced. Each double bond is identified through Δx in the nomenclature of Δx (or delta-x). This represents the xth carbon-carbon bond, originating from the carboxylic end of the molecular backbone.

FAs are the second most important source of energy in humans and are necessary for cellular tissues and membranes [11]. FAs serve as the primary energy source via mitochondria-mediated β-oxidation and tricarboxylic acid (citric acid cycle, TCA) cycle catabolism (Fig. 5.1).

Lipids enter cells via transporters such as CD36 and FATPs. After Once inside, FAs are directed to mitochondria by specific membrane proteins, where they undergos oxidation to produce acetyl-CoA, a key substrate for ATP generation. Glucose transported into the cell also contributes to acetyl-CoA formation, supporting the TCA cycle. The uptake of acetate through MCT provides an additional source of acetyl-CoA. Acetyl-CoA can modulate histone and protein acetylation, influencing epigenetic regulation. VLCFAs and BRCFAs are partially metabolized in peroxisomes, feeding into TCA cycle intermediates. Citrate genrated in the TCA cycle can exit mitochondria to serve as a building block for de novo lipogenesis, including FAs and cholesterol. Palmitate is formed from malonyl-CoA by FA synthase and can be elongated into MUFAs and PUFAs. LCFA are esterified into TGs and stored in lipid droplets. Palmitate can also be converted into CDP-DAG and DAG, which serve as precursors for membrane phospholipids such as PC, PE, PI, and PS. BRCFA, branched-chain fatty acid; CDP-DAG, cytidine diphosphate diacylglycerol; DAG, diacylglycerol; ETC, electron transport chain; FAs, fatty acids; FATP, fatty acid transport protein; MUFA, monounsaturated fatty acid; PA, phosphatidic acid; PC, phosphatidylcholine; PE, phosphatidylethanolamine; PI, phosphatidylinositol; PS, phosphatidylserine; PUFA, polyunsaturated fatty acid; TCA, tricarboxylic acid; VLCFA, very long-chain fatty acid. Image used with kind permission of Anna Greka, Department of Medicine, Brigham and Women's Hospital and Harvard Medical School, Boston, USA [12].

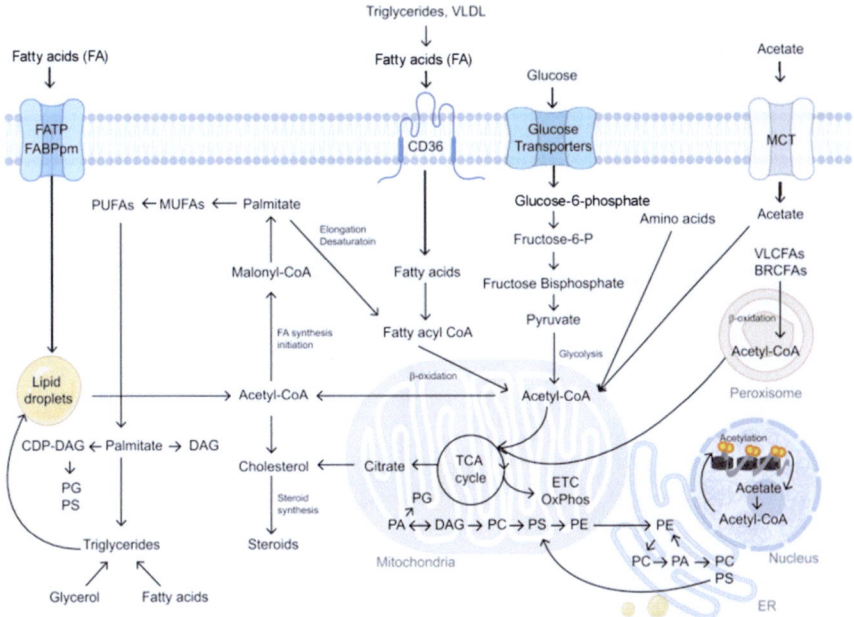

Fig. 5.1 Metabolism of fatty acids

FAs are the primary components of lipids (Yoon et al.). Free fatty acids (FFAs) are lipids released from certain cell types and adipose tissue via lipolysis. FFAs are known to be active players in several biological processes, apart from their activities in the energy supply or as structural elements [13].

5.1.2.1 Lipotoxicity

High levels of circulating lipids have been associated with metabolic disorders [14] and cancer [15]. Exposure to an abundance of lipids over an extended period may result in "lipotoxicity", which is harmful [16]. The molecular pathways involved in lipotoxicity (Fig. 5.2) include inflammation, oxidative stress, endoplasmic reticulum (ER) stress, impaired autophagy, and mitochondrial dysfunction [16]. Efficiently directing free fatty acids (FFAs) toward lipid droplets (LDs), structural lipids, or mitochondria for beta-oxidation could reduce the detrimental effects of lipid accumulation. Growing proof indicates that the fatty acid (FA) composition of lipids and specific (FA) fatty acid concentrations (e.g., odd or even chain saturated fatty acids, ratio of saturated to unsaturated, monounsaturated versus polyunsaturated, omega position, etc.) have unique cellular effects on metabolism [12].

5.1.2.2 Essential Fatty Acids

Polyunsaturated fatty acids (PUFAs) can be obtained through multiple biological pathways. In humans, PUFAs are generated through desaturation of the corresponding alkanoic acid, as they possess a $\Delta 9$-desaturase enzyme that introduces a cis double bond into a saturated fatty acid (FA) [17]. PUFAs can be categorized into $n-3$ FAs and $n-6$ FAs. In Westernized diets, $n-6$ FAs are the most prevalent PUFAs.

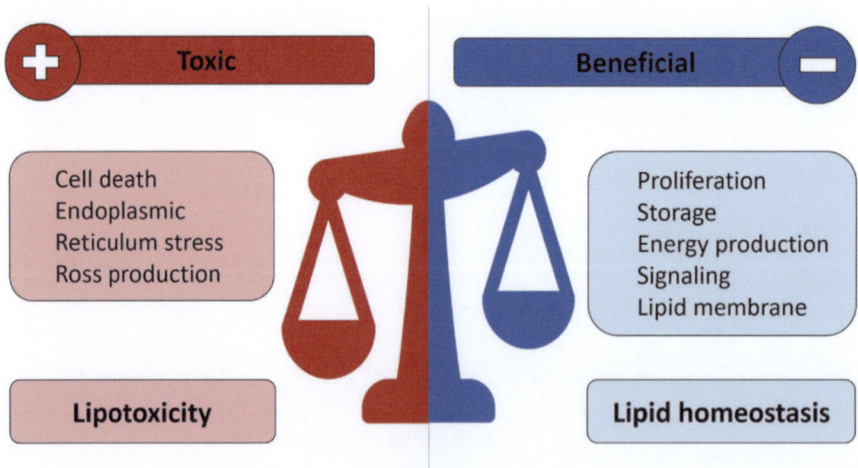

Fig. 5.2 Lipids are beneficial or lipotoxic. (Adapted with kind permission of Anna Greka, Department of Medicine, Brigham and Women's Hospital and Harvard Medical School, Boston, USA [12])

FAs such as linoleic acid ($n - 6$) (LA) (a long-chain, 18-carbon atom fatty acid with two double bonds) and alpha-linolenic acid ($n - 3$) (ALA) (a long-chain, 18-carbon atom FA with three double bonds) are essential for humans because their bodies are unable to synthesize them [17]. This inability arises from the absence of an enzyme that can add a double bond (desaturate) beyond the omega-9 carbon situated at the alpha end of the FAs (i.e., beyond the $n - 6$ and $n - 3$ positions). However, human enzymes can elongate and desaturate essential FAs by adding two carbon atoms and double bonds, respectively, resulting in the formation of other omega-6 and omega-3 FAs. As a result, the majority of polyunsaturated FAs belong to two different families.

The elongation and desaturation of these FAs result in long-chain PUFAs such as eicosapentaenoic acid (EPA) (long-chain PUFAs of 20 carbon atoms and five double bonds), docosahexaenoic acid (DHA) (22 carbon atoms and 6 double bonds), and arachidonic acid (AA) [18]. The conversion of LA into EPA is in the range of 0.2–8%, whereas ALA is converted into DHA in the range of 0–4% of ALA [19]. Hence, it is more effective to consume a diet enriched in $n - 3$ PUFAs, including marine products, to directly obtain the longer-chain FAs EPA and DHA [17].

However, human enzymes can elongate and desaturate essential FAs by adding two carbons and double bonds, respectively, resulting in the formation of other omega-6 and omega-3 FAs. As a result, the majority of polyunsaturated FAs belong to two different families.

5.1.3 Eicosanoids

Polyunsaturated fatty acids (PUFAs) (Fig. 5.3), particularly the $n - 6$ family of linoleic acid (18:2 $n - 6$, LA), gamma-linolenic acid (18:3 $n - 6$, γ-GLA), arachidonic acid ($n - 6$, AA), $n - 3$ family of alpha-linolenic acid (18:3 $n - 3$, ALA), eicosapentaenoic acid (20:5 $n - 3$, EPA), and docosahexaenoic acid (22:6 $n - 3$, DHA), serve as substrates for the synthesis of bioactive lipid mediators, such as eicosanoids (Fig. 5.3), which play a role in inflammatory responses [20].

Eicosanoids are synthesized from omega-3 FAs, including EPA, as well as omega-6 FAs such as dihomo-gamma-linolenic acid and AA. Substrate PUFAs are released from phospholipids within the cell membrane and subsequently metabolized by enzymes such as lipoxygenase (LOX), cyclooxygenase (COX), and cytochrome P450 oxidase (cytP450) [21]. COX pathways produce prostaglandins (PGs) and thromboxanes (TXs), whereas LOX pathways synthesize leukotrienes (LTs) and lipoxins (LXs) and resolvins. Additionally, the cytP450 pathway produces various hydroxy, epoxy, and dihydroxy derivatives [21] that exhibit significant biological activities. However, eicosanoids primarily act locally at their production sites owing to their rapid catabolism. AA is the primary substrate of eicosanoid synthesis.

Eicosanoids are bioactive and operate through cell membrane G protein-linked receptors in various cell types. Some eicosanoids act as ligands for nuclear receptors. Owing to their rapid metabolism, eicosanoids primarily act locally at their production sites. Many eicosanoids are involved in the regulation of female

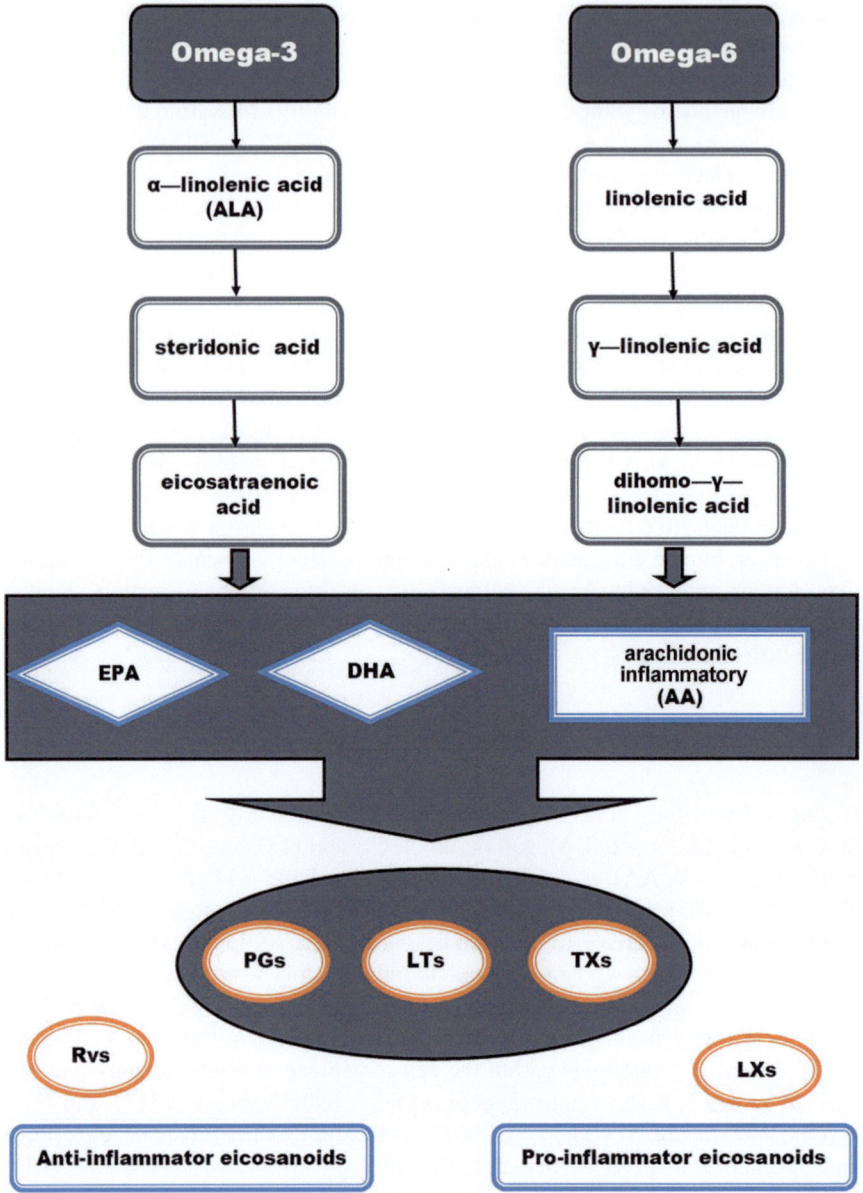

Fig. 5.3 Metabolism of omega-3 and omega-6 fatty acids (FAs). The pathway of omega-3 FAs results in eicosapentaenoic acid (EPA) and docosahexaenoic acid (DHA), while the pathway of omega-6 FAs concludes with aracidonic acid (AA). Eicosanoids, including prostaglandins (PGs), thromboxanes (TXs), and leukotrienes (LTs), are derived from both ARA and EPA. Lipoxins produced from ARA and resolvins produced from EPA are additional members of the eicosanoid family. Docosanoids derived from DHA also form resolvins. It should be emphasized that each FA does not possess a singular, unique functional property, and therefore members of the FA family do not exhibit identical properties. DHA docosahexaenoic acid, EPA eicosapentaenoic acid, TXs thromboxanes, LTs leukotrienes, PGs prostaglandins, LXs lipoxins, Rvs resolvins [20]

reproductive, vascular, gastrointestinal, and renal systems [21], and exhibit various effects on immunity and inflammation [22].

Certain eicosanoids have a significant impact on key indicators of inflammation such as fever, pain, redness, and swelling. However, it is worth noting that while some eicosanoids may be described as pro-inflammatory, they also possess anti-inflammatory functions, and some eicosanoids are involved in resolving inflammation. These activities are linked to the exact signaling mechanisms induced by different eicosanoid receptors and the timing of eicosanoid production. The composition of eicosanoids produced during an inflammatory response is determined by the nature of the stimulus and cell types present. As a result, the effects of PGs on inflammation are complex and involve both pro- and anti-inflammatory actions as well as its role in initiating inflammation resolution.

The main factors that determine the effects and outcomes of omega-6 and omega-3 FA intake are the eicosanoids they produce. There is competition between the $n-3$ and $n-6$ FA families for metabolism because they share the same set of enzymes [23]. Omega-6 FA-derived eicosanoids are more inflammatory than omega-3 FA-derived eicosanoids. DHA- and EPA-derived eicosanoids counteract the pro-inflammatory effects of $n-6$ FAs. However, the ratio of $n-3/n-6$ PUFA in cell and organelle membranes, as well as membrane microdomains, strongly influences membrane function and numerous cellular processes, such as cell death and survival [23]. The recommended dietary ratio of $n-6/n-3$ FAs for health benefits is 1:1–2:1 [20].

5.1.4 Cholesterol

Cholesterol (cholest-5-en-3-ol (3-beta) cholesterol), cholesterol metabolites, and esters are the major components of the plasma membrane and different cell organelles [24]. Cholesterol consists of a sterol backbone, a hydroxy group, a double bond, and a side chain that includes eight carbon atoms. Technical abbreviations will be clearly defined upon first use. The steroid backbone of cholesterol functions is the basic structure of bile acids, with cholic acid and chenodeoxycholic acid as the primary bile acids. Additionally, cholesterol is a precursor of fat-soluble vitamins, including vitamin D3, steroid hormones such as cortisone and aldosterone, and sex hormones such as estradiol and testosterone [25].

Cholesterol in the body emerges from two sources: endogenous sources, which are produced in the peripheral tissues and liver, and dietary sources [26]. Cholesterol can be absorbed into the blood through the digestion of dietary fat via chylomicrons.

The daily cholesterol intake in the Western diet varies from approximately 100–400 mg/day; however, a higher intake of up to 800 mg/day has been investigated [27]. The limitation of cholesterol intake reduces the increase in daily intestinal cholesterol flow, which is 2–4 times larger than the flow of dietary cholesterol [10]. Plant sterols account for approximately 25% of dietary sterol intake or approximately 100–150 mg/day [28]. Compared to omnivores, vegans have a 90%

lower cholesterol intake, which results in a 13% lower serum low density lipoprotein (LDL)-cholesterol concentration [29]. Approximately 50% of cholesterol absorption in the intestine is incomplete, with the remaining amount excreted in feces [30].

5.1.5 Phospholipids

Phospholipids (PLs) are amphipathic lipids that play crucial roles in cell membranes. They are structured as a lipid double layer and are derived from glycerol, which is similar in structure to triglycerides (TGs). They are competent in integrating fatty acids into the cell membrane, as they display better absorption and usage than TGs [31]. In addition to their structural functions, PLs regulate cellular processes. The digestion of PLs is primarily performed by pancreatic phospholipase A2 (pPLA2) and other lipases secreted by the pancreas after food intake [1]. The predominant PL in the intestinal lumen is phosphatidylcholine (PC), which originates from the bile (10–20 g/day in humans) and diet (~1–2 g/day) [1].

5.1.6 Lipoproteins

Owing to the hydrophobic nature of lipids, such as cholesterol and triglycerides (TGs), they must be transported in conjunction with proteins, such as lipoproteins, in circulation [28]. Many fatty acids from daily food intake are transferred as TGs to prevent toxicity [12]. These lipoproteins play major roles in the absorption and transport of dietary lipids by the small intestine, transport of lipids from the liver to peripheral tissues, and transport of lipids from peripheral tissues to the liver and intestine. This process is known as reverse cholesterol transport [28]. A secondary function is to transport bacterial endotoxins from the invaded and infected body parts [32]. Plasma lipoproteins can be classified based on size, lipid composition, and apolipoproteins (Table 5.1).

5.1.7 Lipid Transport System

Lipid transportation involves two separate pathways: an exogenous route for the transport of cholesterol and triglycerides (TGs) absorbed from dietary fat in the intestine and an endogenous system through which cholesterol and TGs gain plasma from the liver and other non-intestinal tissues [33].

5.1.7.1 Exogenous Pathway
The exogenous pathway begins with intestinal absorption of cholesterol and TGs from food sources [33]. The action of gastric enzymes in the stomach ensures that digestion continues. The fat emulsion enters the duodenum in the form of lipid droplets, which are subsequently solubilized through the action of bile acids. Fatty

Table 5.1 Lipoprotein classes [28]

Lipoprotein	Density (g/mL)	Size (nm)	Major lipids	Major apoproteins
Chylomicrons	<0.930	75–1200	Triglycerides	Apo B-48, Apo C, Apo E, Apo A-I, A-II, A-IV
Chylomicron remnants	0.930–1.006	30–80	Triglycerides cholesterol	Apo B-48, Apo E
VLDL	0.930–1.006	30–80	Triglycerides	Apo B-100, Apo E, Apo C
IDL	1.006–1.019	25–35	Triglycerides cholesterol	Apo B-100, Apo E, Apo C
LDL	1.019–1.063	18–25	Cholesterol	Apo B-100
HDL	1.063–1.210	5–12	Cholesterol phospholipids	Apo A-I, Apo A-II, Apo C, Apo E
Lp (a)	1.055–1.085	~30	Cholesterol	Apo B-100, Apo (a)

acids (FAs) in the intestine are mainly dietary, cholesterol in the intestinal lumen is predominantly sourced from bile (around 200–500 mg of cholesterol from diet and 800–1200 mg from bile) [28].

Dietary TGs are further hydrolyzed in the intestinal lumen by pancreatic lipases to produce 2-monoacylglycerol (2-MAG) and long chain fatty acid (LCFA). Pancreatic lipases can hydrolyze 50–70% of total dietary fats [34]. Co-lipase is a necessary cofactor for the full function of the enzyme [35]. The enterocytes absorb the products of digestion and transport them into the endoplasmic reticulum (ER). TG is resynthesized by 2-MAG and LCFA in the ER [7]. This lipid is then coupled with phospholipids, apoproteins and unestrified cholesterol into TG-rich lipoprotein particles called chylomicrons (CMs) for subsequent delivery to peripheral circulation [33]. CMs are shed directly into the lymph before entering the blood stream. In the circulatory system, the triglycerides transported in CMs are metabolized in muscle and adipose tissues by lipoprotein lipase, resulting in the release of free fatty acids (FFAs). These FFAs are subsequently metabolized by adipose and muscle tissues, leading to the formation of CM remnants. These remnants are then taken up by the liver [33]. Nearly 95% of dietary TGs can be absorbed and undergo digestion, uptake, resynthesis, and secretion into circulation in CMs [33, 36, 37].

CMs appear in the plasma following a meal, typically lasting 1–5 h, and giving it a milky appearance. They are usually eliminated from circulation within 12 h of fasting [33].

5.1.7.2 Endogenous Pathway

The endogenous lipoprotein pathway begins in the liver with the formation of very low-density lipoprotein (VLDL) [28]. The remaining TGs present in the CM remnants is transported to the liver [38]. In the liver, TG hydrolysis provides FAs for β-oxidation, signaling, and substrates for the assembly of VLDL TGs within hepatocytes [38]. The TGs transported in VLDL are broken down into free FAs by lipoprotein lipase in both the muscle and adipose tissue, resulting in the formation of intermediate density lipoprotein (IDL). These IDL particles are relatively enriched in cholesterol esters and acquire Apolipoprotein E (Apo E) from high-density lipoprotein (HDL) particles. IDL particles can be removed from circulation by the liver through the binding of Apo E to low-density lipoprotein (LDL) and Low-density lipoprotein receptor-related protein (LRP) receptors. However, while the majority of CM remnants are swiftly cleared by the liver, only a fraction of IDL particles (approximately 50%, though this may vary) undergo clearance. The remaining TGs within IDL particles are hydrolyzed by hepatic lipase, resulting in a further reduction of TG content. Additionally, exchangeable apolipoproteins are transferred from IDL particles to other lipoproteins, culminating in the formation of LDL. Consequently, LDL is considered a product of VLDL metabolism. In individuals with normal metabolism, this pathway can handle substantial amounts of fat ($\geq$100 g/day) without significant increases in plasma TG levels [28].

Recent studies have shown that enterocytes secrete cholesterol, phospholipids, and vitamin E as part of high-density apoB-free/apoAI-containing lipoproteins [1].

5.1.8 Level and Composition of Fat Intake

Daily fat intake should be greater than 10% (as this does not meet the daily requirement of essential FAs) and less than 65–70% (as this would prevent the theoretical minimum daily carbohydrate intake) [39]. Therefore, a middle-ground 30% is recommended as the ideal proportion of daily fat, which should maintain a respiratory quotient in the range of 0.85–0.90. Therefore, the mass of the daily lipid requirement is approximately 1 g/kg/day, or 70 g for a normal-sized person. A direct relationship exists between the amount of fat ingested and the corresponding increase in circulating [28].

According to kinetic studies [40], monounsaturated fatty acids (MUFAs) are preferentially and more rapidly absorbed at the intestinal level than other types of fats. Regarding the FA composition of lipid emulsions, recent expert recommendations [41] indicate that a blend of FAs should be considered, including a source of medium-chain saturated fatty acids, usually from coconut oil (MCTs), omega-9 monounsaturated FAs, and omega-3 polyunsaturated FAs. Soya bean oil contains large quantities of essential FAs (linoleic acid and α-linolenic acid) and is, therefore, a frequently used constituent of parenteral nutrition.

The type of fat consumed depends on the dietary sources, typically including saturated fat from animals and tropical plant oils (coconut, palm), polyunsaturated fat from vegetable oils (such as olive oil for monounsaturated fat, sunflower oil, and corn oil for $n-6$ polyunsaturated fatty acids [PUFAs], flaxseed oil for $n-3$ PUFA), and marine sources (algae and fish oils for LC $n-3$ PUFAs) [18]. Increased consumption of saturated animal fat, in particular, and lower intake of unsaturated fat may have a great effect on the FA composition of human tissues and affect metabolism and health.

5 Lipids in Nutritional Therapy

Moreover, proteins may interfere with the secretion of intestinal TGs by slowing the gastric emptying rate and consequently reducing fat absorption in the intestine [42]. Similarly, polyphenols have been shown to inhibit pancreatic lipase, thus reducing trigacylglyceride digestion and absorption in the intestine [35].

Key Messages

- Fatty acids are the main components of triglycerides and are classified into three types: saturated fatty acids (SFAs), monounsaturated fatty acids (MUFAs), and polyunsaturated fatty acids (PUFAs).
- Polyunsaturated fatty acids (PUFAs) can be derived from multiple biological pathways.
- Lipotoxicity is linked to immunometabolic pathways and cancer.
- Due to their hydrophobic nature, lipids such as cholesterol and triglycerides must be transported in the bloodstream in association with proteins (e.g., lipoproteins).
- It is recommended that 30% of the daily caloric intake should come from fat.

5.2 Fat in the Intensive Care Medicine

5.2.1 Metabolic and Immune Effect in ICU Patients

Patients admitted to the intensive care unit (ICU) often have conditions related to dyslipidemia. In a study group by Stamler and colleagues in 1986, it was estimated that 46% of all coronary heart disease-related deaths were linked to hypercholesterinemia in a cohort of 356,222 patients [43]. The negative impact of hypercholesterolemia and high low density lipoprotein (LDL) levels on health outcomes has been further confirmed by impressive supporting evidence from clinical and genetic studies, as demonstrated by the European Atherosclerosis Society Consensus Panel [44]. Dyslipoproteinemia-related atherosclerosis, which is the underlying pathomechanism, also contributes to the development of conditions, such as ischemic stroke requiring ICU treatment. However, hypertriglyceridemia itself can lead to critical conditions, such as severe pancreatitis with organ failure. Dyslipidemia can also occur during critical illness, increasing the risk of ICU admission.

In contrast, acute critical illnesses have several direct effects on fat metabolism. Initially, triglyceride and very low-density lipoprotein (VLDL) levels increase during the early stage of the disease because of various pathways, such as accelerated lipolysis and pro-inflammatory cytokine-induced fatty acid (FA) synthesis, combined with suppressed FA oxidation [45, 46]. The potential advantage of these altered lipid components may be the enhanced binding of VLDL to lipopolysaccharide (LPS) of gram-negative bacteria in hypertriglyceridemia serum [47]. However, the levels of cholesterol, high-density lipoproteins (HDL), and LDL are reduced in critically ill patients [48–50].

The decreased cholesterol level is a combined effect, including delayed and low-effect LPS-induced cholesterol synthesis and excretion, as well as changes in metabolic pathways that lead to increased production of non-sterol metabolites [45] such as dolichols, an enzyme required for glycosylation of proteins during acute inflammation [51]. Not only the HDL level decreases during critical illness, but also the composition of HDL shifts to acute-phase HDL, which contains more free cholesterol, triglycerides (TGs), free FAs, and less cholesteryl ester. The underlying pathomechanism of HDL reduction is not yet fully understood but involves different metabolic pathways [45]. Increased consumption of pulmonary surfactants, cell regeneration, and pro-inflammatory mediators have been proposed as potential contributing factors [52, 53]. Pro-inflammatory cytokines can directly inhibit cholesterol synthesis and secretion, although the precise mechanism remains unclear [45]. Furthermore, the impaired function of transporters and receptors has been linked to direct pathogenic effects that influence lipid metabolism [53, 54]. HDL has anti-inflammatory properties and can decrease cytokine release [55]. HDL can bind LPS and the gram-positive bacterial component, lipoteichoic acid (LTA) [56]. On one hand, HDL lipoproteins are assumed to possess anti-apoptotic, antithrombotic, anti-inflammatory, and anti-infectious properties [57], on the other hand, increased levels of TGs-rich lipoproteins, such as VLDL or alternated LDL, have proatherogenic properties, which may lead to an increased risk for critical illness [45]. A systematic review and meta-analysis by Hofmaenner et al. revealed a contradictory finding, demonstrating a significantly lower ICU mortality in patients with lower concentrations of total cholesterol, HDL, and LDL [48]. Furthermore, a meta-analysis of 22 studies with 10,122 COVID-19 patients revealed a significant reduction in total cholesterol, LDL, and HDL concentrations in severely ill patients and those with a non-survivor status [50]. The inflammatory effect of omega-3 and omega-6 FAs, along with their metabolic end products, are illustrated in Fig. 5.3.

5.2.2 Fat in Parenteral Nutrition

Parenteral nutrition solutions are a essential therapy option for ICU patients and are endorsed by the ESPEN and ASPEN guidelines. These solutions include all three primary macronutrients: carbohydrates, proteins, and fats. Fat composition has always been a topic of discussion, as FAs play a significant role in providing non-protein and non-carbohydrate calories, particularly during the acute phase of insulin resistance following post-aggression metabolism. Several FAs are used in parenteral lipid emulsions. FAs can be divided into either saturated and unsaturated, with unsaturated further categorized by the number of double-bonds. Monounsaturated fatty acids (MUFA) have one bond, while polyunsaturated fatty acids (PUFA) two or more bonds. The ideal FA balance remains unknown due to inconsistent evidence. Traditionally, parenteral fat emulsions are made from soybean oil containing LCT in a 7:1 ratio of $n-6$ to $n-3$ PUFAs. $n-6$ linoleic acid may have pro-inflammatory properties by converting it to arachidonic acid and eicosanoids such as prostaglandins, thromboxanes, and leukotrienes [58]. In contrast, $n-3$ linolenic acid may exhibit anti-inflammatory and antioxidant effects when metabolized to docosahexaenoic acid (DHA) and eicosapentaenoic acid (EPA) [59]. To enhance the concentration of $n - 3$ FAs, the soybean oil-based emulsion is partly replaced by fish or olive oil, and EPA and DHA at a rate of 0.6–1 g. The consequences of this omega-6 FA-reducing technique were assessed through a meta-analysis, which demonstrated no impact on overall mortality compared to the use of LCT or LCT/MCT (RR: 0.91; 95% CI 0.76–1.10; $p = 0.34$) but a considerably shorter hospital length of stay (LOS) (WMD −6.88; 95% CI −11.27, −2.49; $p = 0.002$). In the subgroup analysis, incorporating eight studies studying fish oil in parenteral nutrition, it was found that there was a more noticeable effect on ICU LOS (WMD −3.53; 95% CI −6.16 to −0.90; $p = 0.009$) and reduction in nosocomial infections (RR 0.65; 95% CI 0.44–0.95; $p = 0.03$), which aligns with the findings of the meta-analysis by Pradelli et al. [60]. Subgroup analysis of three studies employing stand-alone fish-oil-based nutrition revealed a significant reduction in 28-day mortality ($n = 237$; RR, 0.60; 95% CI, 0.36, 0.99; $p = 0.04$) [61].

In such cases, FAs can serve as an effective energy source. Fat metabolism involves the transport of long-chain triglycerides into the mitochondria through carnitine, where LCT is then oxidized to acetyl-CoA, which subsequently enters either the tricarboxylic acid cycle or the ketone pathway. In contrast, medium-chain triglycerides (MCT) can pass through the mitochondrial membrane without requiring active transport [62], making them an essential substrate for critically ill patients, where carnitine depletion may occur [63]. Although only a limited number of studies have explored the metabolism of MCTs, soybean oil-based lipid emulsions mostly consist of $n - 6$ fatty acids. The partial replacement of these emulsions with olive, coconut, or fish oil may increase the amount of MCTs, which is believed to have immune-supporting properties [64, 65]. These findings suggest that the ratio of T-helper (CD4+) to T-suppressor (CD8+) cells was maintained in the MCT soybean oil group compared with that in the soybean group alone [64].

As previously mentioned, omega-3 PUFAs have beneficial properties and are promising components of parenteral nutrition. In the most recent meta-analysis of 49 studies, involving 3641 patients who were electively admitted to either the ICU or non-ICU, the Pradelli study group demonstrated that the use of omega-3 FAs in comparison to standard non-enriched lipid emulsions resulted in a 40% reduction in infection rates (relative risk [RR] 0.61; 95% confidence interval [CI], 0.45–0.84; $p = 0.002$), shorter hospital stay by an average of 2.14 days (95% CI 1.36–2.93; $p < 0.00001$), and an ICU stay that was approximately 2 days shorter (−1.95 days; 95% CI 0.42–3.49; $p = 0.01$). The use of omega-3 FAs in parenteral solutions also has an impact on mortality risk [60]. In a cost-effectiveness analysis that considered results comparable to those of a prior meta-analysis, Pradelli et al. revealed a favorable economic benefit that fully offset therapy costs [66].

In addition to long-chain fatty acids, medium-chain fatty acids (MCFAs) have also been introduced into commercial parenteral solutions. Sandström et al. investigated the safety of chemically produced structured lipids (SL), where MCFAs and LCFAs are related to the glycerol backbone compared to the former standard long-chain triglycerides (LCTs) fat solution. In this small RCT with 20 participants, the authors did not find a significant difference between the groups regarding the observed side effects after receiving one of the solutions for 5–7 days [67]. In a subsequent RCT, Sandström et al. investigated the proposed properties of MCFAs, such as a higher oxidation rate and partly carnitine-independent metabolic pathways. In this study, the researcher investigated whether SL with medium-chain triglycerides (MCTs) and LCTs were metabolized faster than the standard LCT solution. Both patient groups received SLs or LCTs on alternating days, and randomization was used to determine which group started with SLs. The basal rates of intravenous glucose and amino acids were equal in both groups. Energy expenditure was measured using indirect calorimetry each day before and after lipid application. Sandström and colleagues demonstrated that SLs with MCFAs and LCFAs were associated with an increased rate of fat oxidation compared with LCTs [68]. These parenteral lipids were compared with the unique LCTs parenteral solution in 20 postoperative patients. The historical progression of parenteral fat solution use is shown in Fig. 5.4.

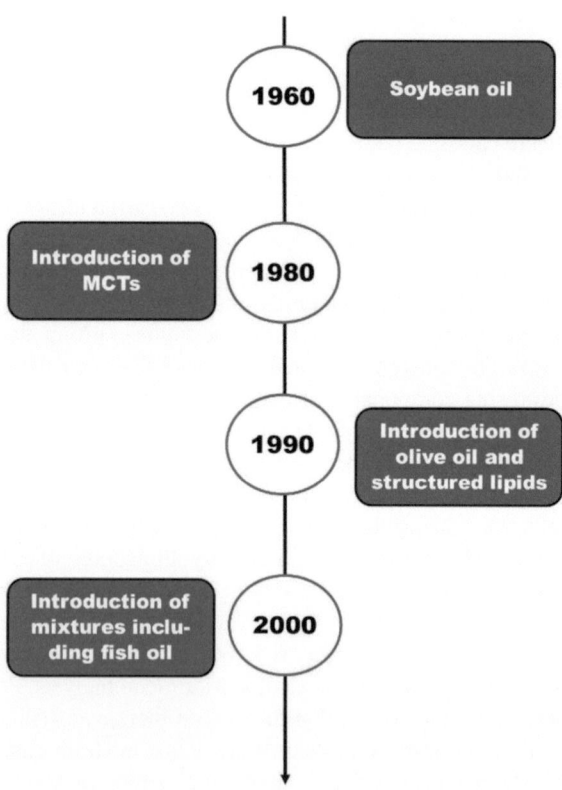

Fig. 5.4 Development of lipid emulsions in parenteral nutrition [69]

5.2.3 Fat in Enteral Nutrition

Fat is one of the three macronutrients found in all commercial enteral solutions. The optimal FA composition is still a matter of debate. Unlike parenteral administration, enteral administration requires proper absorption of fat. However, maldigestion can occur in critically ill patients and can be problematic in enteral nutrition therapy. In a study conducted by Abdelmhamid et al. involving both healthy volunteers and ICU patients, duodenal fat absorption was found to be impaired in critically ill group [70].

FAs can be classified based on a variety of factors, such as chain length, saturation, omega classification, and biological origin (see Sect. 2.2). In a single-center study by Qui et al., fat-modified enteral nutrition, including MCFAs, carnitine, and taurine, was found to have positive effects on feeding tolerance in critically ill patients. Specifically, the intervention group experienced a reduction in complications such as diarrhea, vomiting, and gastric retention by approximately 20% [71]. Similar results were obtained in a pilot trial by Tihista et al. [72]. As previously mentioned, omega-3 FAs have been shown to exert positive anti-inflammatory effects. These immunomodulatory properties were demonstrated in a perioperative cohort where patients were randomly assigned to receive either an enteral formula with arginine, omega-3 FAs, and nucleotides, a standard formula; or a low-fat/low-calorie intravenous solution. After analyzing the 31 study patients, those treated with the immunomodulating solution had lower C-reactive protein (CRP) and leukocytes level as weill as infection rate in surgical patients but not in ICU patients. However, no mortality effect for immunonutrition has been demonstrated, as Heyland et al. found no reduction in mortality with immunonutrition (RR, 1.10; 95% CI, 0.93–1.31).

The classification of immunonutrients encompasses a wide range of substances, beginning with arginine and ending with omega-3 FAs, which makes it difficult to differentiate them with clarity. In contrast to the reduced infection rate in all patients, the mortality was increased in the study cohorts with higher methodical standards (RR, 1.46; 95% CI, 1.01–2.11). These results raise questions regarding whether immunonutrients cause more harm [73]. Regarding the classification of omega FAs, the optimail ratio of omega-3 to omega-6 remains uncertain. The increasing amount of omega-6 FAs over the past century, due to dietary habits and industrial changes, has shifted omega-6 to omega-3 ratio in Western population from 1–2:1 to 20–30:1 [74]. Given this, a higher omega-6 to omega-3 FA ratio disrupts the balance of arachidonic acid (AA), thereby enhancing the production of AA-derived pro-inflammatory eicosanoids. In a small RCT involving 41 postoperative patients, three different nutrition formulas were tested for their effects on the immune response and inflammation. The study included a mixed immunonutrient formula with arginine, omega-3 FAs, and nucleotides (designated as "A", $n = 14$), a standard enteral formula (designated as "B", $n = 14$), and a low-calorie and low-fat IV solution (designated as "C", $n = 13$). The results indicated that enteral mixed immunonutrients were associated with a reduced number of leukocytes compared to both standard enteral and intravenous solutions. (A, 9.0 ± 2.9; B, 8.0 ± 2.4; C, $11.1 \pm 3.5 \times 106$ cells/mL; A versus C, B versus C; $p < 0.05$). The median CRP level was significantly lower in the immunonutrient (A) and enteral standard nutrition (B) groups (A, 80.4 [69.9] mg/L; B, 70 [74] mg/L; C, 88.5 [142] mg/L; A versus C, $p < 0.05$; B) [75].

In addition to omega-3 FAs, gamma-linolenic acid (GLA), an omega-6 derivative, can modulate cellular lipid composition, resulting in anti-inflammatory effects. In a RCT of patients with acute respiratory distress syndrome (ARDS), the use of fish oil eicosapentaenoic acid (EPA) and borage oil-derived GLA significantly reduced levels of the pro-inflammatory interleukin-8 (IL-8) in the bronchoalveolar lavage fluid [76]. However, a meta-analysis of eight studies cited in the ESPEN guideline, examining supplementation with EPA (with or without GLA), found no significant differences in mortality (RR 0.9, 95% CI [0.61–1.33]; $p = 0.6$), length of ICU stay (mean difference, -0.82; 95% CI [-7.73–1.08] $p = 0.4$), or length of ventilation (mean difference, -0.58; 95% [-3.71–2.56]; $p = 0.72$) [77, 78]. Due to these mixed findings, the current ESPEN guideline does not recommend routine use of high-dose omega-3 enriched formulas. However, they emphasize that omega-3-containing solutions may be used if they provide the recommended daily requirement of 500 mg EPA [78].

Structured lipids (SLs) have been developed for industrial production of improved fat molecules in enteral feeding solutions. Unlike natural triglycerides, which contain a random distribution of LCFAs and MCFAs based on their natural soureces, SLs are designed to position specific proportion of SCFAs, MCFAs, and LCFAs on a glycerol backbone through esterification. This rearrangement may lead to improved fat adsorption, FA profile, and pharmacological properties. Tso et al. compared the adsorption of fish oil–MCT structured lipids with that of a physical mixture of the same components in an animal model, evaluating how the different molecular arrangements on the glycerol backbone affected fat uptake. After inducing intestinal ischemia with temporary arterial clamping, lymph composition was analyzed. Rats fed SLs displayed significantly better fat adsorption than those fed a physical mixture of FAs [79]. In an early RCT by Kenler et al. in 1995, patients receiving fish oil-SLs experienced 31% fewer gastrointestinal complications, without adverse effects, compared with those receiving a standard solution lacking structured omega-3 FAs. Furthermore, the fish oil group showed a higher level of erythrocyte incorporation of omega-3 FAs after 7 days (%; standard vs. fish oil; 5.78 ± 0.66 vs. 8.64 ± 0.78; $p < 0.01$) and a significantly lower number of infections (5/18 vs. 1/17; $p = 0.090$). However, it should be noted that the standard enteral solution in this trial contained 16% less omega-3 FAs (1.54% vs. 17.68%) [80]. Encouraging results were also observed in a small RCT ($n = 20$) on postoperative patients by Swails et al. In this study, patients received either fish oil-SLs or a standard solution without SLs. On day 7, peripheral blood mononuclear cells (PBMC) were collected, and a radioimmune assay for eicosanoid products (prostaglandin E_2 [PGE_2], 6-keto $PGF_{1\alpha}$; and thromboxane B_2) was performed to determine prostaglandin concentrations in stimulated and unstimulated PBMCs. Apart from good tolerability and no significant side effects, the authors found a significant reduction in PGE_2 ($p < 0.03$) and 6–6-keto $PGF_{1\alpha}$ ($p < 0.01$) in patients receiving FOSL-HN [81].

The use of SLs enables the combination of SCFAs and LCFAs, thereby integrating their respective properties. In a mouse model, Yue et al. examined the effects of combined SLs on lipid distribution compared to high-fat-diet. Mice in the study were assigned to either a low- or high-fat diet, with the high-fat groups supplemented with 0% SLs, 10% SLs, or 50% SLs. After a 10-week feeding period, the authors reported an improvement in dyslipidemia in the high-fat group supplemented with 50% SLs. Additionally, increasing proprotions of SLs were associated with smaller lipid droplets in adipocytes. Beneficial effects were also observed on hepatic lipid accumulation, liver injury, and inflammation in obese mice [82]. In an early animal study, Swenson et al. fed two groups of rats either SLs or omega-6 FAs, including safflower oil, for 42 days. Following experimentally induced dorsal scald burns, the authors observed beneficial effects in the SL group, including reduced level of pro-inflammatory arachidonic acid metabolites and increased omega-3 FA levels [83].

SLs have several beneficial physicochemical properties compared to non-structured lipids. For instance, SLs have a reduced caloric value. Zhow et al. reported a 21.41% decrease in total calorie load ($p < 0.05$). The glycerol backbone of SL allows different FAs to be esterified at three distinct carbon atoms, resulting in four possible configurations: medium–long–medium (MLM), medium–medium–long (MML), long–medium–long (LML), and long–long–medium (LLM). According to a review of SLs by Lopes et al., the MLM configuration appears to be the most health-promoting among these arrangements [84].

MCTs are triglycerides composed of MCFAs esterified to a glycerol backbone. They are industrially produced and, like SCFAs, are rapidly and easily absorbed. Because they can be directly absorbed into the lymphatic system without prior enzymatic splitting. MCTs are commonly used in critical care for conditions involving intestinal fat malabsorption, such as chronic pancreatitis with pancreatic insufficiency, lymphatic drainage disorders, such as fistula and leaks, short bowel syndrome, and biliary atresia. Despite their reputation for promoting weight loss, robust scientific evidence is lacking and remains debated [85]. Some authors have suggested that MCTs may serve as a rapid source of energy [84, 85], but these claims have not been consistently confirmed. While several studies reported no benefit, a small RCT ($n = 19$) by Tsjui et al. found that a mixture of SLs with EPA and MCTs enhanced endurance in healthy volunteers compared to the group receiving the same components in physically mixed oil.

5.3 Special Cases in the ICU

5.3.1 Fat-Overload Syndrome

In light of the emergence of intravenous fat emulsions for nutritional purposes, case of fat overload syndrome have been documented, particularly in pediatric patients [86, 87]. This syndrome arises from the rapid infusion of soya-based or fish oil-containing solutions [88], leading to various symptoms that, in severe cases, result in multiorgan failure or even death. A group of researchers led by Hayes systematically reviewed different case reports and studies to identify adverse events associated with fat emulsions used for therapeutic or nutritional purposes. They identified 87 articles on human studies and grouped the key features of fat overload syndrome according to the affected organs. The researchers reported cardiovascular, respiratory, renal, neurological, pancreatic, allergic, and haemato-immunological side effects, as well as issues with medical devices, such as obstruction of the extracorporeal circuits. The qualitys of evidence from studies ranged from low to moderate, which may explain the variability in symptoms. For instance, cardiovascular manifestations included increased or decreased cardiac output, with different theories proposed to explain the underlying pathophysiology. In patients with ARDS, the findings ranged from elevated pulmonary resistance and cardiogenic output to reduced pulmonary and systemic vascular resistance. It has been hypothesized that metabolites of arachidonic acids, such as prostaglandins and thromboxanes, may contribute to ARDS by promoting thromboembolic and inflammatory events [89]. In addition to these pulmonary adverse events, liver failure with coagulopathy and impaired hepatic function has also been described. Studies have identified fat droplets not only in the liver but also in the brain, spleen, kidney, and lung [89, 90]. Neurological symptoms such as seizures may also occur [89]. Laboratory tests have revealed increased triglyceride levels and fat droplets in white blood cells [86] and platelets [91], which resolve once infusion is stopped. If discontinuation of the infusion is unsuccessful, plasmapheresis may be a potential treatment, as described in patients with hypertriglyceridemia-induced pancreatitis [92]. These findings suggest that the infusion rate should not exceed the daily dosage of >1.5 g/kg [93].

5.3.2 Carnitine Depletion

Carnitine plays a crucial role in transporting long-chain fatty acids across the mitochondrial membrane through esterification. In addition to enzyme deficiencies, severe malnourishment, and significant weight loss can lead to low carnitine levels. However, small prevalence studies in critically ill patients reported a carnitine deficiency rate of approximately 20% in this population [63, 94]. Several factors, such as unexplained hypertriglyceridemia, fatty liver, hyperlactatemia, severe cardiomyopathy, myopathy, or hyperammonemia in patients with risk factors, including chronic parenteral nutrition, renal replacement therapy, concurrent renal and hepatic insufficiency, and valproic acid use, can indicate carnitine deficiency. In such cases, carnitine supplementation can be considered after confirming the diagnosis through a complete laboratory carnitine assessment [62]. Although evidence of reduced inflammatory biomarkers [95] had suggested limited benefit, an RCT by Yahaypoor et al. investigated the effect of a 7-day supplementation of 3 g/day compared with placebo in ICU patients. In addition to a reduction in inflammatory biomarkers, this study also showed reduced 28-day mortality as a secondary outcome [96].

5.3.3 Lung Dysfunction—Acute Respiratory Distress Syndrome (ARDS)

The causes of ARDS can be classified as direct, such as pneumonia or trauma, or indirect, such as sepsis or pancreatitis. Additionally, lipid metabolites may influence ARDS pathology. In 1987, Deby-Dupont et al. discovered that an imbalance of thromboxane and prostacyclin exists in ARDS patients, implying that pro-inflammatory and thrombocyte-activating thromboxanes may play a crucial role in ARDS development [97]. Conversely, the omega-3 fatty acids (FAs) eicosapentaenoic acid (EPA) and doxosahexaenoic acid (DHA), with their anti-inflammatory properties, could benefit the adult ARDS population with respiratory distress. In a landmark study by Gadek et al. in 1999, the anti-inflammatory properties of EPA and gamma-linolenic acid (GLA) were investigated in ARDS patients. The authors examined the inhibitory effect of dihomo-gamma-linolenic acid (DGLA), a metabolic product of GLA, on thrombocyte aggregation [98] and oxygen radical release [99]. During the 4-year recruitment period, 146 ARDS patients were randomly assigned to receive an enteral formula enriched with EPA and GLA or a standard formula. The results showed a significantly decreased number of neutrophils in the bronchial alveolar lavage, improved oxygenation with a decreased need for mechanical ventilation, and reduced ICU days [100]. In the first meta-analysis in 2009, which included only three RCTs, the risk of mortality was reduced in patients who received omega-3 polyunsaturated fatty acids (PUFA) (odds ratio [OR] = 0.40; 95% confidence interval [CI] = 0.24–0.68; $p = 0.001$) [101]. However, subsequent RCTs did not demonstrate these positive effects [102, 103]. A possible explanation for these contradictory results could be the use of outdated, non-standard nutritional solutions. Li et al. conducted an updated meta-analysis that included six RCTs and did not show a reduced mortality risk (RR, 0.81; 95% CI, 0.50–1.31; $p = 0.38$; 6 trials, $n = 717$) [104]. In 2021, Singer and colleagues conducted an single-center RCT to examine the effects of omega-3 PUFA supplementation. After enrolling 128 mechanically ventilated patients, the authors did not find any significant improvement in blood oxygenation. However, patients receiving omega-3 FAs could were able to wean off catecholamines significantly earlier than controls [105]. The meta-analysis by Dushinanthan et al. detected a significantly improved PO_2/FiO_2 at day 4 (mean difference 38.88 mmHg; 95% CI [10.75, 67.02], $p = 0.01$) and day 7 (MD 23.44 mmHg; 95% CI [1.73, 45.15]; $p = 0.03$). However, due to the high heterogeneity among the included studies, the authors cautioned against overinterpreting this positive effect [106]. This uncertainty is also reflected in the guideline recommendations, where the widespread use of omega-3 enriched formula in patients with ARDS is not recommended by ASPEN [107] or ESPEN [78].

Furthermore, the use of lipid components may influence ARDS onset. In a prospective randomized crossover study, Suchner et al. demonstrated that the infusion rate of soybean-based fat emulsions modulates thromboxane production. This occurs because soybean-based fat emulsions contain a high proportion of linoleic acid, which increases arachidonic acids availability, leading to higher levels of thromboxane and prostacyclin. The authors investigated the effect of different infusion rates and found that elevated linoleic acid intake was associated with increased thromboxane production, particularly in patients with ARDS. As the lungs can directly absorb thromboxane, these findings underscore the importance of carefully administrating lipid emulsions [108]. Based on current evidence, international guidelines do not recommend omega-3-enriched formulas as the sole lipid source. However, formulas containing moderate amounts of omega-3-lipids at appropriate nutritional doses are considered acceptable [41].

5.3.4 Cardiovascular Dysfunction

Nutritional habits have a significant impact on the development of cardiovascular diseases, particularly coronary heart disease (CHD). Fish containing $n-3$-PUFAs have shown positive effects in this regard. $n-3$-PUFAs have been extensively studied for their beneficial effects on cardiovascular health. In a study by Burr et al., a 29% reduction in 2-year all-cause mortality was observed in 2,033 randomized men after myocardial infarcts through a specialized diet that included a reduction in fat intake, increased fatty fish consumption, and high-fiber products [109]. A recent meta-analysis of 47 studies with a total of approximately one million participants demonstrated that higher fish consumption was significantly associated with a lower incidence of CHD [RR: 0.91, 95% CI: 0.84, 0.97; I2 = 47.4%] and reduced mortality [RR: 0.85, 95% CI: 0.77, 0.94; I2 = 51.3%] [110]. However, the effect of $n-6$ PUFAs on cardiovascular diseases remains unclear. Ouchi et al. investigated the association of omega-6 PUFA with outcome parameters in a cohort of 417 patients with acute cardiovascular diseases treated in the ICU. In this study, the concentrations of dihomo-gamma-linolenic acid (DGLA), arachidonic acid (AA), and the DGLA/AA ratio were measured in blood samples. The authors observed higher levels of DGLA and AA in the survivor group. Additionally, DGLA and DGLA/ASS were associated with decreased mortality (DGLA: HR, 0.94; 95% CI, 0.89–0.99; $p = 0.03$; DGLA/AA: HR, 0.87; 95% CI, 0.78–0.98; $p = 0.02$) [111]. Despite the potential benefits of omega-3 fatty acids in preventing cardiovascular diseases, there is a lack of studies investigating their use in ICU patients. Consequently, recommendations for nutrition therapy in this special patient group are limited. At the same time, concerns have been raised about a possible increased risk of atrial fibrillation, prompting meta-analysis to assess the association between $n-3$ PUFA supplements, in the form of "fish oil," and atrial fibrillation. It is important to note that these omega-3 FAs in supplements are purified by synthesis in the ester form from fish oil [112]. In a meta-analysis conducted in 2021, seven RCTs with 81,210 patients revealed a higher risk of AF in those receiving fish oil supplements (HR 1.25, 95% CI 1.07–1.46; $p = 0.013$). This hazard ratio was even higher in trials providing a dosage >1 g/day (HR 1.49, 95% CI, 1.04–2.15; $p = 0.042$) than in those with a dosage <1 g/day (HR 1.12, 95% CI, 1.03–1.22; $p = 0.024$). In a subsequent meta-analysis by Lombardi et al., five RCTs were analyzed again showing an increased risk of AF in patients receiving $n - 3$ PUFA supplements [IRR 1.37, 95% CI 1.22–1.54; $p < 0.001$] [113]. Comparable findings have recently been reported in meta-analyses, including the five latest large RCTs on $n - 3$ PUFA fish oil supplements. According to these studies fish oil supplementation can, on the one hand, significantly reduce the risk of myocardial infarction (RR 0.85, 95% CI 0.72–0.99; $p = 0.04$), but on the other hand, is associated with an increased risk for AF (RR 1.32, 95% CI 1.11–1.58; $p = 0.002$) [114]. Based on these findings, the Pharmacovigilance Risk Assessment Committee (PRAC) of the European Medicines Agency (EMA) announced in September 2023 that the increased risk of AF is a potential side effect of omega-3 PUFA supplements, with the highest risk occurring when the dosage exceeds 4 g/day [115]. However, it should be noted that in these studies the omega-3 FAs were given in the form of fish oil-synthesized ethyl esters, and not in the natural triglyceride form of fish oil. In ICUS, fish oil is typically administered intravenously or enteraly. Therefore, the EMA safety warning initially applies only to supplements containing ethyl ester omega-3 FAs. Further investigations into the effects of fish oil are still required.

5.3.5 Brain Dysfunction—Delirium

The brain can be affected in the ICU in various ways. Direct damage to brain tissue may occur, for example through stroke and traumatic injury. Additionally, indirect damage can result from metabolic or inflammatory disturbances. The role of FAs in these pathologies is multifaceted.

The primary causes of direct cell damage are ischemia and reperfusion, which occur after an interruption in blood supply. This leads to the activation of death signals such as necrosis, necroptosis, apoptosis, and autophagy, which interact with each other. Apoptosis can be divided into two pathways, extrinsic and intrinsic. In the extrinsic pathway, activated "death" receptors activate proteases and subsequent cell protein proteolysis. In contrast, the intrinsic pathway is activated by cytotoxic stimuli, leading to the insertion of pro-death proteins into the outer mitochondrial membrane, causing the it to become permeable [116]. Here, the potential beneficial effects of omega-3 FAs have been investigated in several animal models. King et al. demonstrated a neuroprotective effect in traumatic brain injury in rats. After applying a bolus of DHA 30 min after injury, a reduction in apoptosis, and consequently, in the loss of oligodendrocytes, was obeserved [117]. Other animal studies have demonstrated similar neuroprotective effects though the modulation of autophagy [118].

In addition to cell death that occurs following ischemic circumstances, poorly defined structural alterations, such as delirium an acute and fluctuating brain dysfunction, are highly prevalent in ICUs and are associated with poor outcomes [119, 120]. Mouse models have demonstrated that nutritional factors may play a crucial role in the pathology of delirium. Farr et al. showed in their animal model that leptin, produced by adipose tissue, improved cognitive function [121]. However, hypertriglyceridemia is associated with cognitive impairment in mice and this negative effect can be reversed by gemfibrozil [122]. High triglyceride levels inhibit leptin transport across the blood-brain barrier and impair brain function [123]. There is a possible association between hypertriglyceridemia and cognitive function in humans [124], and patients with hypertriglyceridemia display a decline in memory function over 10 years [125]. Based on this evidence, an RCT was conducted to investigate the nutritional effects on delirium in the ICU setting. Naghibi et al. conducted a trial with 161 mechanically ventilated ICU patients, showing a significantly decreased number of delirium episodes by approximately 2 days (2.71 ± 2.01 days; mean $\pm$ SD) in the cohort receiving 2 g of omega-FAs syrup compared to the placebo group (4.72 ± 2.19 days; mean $\pm$ SD; $p = 0.032$) [126]. However, due to an insufficient description of the study cohorts and the small sample size, these optimistic results should be interpreted with caution. There is currently a lack of evidence concerning delirium and additional supplementation with omega-3 fatty acids. In contrast, in a RCT by Burkhart et al., 50 patients were randomized to receive either a parenteral omega 3-FAs or placebo. In addition to non-significant findings in inflammatory markers, no significant difference in septic encephalopathy was found between the two groups [127]. For patients who have experienced a stroke, the available evidence does not allow for the determination of the superior effectiveness of any treatment. A meta-analysis of both prospective cohort studies and RCTs has produced inconclusive results. While prospective cohorts indicated a modest-to-moderate risk reduction for cerebrovascular diseases, RCTs were unable to confirm these findings due to design limitation [128].

5.3.6 Sepsis

Since the Third International Consensus Conference in 2016, definitions of sepsis and septic shock have undergone further refinement. To diagnose sepsis, it is essential to differentiate between sepsis and simple infection by identifying organ dysfunction resulting from a systemic infection [129]. Sepsis is a complex syndrome involving various contributing factors that can lead to organ failure. The inflammatory stress response triggers the breakdown of lipid stores for glucose production (Wischmeyer). Although certain FAs have a specific effects on the immune system, the overall scientific picture of this issue remains inconsistent. In an RCT involving 165 patients with severe sepsis and septic shock in Brazil, Pontes-Arruda et al. demonstrated that enteral nutrition with EPA, GLA, and other antioxidants resulted in a 19.4% reduction in mortality and improved oxygenation [130]. Despite this positive example, the current sepsis guideline from the Surviving Sepsis Campaign does not recommend a special lipid-modified therapy. However, evidence from a meta-analysis showed a reduced infection risk and shorter length of stay with the application of fish oil-containing parenteral solutions. According to the ASPEN and ESPEN guidelines, these solutions can be prescribed to critically ill patients, including those with sepsis [78, 107].

Key Messages

- Dyslipidemia, including hypercholesterolemia and hypertriglyceridemia, is common in ICU patients and is associated with critical illness requiring intensive care.
- Acute critical illnesses disrupt fat metabolism, alter lipid components and pathways, and thereby affect outcomes through the inflammatory response.
- Parenteral and enteral nutrition solutions containing fats are essential in ICU nutrient therapy. The optimal fatty acid composition remains debated. Fat-modified enteral solutions may improve feeding tolerance and reduce complications. While omega-3 fatty acids show anti-inflammatory potential, their effect on mortality remains uncertain.
- Fat overload syndrome from intravenous fat emulsions can lead to multiorgan failure, underscoring the importance of cautious administration.
- Omega-3 fatty acids may exert neuroprotective effects, but their role in delirium and cognitive function is inconclusive.
- Due to the anti-inflammatory properties of omega-3 fatty acids, fish oil-containing solutions can be used, provided that recommended daily dosages are carefully observed.

References

1. Iqbal J, Hussain MM. Intestinal lipid absorption. Am J Physiol Endocrinol Metab. 2009;296:E1183–94.
2. Bell SJ, Bradley D, Forse RA, Bistrian BR. The new dietary fats in health and disease. J Am Diet Assoc. 1997;97:280–6; quiz 287–8
3. St-Onge MP, Jones PJ. Physiological effects of medium-chain triglycerides: potential agents in the prevention of obesity. J Nutr. 2002;132(3):329–32. https://doi.org/10.1093/jn/132.3.329. PMID: 11880549
4. Koruda MJ, Rolandelli RH, Settle RG, Saul SH, Rombeau JL. Harry M. Vars award. The effect of a pectin-supplemented elemental diet on intestinal adaptation to massive small bowel resection. JPEN J Parenter Enteral Nutr. 1986;10:343–50.
5. Azam S, Haque ME, Balakrishnan R, Kim IS, Choi DK. The ageing brain: molecular and cellular basis of neurodegeneration. Front Cell Dev Biol. 2021;9:683459.
6. Panickar KS, Bhathena SJ. Control of fatty acid intake and the role of essential fatty acids in cognitive function and neurological disorders. In: Montmayeur JP, Le Coutre J, editors. Fat detection: taste, texture, and post ingestive effects. Boca Raton: CRC/Tayor & Francis; 2010.
7. Li X, Liu Q, Pan Y, Chen S, Zhao Y, Hu Y. New insights into the role of dietary triglyceride absorption in obesity and metabolic diseases. Front Pharmacol. 2023;14:1097835.
8. Guyton AC, Hall JE. Medical physiology. Gökhan N, Çavuşoğlu H (Çeviren). 2006;3.
9. Raghu P. Functional diversity in a lipidome. Proc Natl Acad Sci USA. 2020;117:11191–3.
10. Stellaard F. From dietary cholesterol to blood cholesterol, physiological lipid fluxes, and cholesterol homeostasis. Nutrients. 2022;14:1643.

11. Jacenik D, Bagues A, Lopez-Gomez L, Lopez-Tofino Y, Iriondo-Dehond A, Serra C, Banovcanova L, Galvez-Robleno C, Fichna J, Del Castillo MD, Uranga JA, Abalo R. Changes in fatty acid dietary profile affect the brain-gut axis functions of healthy young adult rats in a sex-dependent manner. Nutrients. 2021;13(6):1864.
12. Yoon H, Shaw JL, Haigis MC, Greka A. Lipid metabolism in sickness and in health: emerging regulators of lipotoxicity. Mol Cell. 2021;81:3708–30. https://doi.org/10.1016/j.molcel.2021.08.027. PMID: 34547235; PMCID: PMC8620413.
13. Rodriguez-Carrio J, Salazar N, Margolles A, Gonzalez S, Gueimonde M, De Los Reyes-Gavilan CG, Suarez A. Free fatty acids profiles are related to gut microbiota signatures and short-chain fatty acids. Front Immunol. 2017;8:823.
14. Musunuru K, Kathiresan S. Genetics of common, complex coronary artery disease. Cell. 2019;177:132–45.
15. Beloribi-Djefaflia S, Vasseur S, Guillaumond F. Lipid metabolic reprogramming in cancer cells. Oncogene. 2016;5:e189.
16. Lytrivi M, Castell AL, Poitout V, Cnop M. Recent insights into mechanisms of beta-cell lipo- and glucolipotoxicity in type 2 diabetes. J Mol Biol. 2020;432:1514–34.
17. Tapiero H, Ba GN, Couvreur P, Tew KD. Polyunsaturated fatty acids (PUFA) and eicosanoids in human health and pathologies. Biomed Pharmacother. 2002;56:215–22.
18. Tvrzicka E, Kremmyda LS, Stankova B, Zak A. Fatty acids as biocompounds: their role in human metabolism, health and disease – a review. Part 1: classification, dietary sources and biological functions. Biomed Pap Med Fac Univ Palacky Olomouc Czech Repub. 2011;155:117–30.
19. Arterburn LM, Hall EB, Oken H. Distribution, interconversion, and dose response of n-3 fatty acids in humans. Am J Clin Nutr. 2006;83:1467S–76S.
20. Saini RK, Keum YS. Omega-3 and omega-6 polyunsaturated fatty acids: dietary sources, metabolism, and significance – a review. Life Sci. 2018;203:255–67. https://doi.org/10.1016/j.lfs.2018.04.049. Epub 2018 Apr 30. PMID: 29715470.
21. Calder PC. Eicosanoids. Essays Biochem. 2020;64:423–41. https://doi.org/10.1042/EBC20190083. PMID: 32808658.
22. Calder PC. n-3 PUFA and inflammation: from membrane to nucleus and from bench to bedside. Proc Nutr Soc. 2020;79(4):404–16.
23. Schmitz G, Ecker J. The opposing effects of n-3 and n-6 fatty acids. Prog Lipid Res. 2008;47:147–55.
24. Arnold DR, Kwiterovich PO. Cholesterol | absorption, function, and metabolism. In: Caballero B, editor. Encyclopedia of food sciences and nutrition. 2nd ed. Oxford: Academic Press; 2003.
25. Arnold DR, Kwiterovich PO. CHOLESTEROL | absorption, function, and metabolism. In: Caballero B, editor. Encyclopedia of food sciences and nutrition. 2nd ed. Oxford: Academic Press; 2003. p. 1226–37.
26. van Heek M, Farley C, Compton DS, Hoos L, Alton KB, Sybertz EJ, Davis HR Jr. Comparison of the activity and disposition of the novel cholesterol absorption inhibitor, SCH58235, and its glucuronide, SCH60663. Br J Pharmacol. 2000;129:1748–54.
27. Pan XF, Yang JJ, Lipworth LP, Shu XO, Cai H, Steinwandel MD, Blot WJ, Zheng W, Yu D. Cholesterol and egg intakes with cardiometabolic and all-cause mortality among Chinese and low-income Black and White Americans. Nutrients. 2021;13(6):2094.
28. Feingold KR. Introduction to lipids and lipoproteins. South Dartmouth: MDText.com, Inc.; 2000.
29. Lutjohann D, Meyer S, von Bergmann K, Stellaard F. Cholesterol absorption and synthesis in vegetarians and omnivores. Mol Nutr Food Res. 2018;62:e1700689.
30. Cohn JS, Kamili A, Wat E, Chung RW, Tandy S. Dietary phospholipids and intestinal cholesterol absorption. Nutrients. 2010;2:116–27.
31. Torres Garcia J, Duran Aguero S. Phospholipids: properties and health effects. Nutr Hosp. 2014;31:76–83.

32. Feingold KR, Grunfeld C. Lipids: a key player in the battle between the host and microorganisms. J Lipid Res. 2012;53:2487–9.
33. Cox RA, García-Palmieri M. Chapter 31 Cholesterol, triglycerides, and associated lipoproteins. In: Walker HK, Dallas Hall W, Hurst JW, editors. Clinical methods: the history, physical, and laboratory examinations. 3rd ed. Boston: Butterworths; 1990.
34. Birari RB, Bhutani KK. Pancreatic lipase inhibitors from natural sources: unexplored potential. Drug Discov Today. 2007;12:879–89.
35. Buchholz T, Melzig MF. Polyphenolic compounds as pancreatic lipase inhibitors. Planta Med. 2015;81:771–83.
36. Mansbach CM 2nd, Siddiqi S. Control of chylomicron export from the intestine. Am J Physiol Gastrointest Liver Physiol. 2016;310:G659–68.
37. Zembroski AS, Xiao C, Buhman KK. The roles of cytoplasmic lipid droplets in modulating intestinal uptake of dietary fat. Annu Rev Nutr. 2021;41:79–104.
38. Alves-Bezerra M, Cohen DE. Triglyceride metabolism in the liver. Compr Physiol. 2017;8:1–8.
39. Bier DM, Brosnan JT, Flatt JP, Hanson RW, Heird W, Hellerstein MK, Jequier E, Kalhan S, Koletzko B, Macdonald I, Owen O, Uauy R. Report of the IDECG Working Group on lower and upper limits of carbohydrate and fat intake. International Dietary Energy Consultative Group. Eur J Clin Nutr. 1999;53 Suppl 1:S177–8.
40. Hodson L, McQuaid SE, Karpe F, Frayn KN, Fielding BA. Differences in partitioning of meal fatty acids into blood lipid fractions: a comparison of linoleate, oleate, and palmitate. Am J Physiol Endocrinol Metab. 2009;296:E64–71.
41. Singer P, Blaser AR, Berger MM, Calder PC, Casaer M, Hiesmayr M, Mayer K, Montejo-Gonzalez JC, Pichard C, Preiser JC, Szczeklik W, van Zanten ARH, Bischoff SC. ESPEN practical and partially revised guideline: clinical nutrition in the intensive care unit. Clin Nutr. 2023;42:1671–89.
42. Karamanlis A, Chaikomin R, Doran S, Bellon M, Bartholomeusz FD, Wishart JM, Jones KL, Horowitz M, Rayner CK. Effects of protein on glycemic and incretin responses and gastric emptying after oral glucose in healthy subjects. Am J Clin Nutr. 2007;86:1364–8.
43. Stamler J, Wentworth D, Neaton JD. Is relationship between serum cholesterol and risk of premature death from coronary heart disease continuous and graded? Findings in 356,222 primary screenees of the Multiple Risk Factor Intervention Trial (MRFIT). JAMA. 1986;256:2823–8.
44. Ference BA, Ginsberg HN, Graham I, Ray KK, Packard CJ, Bruckert E, Hegele RA, Krauss RM, Raal FJ, Schunkert H, Watts GF, Borén J, Fazio S, Horton JD, Masana L, Nicholls SJ, Nordestgaard BG, van de Sluis B, Taskinen MR, Tokgözoglu L, Landmesser U, Laufs U, Wiklund O, Stock JK, Chapman MJ, Catapano AL. Low-density lipoproteins cause atherosclerotic cardiovascular disease. 1. Evidence from genetic, epidemiologic, and clinical studies. A consensus statement from the European Atherosclerosis Society Consensus Panel. Eur Heart J. 2017;38:2459–72.
45. Khovidhunkit W, Kim MS, Memon RA, Shigenaga JK, Moser AH, Feingold KR, Grunfeld C. Effects of infection and inflammation on lipid and lipoprotein metabolism: mechanisms and consequences to the host. J Lipid Res. 2004;45:1169–96.
46. Wendel M, Paul R, Heller AR. Lipoproteins in inflammation and sepsis. II Clinical aspects. Intensive Care Med. 2007;33:25–35.
47. Kitchens RL, Thompson PA, Munford RS, O'Keefe GE. Acute inflammation and infection maintain circulating phospholipid levels and enhance lipopolysaccharide binding to plasma lipoproteins. J Lipid Res. 2003;44:2339–48.
48. Hofmaenner DA, Arina P, Kleyman A, Page Black L, Salomao R, Tanaka S, Guirgis FW, Arulkumaran N, Singer M. Association between hypocholesterolemia and mortality in critically ill patients with sepsis: a systematic review and meta-analysis. Crit Care Explor. 2023;5:e0860.
49. Sammalkorpi K, Valtonen V, Kerttula Y, Nikkilä E, Taskinen MR. Changes in serum lipoprotein pattern induced by acute infections. Metabolism. 1988;37:859–65.

50. Zinellu A, Paliogiannis P, Fois AG, Solidoro P, Carru C, Mangoni AA. Cholesterol and triglyceride concentrations, COVID-19 severity, and mortality: a systematic review and meta-analysis with meta-regression. Front Public Health. 2021;9:705916.
51. Sarkar M, Mookerjea S. Differential effect of inflammation and dexamethasone on dolichol and dolichol phosphate synthesis. Biochem Cell Biol. 1988;66:1265–9.
52. Feingold KR, Spady DK, Pollock AS, Moser AH, Grunfeld C. Endotoxin, TNF, and IL-1 decrease cholesterol 7 alpha-hydroxylase mRNA levels and activity. J Lipid Res. 1996;37:223–8.
53. Mujawar Z, Rose H, Morrow MP, Pushkarsky T, Dubrovsky L, Mukhamedova N, Fu Y, Dart A, Orenstein JM, Bobryshev YV, Bukrinsky M, Sviridov D. Human immunodeficiency virus impairs reverse cholesterol transport from macrophages. PLoS Biol. 2006;4:e365.
54. Qin C, Minghan H, Ziwen Z, Yukun L. Alteration of lipid profile and value of lipids in the prediction of the length of hospital stay in COVID-19 pneumonia patients. Food Sci Nutr. 2020;8:6144–52.
55. Pajkrt D, Doran JE, Koster F, Lerch PG, Arnet B, van der Poll T, Ten Cate JW, van Deventer SJ. Antiinflammatory effects of reconstituted high-density lipoprotein during human endotoxemia. J Exp Med. 1996;184:1601–8.
56. Levels JH, Abraham PR, van Barreveld EP, Meijers JC, van Deventer SJ. Distribution and kinetics of lipoprotein-bound lipoteichoic acid. Infect Immun. 2003;71:3280–4.
57. Tanaka S, Couret D, Tran-Dinh A, Duranteau J, Montravers P, Schwendeman A, Meilhac O. High-density lipoproteins during sepsis: from bench to bedside. Crit Care. 2020;24:134.
58. Wanten GJ, Calder PC. Immune modulation by parenteral lipid emulsions. Am J Clin Nutr. 2007;85:1171–84.
59. Gutiérrez S, Svahn SL, Johansson ME. Effects of omega-3 fatty acids on immune cells. Int J Mol Sci. 2019;20(20):5028.
60. Pradelli L, Mayer K, Klek S, Omar Alsaleh AJ, Clark RA, Rosenthal MD, Heller AR, Muscaritoli M. ω-3 fatty-acid enriched parenteral nutrition in hospitalized patients: systematic review with meta-analysis and trial sequential analysis. J Parenter Enter Nutr. 2020;44:44–57.
61. Notz Q, Lee ZY, Menger J, Elke G, Hill A, Kranke P, Roeder D, Lotz C, Meybohm P, Heyland DK, Stoppe C. Omega-6 sparing effects of parenteral lipid emulsions-an updated systematic review and meta-analysis on clinical outcomes in critically ill patients. Crit Care. 2022;26:23.
62. Bonafé L, Berger MM, Que YA, Mechanick JI. Carnitine deficiency in chronic critical illness. Curr Opin Clin Nutr Metab Care. 2014;17:200–9.
63. Oami T, Oshima T, Hattori N, Teratani A, Honda S, Yoshida T, Oda S. L-carnitine in critically ill patients—a case series study. Renal Replace Ther. 2018;4:1–8.
64. Gogos CA, Kalfarentzos FE, Zoumbos NC. Effect of different types of total parenteral nutrition on T-lymphocyte subpopulations and NK cells. Am J Clin Nutr. 1990;51:119–22.
65. Sedman PC, Somers SS, Ramsden CW, Brennan TG, Guillou PJ. Effects of different lipid emulsions on lymphocyte function during total parenteral nutrition. Br J Surg. 1991;78:1396–9.
66. Pradelli L, Eandi M, Povero M, Mayer K, Muscaritoli M, Heller AR, Fries-Schaffner E. Cost-effectiveness of omega-3 fatty acid supplements in parenteral nutrition therapy in hospitals: a discrete event simulation model. Clin Nutr. 2014;33:785–92.
67. Sandström R, Hyltander A, Körner U, Lundholm K. Structured triglycerides to postoperative patients: a safety and tolerance study. JPEN J Parenter Enteral Nutr. 1993;17:153–7.
68. Sandström R, Hyltander A, Körner U, Lundholm K. Structured triglycerides were well tolerated and induced increased whole body fat oxidation compared with long-chain triglycerides in postoperative patients. JPEN J Parenter Enteral Nutr. 1995;19:381–6.
69. Calder PC, Adolph M, Deutz NE, Grau T, Innes JK, Klek S, Lev S, Mayer K, Michael-Titus AT, Pradelli L, Puder M, Vlaardingerbroek H, Singer P. Lipids in the intensive care unit: recommendations from the ESPEN Expert Group. Clin Nutr. 2018;37:1–18.
70. Ali Abdelhamid Y, Cousins CE, Sim JA, Bellon MS, Nguyen NQ, Horowitz M, Chapman MJ, Deane AM. Effect of critical illness on triglyceride absorption. JPEN J Parenter Enteral Nutr. 2015;39:966–72.

71. Qiu C, Chen C, Zhang W, Kou Q, Wu S, Zhou L, Liu J, Ma G, Chen J, Chen M, Luo H, Zhang X, Lai J, Yu Z, Yu X, Liao W, Guan X, Ouyang B. Fat-modified enteral formula improves feeding tolerance in critically ill patients: a multicenter, single-blind, randomized controlled trial. JPEN J Parenter Enteral Nutr. 2017;41:785–95.
72. Tihista S, Echavarria E. Effect of omega 3 polyunsaturated fatty acids derived from fish oil in major burn patients: a prospective randomized controlled pilot trial. Clin Nutr. 2018;37:107–12.
73. Heyland DK, Novak F, Drover JW, Jain M, Su X, Suchner U. Should immunonutrition become routine in critically ill patients? A systematic review of the evidence. JAMA. 2001;286:944–53.
74. Simopoulos AP. Essential fatty acids in health and chronic disease. Am J Clin Nutr. 1999;70:560S–9S.
75. Schilling J, Vranjes N, Fierz W, Joller H, Gyurech D, Ludwig E, Marathias K, Geroulanos S. Clinical outcome and immunology of postoperative arginine, omega-3 fatty acids, and nucleotide-enriched enteral feeding: a randomized prospective comparison with standard enteral and low calorie/low fat i.v. solutions. Nutrition. 1996;12:423–9.
76. Pacht ER, Demichele SJ, Nelson JL, Hart J, Wennberg AK, Gadek JE. Enteral nutrition with eicosapentaenoic acid, gamma-linolenic acid, and antioxidants reduces alveolar inflammatory mediators and protein influx in patients with acute respiratory distress syndrome. Crit Care Med. 2003;31:491–500.
77. International Society for the Study of Fatty Acids and Lipids. Intake of PUFA in healthy adults [Online]. 2024. Available: https://www.issfal.org/statement-3. Accessed 27 Mar 2024.
78. Singer P, Blaser AR, Berger MM, Alhazzani W, Calder PC, Casaer MP, Hiesmayr M, Mayer K, Montejo JC, Pichard C, Preiser JC, van Zanten ARH, Oczkowski S, Szczeklik W, Bischoff SC. ESPEN guideline on clinical nutrition in the intensive care unit. Clin Nutr. 2019;38:48–79.
79. Tso P, Lee T, Demichele SJ. Lymphatic absorption of structured triglycerides vs. physical mix in a rat model of fat malabsorption. Am J Phys. 1999;277:G333–40.
80. Kenler AS, Swails WS, Driscoll DF, Demichele SJ, Daley B, Babineau TJ, Peterson MB, Bistrian BR. Early enteral feeding in postsurgical cancer patients. Fish oil structured lipid-based polymeric formula versus a standard polymeric formula. Ann Surg. 1996;223:316–33.
81. Swails WS, Kenler AS, Driscoll DF, Demichele SJ, Babineau TJ, Utsunamiya T, Chavali S, Forse RA, Bistrian BR. Effect of a fish oil structured lipid-based diet on prostaglandin release from mononuclear cells in cancer patients after surgery. JPEN J Parenter Enteral Nutr. 1997;21:266–74.
82. Yue C, Tang Y, Chang M, Wang Y, Peng H, Wang X, Wang Z, Zang X, Ben H, Yu G. Dietary supplementation with short- and long-chain structured lipids alleviates obesity via regulating hepatic lipid metabolism, inflammation and gut microbiota in high-fat-diet-induced obese mice. J Sci Food Agric. 2024;104(9):5089–103.
83. Swenson ES, Selleck KM, Babayan VK, Blackburn GL, Bistrian BR. Persistence of metabolic effects after long-term oral feeding of a structured triglyceride derived from medium-chain triglyceride and fish oil in burned and normal rats. Metabolism. 1991;40:484–90.
84. Lopes PA, Alfaia CM, Pestana JM, Prates JAM. Structured lipids engineering for health: novel formulations enriched in n-3 long-chain polyunsaturated fatty acids with potential nutritional benefits. Metabolites. 2023;13(10):1060.
85. Munroe C, Frantz D, Martindale RG, McClave SA. The optimal lipid formulation in enteral feeding in critical illness: clinical update and review of the literature. Curr Gastroenterol Rep. 2011;13:368–75.
86. Belin RP, Bivins BA, Jona JZ, Young VL. Fat overload with a 10% soybean oil emulsion. Arch Surg. 1976;111:1391–3.
87. Heyman MB, Storch S, Ament ME. The fat overload syndrome. Report of a case and literature review. Am J Dis Child. 1981;135:628–30.
88. Moon HJ, Hwang IW, Lee JW, Hong SY. A case of fat overload syndrome after rapid infusion of SMOFlipid emulsion in an adult. Am J Emerg Med. 2017;35:660.e3–4.

89. Hayes BD, Gosselin S, Calello DP, Nacca N, Rollins CJ, Abourbih D, Morris M, Nesbitt-Miller A, Morais JA, Lavergne V. Systematic review of clinical adverse events reported after acute intravenous lipid emulsion administration. Clin Toxicol (Phila). 2016;54:365–404.
90. Haber LM, Hawkins EP, Seilheimer DK, Saleem A. Fat overload syndrome. An autopsy study with evaluation of the coagulopathy. Am J Clin Pathol. 1988;90:223–7.
91. Campbell AN, Freedman MH, Pencharz PB, Zlotkin SH. Bleeding disorder from the "fat overload" syndrome. JPEN J Parenter Enteral Nutr. 1984;8:447–9.
92. Wu C, Xu T, Yi Z, Song N, Zhou Y, Liang F, Zhang B. Double filtration plasmapheresis for hypertriglyceridemic acute pancreatitis caused by fat overload syndrome. J Clin Pharm Ther. 2022;47:1885–7.
93. Singer P, Berger MM, van den Berghe G, Biolo G, Calder P, Forbes A, Griffiths R, Kreyman G, Leverve X, Pichard C, ESPEN. ESPEN guidelines on parenteral nutrition: intensive care. Clin Nutr. 2009;28:387–400.
94. Wennberg A, Hyltander A, Sjoberg A, Arfvidsson B, Sandstrom R, Wickstrom I, Lundholm K. Prevalence of carnitine depletion in critically ill patients with undernutrition. Metabolism. 1992;41:165–71.
95. Haghighatdoost F, Jabbari M, Hariri M. The effect of L-carnitine on inflammatory mediators: a systematic review and meta-analysis of randomized clinical trials. Eur J Clin Pharmacol. 2019;75:1037–46.
96. Yahyapoor F, Sedaghat A, Feizi A, Bagherniya M, Pahlavani N, Khadem-Rezaiyan M, Safarian M, Islam MS, Zarifi SH, Arabi SM, Norouzy A. The effects of l-Carnitine supplementation on inflammatory markers, clinical status, and 28 days mortality in critically ill patients: a double-blind, randomized, placebo-controlled trial. Clin Nutr ESPEN. 2022;49:61–7.
97. Deby-Dupont G, Braun M, Lamy M, Deby C, Pincemail J, Faymonville ME, Damas P, Bodson L, Lecart MP, Goutier R. Thromboxane and prostacyclin release in adult respiratory distress syndrome. Intensive Care Med. 1987;13:167–74.
98. Yeung J, Tourdot BE, Adili R, Green AR, Freedman CJ, Fernandez-Perez P, YU J, Holman TR, Holinstat M. 12(S)-HETrE, a 12-lipoxygenase oxylipin of dihomo-γ-linolenic acid, inhibits thrombosis via gαs signaling in platelets. Arterioscler Thromb Vasc Biol. 2016;36:2068–77.
99. Suzuki N, Sawada K, Takahashi I, Matsuda M, Fukui S, Tokuyasu H, Shimizu H, Yokoyama J, Akaike A, Nakaji S. Association between polyunsaturated fatty acid and reactive oxygen species production of neutrophils in the general population. Nutrients. 2020;12:3222.
100. Gadek JE, Demichele SJ, Karlstad MD, Pacht ER, Donahoe M, Albertson TE, Van Hoozen C, Wennberg AK, Nelson JL, Noursalehi M. Effect of enteral feeding with eicosapentaenoic acid, gamma-linolenic acid, and antioxidants in patients with acute respiratory distress syndrome. Enteral Nutrition in ARDS Study Group. Crit Care Med. 1999;27:1409–20.
101. Pontes-Arruda A, Demichele S, Seth A, Singer P. The use of an inflammation-modulating diet in patients with acute lung injury or acute respiratory distress syndrome: a meta-analysis of outcome data. JPEN J Parenter Enteral Nutr. 2008;32:596–605.
102. Kagan I, Cohen J, Stein M, Bendavid I, Pinsker D, Silva V, Theilla M, Anbar R, Lev S, Grinev M, Singer P. Preemptive enteral nutrition enriched with eicosapentaenoic acid, gamma-linolenic acid and antioxidants in severe multiple trauma: a prospective, randomized, double-blind study. Intensive Care Med. 2015;41:460–9.
103. Rice TW, Wheeler AP, Thompson BT, Deboisblanc BP, Steingrub J, Rock P, NIH NHLBI Acute Respiratory Distress Syndrome Network of Investigators. Enteral omega-3 fatty acid, gamma-linolenic acid, and antioxidant supplementation in acute lung injury. JAMA. 2011;306:1574–81.
104. Li C, Bo L, Liu W, Lu X, Jin F. Enteral immunomodulatory diet (Omega-3 fatty acid, gamma-linolenic acid and antioxidant supplementation) for acute lung injury and acute respiratory distress syndrome: an updated systematic review and meta-analysis. Nutrients. 2015;7:5572–85.

105. Singer P, Bendavid I, Mesilati-Stahy R, Green P, Rigler M, Lev S, Schif-Zuck S, Amiram A, Theilla M, Kagan I. Enteral and supplemental parenteral nutrition enriched with omega-3 polyunsaturated fatty acids in intensive care patients – a randomized, controlled, double-blind clinical trial. Clin Nutr. 2021;40:2544–54.
106. Dushianthan A, Cusack R, Burgess VA, Grocott MP, Calder PC. Immunonutrition for acute respiratory distress syndrome (ARDS) in adults. Cochrane Database Syst Rev. 2019;1:CD012041.
107. McClave SA, Taylor BE, Martindale RG, Warren MM, Johnson DR, Braunschweig C, McCarthy MS, Davanos E, Rice TW, Cresci GA, Gervasio JM, Sacks GS, Roberts PR, Compher C, Society of Critical Care Medicine & American Society for Parenteral and Enteral Nutrition. Guidelines for the provision and assessment of nutrition support therapy in the adult critically ill patient: Society of Critical Care Medicine (SCCM) and American Society for Parenteral and Enteral Nutrition (A.S.P.E.N.). JPEN J Parenter Enteral Nutr. 2016;40:159–211.
108. Suchner U, Katz DP, Furst P, Beck K, Felbinger TW, Thiel M, Senftleben U, Goetz AE, Peter K. Impact of sepsis, lung injury, and the role of lipid infusion on circulating prostacyclin and thromboxane A(2). Intensive Care Med. 2002;28:122–9.
109. Burr ML, Fehily AM, Gilbert JF, Rogers S, Holliday RM, Sweetnam PM, Elwood PC, Deadman NM. Effects of changes in fat, fish, and fibre intakes on death and myocardial reinfarction: diet and reinfarction trial (DART). Lancet. 1989;2:757–61.
110. Zhang B, Xiong K, Cai J, Ma A. Fish consumption and coronary heart disease: a meta-analysis. Nutrients. 2020;12(8):2278.
111. Ouchi S, Miyazaki T, Shimada K, Sugita Y, Shimizu M, Murata A, Kato T, Aikawa T, Suda S, Shiozawa T, Hiki M, Takahashi S, Kasai T, Miyauchi K, Daida H. Decreased circulating dihomo-gamma-linolenic acid levels are associated with total mortality in patients with acute cardiovascular disease and acute decompensated heart failure. Lipids Health Dis. 2017;16:150.
112. Bays H. Rationale for prescription omega-3-acid ethyl ester therapy for hypertriglyceridemia: a primer for clinicians. Drugs Today (Barc). 2008;44:205–46.
113. Lombardi M, Carbone S, Del Buono MG, Chiabrando JG, Vescovo GM, Camilli M, Montone RA, Vergallo R, Abbate A, Biondi-Zoccai G, Dixon DL, Crea F. Omega-3 fatty acids supplementation and risk of atrial fibrillation: an updated meta-analysis of randomized controlled trials. Eur Heart J Cardiovasc Pharmacother. 2021;7:e69–70.
114. Yan J, Liu M, Yang D, Zhang Y, An F. The most important safety risk of fish oil from the latest meta-analysis? Eur J Prev Cardiol. 2022;29:zwac056.186.
115. Pharmacovigilance Risk Assessment Committee (PRAC) of the European Medicines Agency (EMA). Meeting highlights from the Pharmacovigilance Risk Assessment Committee (PRAC) 25–28 September 2023 [Online]. 2023. Available: https://www.ema.europa.eu/en/news/meeting-highlights-pharmacovigilance-risk-assessment-committee-prac-25-28-september-2023. Accessed 19 May 2024.
116. Kalogeris T, Baines CP, Krenz M, Korthuis RJ. Cell biology of ischemia/reperfusion injury. Int Rev Cell Mol Biol. 2012;298:229–317.
117. King VR, Huang WL, Dyall SC, Curran OE, Priestley JV, Michael-Titus AT. Omega-3 fatty acids improve recovery, whereas omega-6 fatty acids worsen outcome, after spinal cord injury in the adult rat. J Neurosci. 2006;26:4672–80.
118. Zirpoli H, Chang CL, Carpentier YA, Michael-Titus AT, Ten VS, Deckelbaum RJ. Novel approaches for omega-3 fatty acid therapeutics: chronic versus acute administration to protect heart, brain, and spinal cord. Annu Rev Nutr. 2020;40:161–87.
119. Gleason LJ, Schmitt EM, Kosar CM, Tabloski P, Saczynski JS, Robinson T, Cooper Z, Rogers SO Jr, Jones RN, Marcantonio ER, Inouye SK. Effect of delirium and other major complications on outcomes after elective surgery in older adults. JAMA Surg. 2015;150:1134–40.
120. Pun BT, Badenes R, Heras La Calle G, Orun OM, Chen W, Raman R, Simpson BK, Wilson-Linville S, Hinojal Olmedillo B, Vallejo de la Cueva A, van der Jagt M, Navarro Casado R, Leal Sanz P, Orhun G, Ferrer Gomez C, Nunez Vazquez K, Pineiro Otero P, Taccone FS,

Gallego Curto E, Caricato A, Woien H, Lacave G, O'Neal HR Jr, Peterson SJ, Brummel NE, Girard TD, Ely EW, Pandharipande PP, COVID-19 Intensive Care International Study Group. Prevalence and risk factors for delirium in critically ill patients with COVID-19 (COVID-D): a multicentre cohort study. Lancet Respir Med. 2021;9:239–50.
121. Farr SA, Banks WA, Morley JE. Effects of leptin on memory processing. Peptides. 2006;27:1420–5.
122. Farr SA, Yamada KA, Butterfield DA, Abdul HM, XU L, Miller NE, Banks WA, Morley JE. Obesity and hypertriglyceridemia produce cognitive impairment. Endocrinology. 2008;149:2628–36.
123. Banks WA, Farr SA, Morley JE. The effects of high fat diets on the blood-brain barrier transport of leptin: failure or adaptation? Physiol Behav. 2006;88:244–8.
124. Sims RC, Madhere S, Gordon S, Clark E Jr, Abayomi KA, Callender CO, Campbell AL Jr. Relationships among blood pressure, triglycerides and verbal learning in African Americans. J Natl Med Assoc. 2008;100:1193–8.
125. De Frias CM, Bunce D, Wahlin A, Adolfsson R, Sleegers K, Cruts M, Van Broeckhoven C, Nilsson LG. Cholesterol and triglycerides moderate the effect of apolipoprotein E on memory functioning in older adults. J Gerontol B Psychol Sci Soc Sci. 2007;62:P112–8.
126. Naghibi T, Shafigh N, Mazloomzadeh S. Role of omega-3 fatty acids in the prevention of delirium in mechanically ventilated patients. J Res Med Sci. 2020;25:10.
127. Burkhart CS, Dell-Kuster S, Siegemund M, Pargger H, Marsch S, Strebel SP, Steiner LA. Effect of n-3 fatty acids on markers of brain injury and incidence of sepsis-associated delirium in septic patients. Acta Anaesthesiol Scand. 2014;58:689–700.
128. Chowdhury R, Stevens S, Gorman D, Pan A, Warnakula S, Chowdhury S, Ward H, Johnson L, Crowe F, Hu FB, Franco OH. Association between fish consumption, long chain omega 3 fatty acids, and risk of cerebrovascular disease: systematic review and meta-analysis. BMJ. 2012;345:e6698.
129. Singer M, Deutschman CS, Seymour CW, Shankar-Hari M, Annane D, Bauer M, Bellomo R, Bernard GR, Chiche J-D, Coopersmith CM, Hotchkiss RS, Levy MM, Marshall JC, Martin GS, Opal SM, Rubenfeld GD, van der Poll T, Vincent J-L, Angus DC. The third international consensus definitions for sepsis and septic shock (sepsis-3). JAMA. 2016;315:801.
130. Pontes-Arruda A, Aragao AM, Albuquerque JD. Effects of enteral feeding with eicosapentaenoic acid, gamma-linolenic acid, and antioxidants in mechanically ventilated patients with severe sepsis and septic shock. Crit Care Med. 2006;34:2325–33.

Part II
Clinical Application

Nutritional Adjustment

Thomas W. Felbinger, Konstantin Mayer, and Andreas Rümelin

During the early post-traumatic phase or in the early phase after ICU admission, it is of utmost importance to avoid overfeeding as hyperalimentation is associated with worsened outcome [1–3]. Overfeeding increases hyperglycemia, hyperlipidemia, and hypercarbia which may lead to liver dysfunction, electrolyte disturbances, and immune dysfunction. The so-called full energy- and protein-goal of nutritional therapy in critically ill patients should only be reached after about 1 week after admission to the ICU. For many critically ill patients, the goal of 70% of protein and energy goal during the first week in the ICU is sufficient.

On the other side, providing no or insufficient nutrients in the metabolic stable patients also must be avoided for the long-term ICU patient as prolonged energy deficit also might be associated with negative effects. Prolonged weaning from the ventilator, prolonged immobilization, and longer stay in the ICU and the hospital might be the negative consequences of prolonged energy deficit in the metabolically stable long-term ICU patient. An inadequate supply of nutrients exacerbates an already catabolic metabolic state. Nutrient deficiencies that accumulate over the course of days represent an independent parameter for worsened outcome [4, 5].

T. W. Felbinger
Department of Anesthesiology, Perioperative and Pain Medicine, Harlaching and Neuperlach Medical Centers, The Munich Municipal Hospitals Group Ltd, München, Germany
e-mail: thomas.felbinger@muenchen-klinik.de

K. Mayer (✉)
Department of Pneumology, Infectiology, and Sleep Medicine, ViDia Hospitals, Karlsruhe, Germany

Faculty of Medicine, University of Giessen, Giessen, Germany
e-mail: pneumologie@vincentius-ka.de

A. Rümelin
Department of Anesthesiology, Hospital "Land Hadeln", Otterndorf, Germany

© The Author(s), under exclusive license to Springer Nature Switzerland AG 2025
A. Rümelin et al. (eds.), *Nutrition in ICU Patients*,
https://doi.org/10.1007/978-3-032-00818-3_6

Because of the heterogeneity of the critically ill patients in our ICUs, no convincing study has demonstrated a single superior strategy for nutritional adjustment that fits all patient subpopulations for improving patients' outcome. Therefore, an ideal strategy for the nutritional adjustment depends on the metabolic condition of the treated patients.

In relatively stable conditions, a straightforward adjustment of calories and protein as recommended by the DGEM (German Society for Nutritional Medicine) might be preferable (see Fig. 6.1). In those patients, the caloric and protein goal may be reached within few days.

For more metabolically compromised patients, a slower increase in calories and protein may be more suited to fit patients' needs and to avoid early hyperalimentation. Many similar protocols have been recommended. Figure 6.2 shows one possible algorithm as recommended by Zanten et al. It must be taken into account that adjustment is an increase in calories and protein based on clinical improvements of patients' status, but also a decrease of calories and protein if patients' clinical status deteriorates. This is, in particular, true for patients with complicated abdominal sepsis. These patients often present with ups and downs in their clinical course.

In case of severe gastro-intestinal dysfunction, an even more slowed-down approach of adjustment of enteral nutrition may be preferable. Lacking prospective randomized controlled trials, many clinicians use a daily increase of 10 mL/h in this high-risk ICU subpopulation, if no side effects such as increase in lactic acid, increase in renal retention parameters as a sign of hyperalimentation, or deterioration of abdominal discomfort will occur. Using this approach, severe regurgitation or even small bowel ischemia may be avoided.

Finally, one must always adapt the published algorithms to one's own patient subpopulations, local conditions, and the clinical experience within the team.

6 Nutritional Adjustment

Individual control of the substrate supply based on the degree of insulin resistance

Day 0 substrate supply	0 kcal/kg day		

Day 1 substrate supply	16 kcal/kg day; of which 0.75 g protein/kg day ~ 3kcal/kg day		

Day 2	\multicolumn{3}{l}{maximum (max.) insulin requirement on day 1}
	max. 1 IE/h	max. 4 IE/h	> 4 IE/h
substrate supply	24 kcal/kg day	12 kcal/kg day	6 kcal/kg day

Following days	maximum (max.) insulin requirement on the day before		
	max. 1 IE/h	max. 4 IE/h	> 4 IE/h
	feed rate the day before	feed rate the day before	feed rate the day before
substrate supply	plus 4 kcal/kg day	minus 4 kcal/kg day	minus 12 kcal/kg day
	(max. 24 kcal/kg day)	(max. 0 kcal/kg day)	(max. 0 kcal/kg day)

Day 0 refers to the day of the homeostasis disorder. The goal is to maintain a blood glucose concentration < 180 mg/dl.

Individual control of the substrate supply based on the phosphate concentration

Day 0 substrate supply	0	

Day 1 substrate supply	16 kcal/kg day; of which 0.75 g protein/kg day ~ 3kcal/kg day	

Day 2	phosphate concentration in the morning of the day	
	≥ 0.65 mmol/l	< 0.65 mmol/l
substrate supply	24 kcal/kg day	6 kcal/kg day + phosphate substitution

Following days	phosphate concentration in the morning of the day	
	≥ 0.65 mmol/l	< 0.65 mmol/l
	feed rate the day before	feed rate the day before
substrate supply	plus 4 kcal/kg day	6 kcal/kg day + phosphate sustitution
	(max. 24 kcal/kg day)	

Day 0 refers to the day of the homeostasis disorder. This scheme is not applicable to patients undergoing renal replacement therapy.

Fig. 6.1 Algorithms for nutritional composition taking into account the glucose and phosphate concentration. (Adapted from Elke et al. [6])

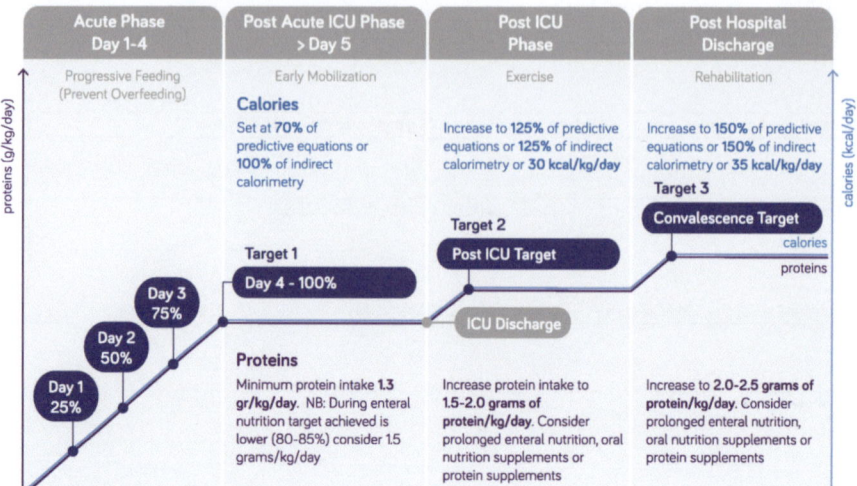

Fig. 6.2 Substrate supply for the critically ill. (Proposed scheme of gradual increase in substrate supply as proposed by Zanten el al [7])

References

1. Singer P, Blaser AR, Berger MM, Calder PC, Casaer M, Hiesmayr M, et al. ESPEN practical and partially revised guideline: clinical nutrition in the intensive care unit. Clin Nutr. 2023;42(9):1671–89.
2. Reignier J, Boisrame-Helms J, Brisard L, Lascarrou JB, Ait Hssain A, Anguel N, et al. Enteral versus parenteral early nutrition in ventilated adults with shock: a randomised, controlled, multicentre, open-label, parallel-group study (NUTRIREA-2). Lancet. 2018;391(10116):133–43.
3. Reignier J, Plantefeve G, Mira JP, Argaud L, Asfar P, Aissaoui N, et al. Low versus standard calorie and protein feeding in ventilated adults with shock: a randomised, controlled, multicentre, open-label, parallel-group trial (NUTRIREA-3). Lancet Respir Med. 2023;11(7):602–12.
4. Siqueira-Paese MC, Dock-Nascimento DB, De Aguilar-Nascimento JE. Critical energy deficit and mortality in critically ill patients. Nutr Hosp. 2016;33(3):253.
5. Faisy C, Lerolle N, Dachraoui F, Savard JF, Abboud I, Tadie JM, et al. Impact of energy deficit calculated by a predictive method on outcome in medical patients requiring prolonged acute mechanical ventilation. Br J Nutr. 2009;101(7):1079–87.
6. Elke G, Hartl WH, Kreymann KG, Adolph M, Felbinger TW, Graf T, et al. Clinical nutrition in critical care medicine – guideline of the German Society for Nutritional Medicine (DGEM). Clin Nutr ESPEN. 2019;33:220–75.
7. van Zanten ARH, De Waele E, Wischmeyer PE. Nutrition therapy and critical illness: practical guidance for the ICU, post-ICU, and long-term convalescence phases. Crit Care. 2019;23(1):368.

Enteral and Parenteral Nutrition in the ICU

Arved Weimann and Geraldine de Heer

As a basic principle, nutritional therapy in the critically ill is aiming on avoidance of malnutrition in primarily well-nourished patients and at least further deterioration in malnourished patients at the time of admission to the ICU.

However, there is currently limited high-quality evidence to clearly define the association between energy and/or protein delivery and skeletal muscle mass changes in acute critical illness [1]. In a recent multicentric observational study in 1172 patients staying in ICU ≥5 days, early moderate daily calorie and protein intakes were associated with improved clinical outcomes [2].

7.1 The Gastro-Intestinal Barrier

According to a classical concept, the gut is considered to be "the origin of multiorgan failure," which is also the rationale for early enteral nutrition [3].

Plenty of experimental data have established the concept that enteral nutrition is pivotal for the gut-associated immune system, and protective against shock-induced gut dysfunction as a "starter" of subsequent distant organ injury. A new dimension for our understanding of sepsis in the critically ill is the emerging role of the colonizing physiological intestinal microbiome and its interaction with the intestinal immune cells [4]. Under healthy conditions, the commensal microbiome has a

A. Weimann (✉)
Department of General, Visceral and Oncological Surgery, St. George Hospital, Leipzig, Germany
e-mail: Arved.Weimann@sanktgeorg.de

G. de Heer
Department Intensive Care Medicine, University Hospital Hamburg Eppendorf (UKE), Hamburg, Germany
e-mail: deheer@uke.de

© The Author(s), under exclusive license to Springer Nature Switzerland AG 2025
A. Rümelin et al. (eds.), *Nutrition in ICU Patients*,
https://doi.org/10.1007/978-3-032-00818-3_7

colonizing and symbiotic relationship with the host maintaining gut homeostasis. An intact microbiome in crosstalk with the host may also govern the immune response after injury. Short-chain fatty acids are produced by microbes and are considered a key mediator. However, stress and catabolism, as well as prolonged administration of antibiotics lead to a change of bacteria colonization and metabolism while decreased host resilience and cytokines as well as signals from the surrounding bacteria microenvironment ("sensing") induce a selected increase of virulence in special bacteria. This shift of the physiological microbiome to a pathobiome is accompanied by a loss of diversification of bacteria. Virulent bacteria may interact with a loss of function of the intestinal barrier with subsequent maladaptation of the immune response. Focusing on the microbiome, the shift to a dysbiome and the loss of bacteria diversification have become an important mechanism for disruption of the intestinal barrier with bacterial translocation inducing inflammatory mediators in the bowel wall leading to sepsis [4–6]. Therefore, the maintenance of the microbiome and the integrity of the intestinal barrier is a strong argument for early enteral nutrition in the critically ill. Many clinical studies and meta-analyses have confirmed the feasibility and the benefits of enteral feeding in the critically ill as well.

7.2 Is Enteral Nutrition Really Better than Parenteral Nutrition?

For a long time, the issue of "enteral or parenteral" has been controversially discussed with a lot of emotions [7]. The traditional argument for the physiological enteral route has been "Use the gut or lose it." Furthermore, enteral nutrition is less expensive.

Recent evidence has come up from a large multicenter randomized clinical trial (Calories) from the UK which raised some questions about the superiority of enteral over parenteral nutrition and the concept of early gut feeding in any case of critical illness. Almost 2400 critically ill patients were randomized for early enteral or parenteral nutrition. Regarding 30-day mortality as the primary end point, no significant difference could be found [parenteral 393/1188 (33.1%) vs. enteral 409/1195 (34.2%), $p = 0.57$]. ICU mortality, length of stay in acute care, and mortality by 90 days were also without significant difference [8]. Unless the study had some considerable limitations, it reflected the real-life situation and defused the discussion about early enteral vs. parenteral. In a retrospective analysis of 2270 critically ill septic patients from an international database, Elke et al. [9] demonstrated that the amount of calorie and protein intake close to the recommendations may significantly improve outcome.

Comparing (early) enteral and parenteral nutrition, four recent meta-analyses [10–13] including 16 up to 25 studies with 3325 up to 3816 patients provide these results:

- *In general, early enteral nutrition has no significant impact on mortality, but this may be considered in high-risk subgroups.*
- *Early enteral nutrition significantly decreases the risk for infectious complications.*

It has been pointed out by Elke et al. [10] that the reduced infection rate may be related even more to a lesser provision of calories than by the enteral route itself.

A recent randomized multicenter trial (Nutrirea-2) in 2410 ventilated adults with shock did not reveal benefits of early isocaloric enteral (n = 1202) versus parenteral (n = 1208) nutrition regarding mortality or secondary complications. On day 28, 443 (37%) of the enterally fed patients and 422 (35%) of the parenterally fed patients had died (absolute difference estimate 2% (95% CI −1.9 to 5.8); p = 0.33. The cumulative incidence of ICU-acquired infections was not different (enteral: 174 −14%, parenteral: 194 −16%) HR 0.89 (95% CI 0.72–1.09); p = 0.25. However, the enteral group had significantly higher cumulative incidences of vomiting, diarrhea, bowel ischemia, and pseudo-obstruction [14].

The recent ASPEN guideline states: "Because similar energy intake provided as PN is not superior to EN and no differences in harm were identified, we recommend that either PN or EN is acceptable" [15].

Although clear benefits are lacking regarding the optimal nutritional route, there is still some consensus among experts about a cautious individualized approach with "trophic feeding" in high-risk patients without absolute contraindication [16] aiming on prevention of mucosal atrophy in the gut. While severe critical illness is frequently associated with considerable gastrointestinal dysfunction, even severe sepsis or septic shock have not been considered clear contraindications [17–19].

Contraindications for enteral nutrition according to the ESICM Clinical Practice Guidelines [17].

In the absence of evidence, delaying enteral nutrition in critically ill patients is suggested under certain conditions—see Table 7.1.

Table 7.1 Contraindications for enteral nutrition according to Reintam-Blaser et al. [17]

Uncontrolled shock
Uncontrolled hypoxemia and acidosis
Uncontrolled upper GI bleeding
Gastric aspirate >500 mL/6 h
Bowel ischemia
Bowel obstruction
Abdominal compartment syndrome
High-output fistula without distal feeding access.

7.3 How Early Is Early?

Bearing in mind that the gut may be the "motor" for multi-organ failure, enteral feeding should be started within 24–48 h with a low feeding rate (5–10 mL) adopted to haemodynamic stability.

The ESPEN guideline states as a B recommendation: *If oral intake is not possible, early enteral nutrition (within 48 h) in critically ill adult patients should be performed/initiated rather than delaying enteral nutrition* [19].

7.4 GI Intolerance and Dysfunction

7.4.1 Feeding Intolerance

Motility disorders include delayed passage with slow gastric emptying and constipation and accelerated passage with impaired small intestinal nutrient absorption or nutrition-related diarrhea [20]. There are no clear definitions regarding gastrointestinal dysfunction, gastric dysmotility, and feeding intolerance. Feeding intolerance can be considered as a sign of gastrointestinal dysfunction [21].

Recently, an international expert consensus has defined *intestinal failure* as the

> reduction of gut function below the minimum necessary for the absorption of macronutrients and/or water and electrolytes, such that intravenous supplementation is required to maintain health and/or growth [22].

Functionally, acute (type I) and prolonged acute intestinal failure (type II) can be differentiated [22].

In a review of 72 studies, the authors found 43 definitions of feeding intolerance, which were classified into three main categories: increased gastric residual volumes, presence of abnormal clinical gastrointestinal symptoms, and inadequate high delivery of enteral nutrition. The prevalence of gastrointestinal dysfunction in that study was in a range of 2–75% and also in association with adverse outcome. In a retrospective observational study from the same authors, a definition of feeding intolerance based on the presence of at least three out of five gastrointestinal symptoms was strongly related to ICU mortality (6.3% prevalence in survivors vs. 23.5% in non-survivors, $P < 0.001$, odds ratio [95% confidence interval (CI) 3.39 (2.23–5.14)]), whereas enteral underfeeding less than 23% of caloric target was the strongest predictor for mortality 90 days after admission [50.7% prevalence among survivors vs. 75.2% in non-survivors, $P < 0.001$, odds ratio (95% CI) 2.34 (1.80–3.04)] (Reintam Blaser et al. 2014). Martinez et al. [23] reviewed the literature in critically ill children with gastric dysmotility, which was observed in up to 50% of all cases, associated with feeding intolerance, aspiration, ventilator-associated pneumonia, and a risk for poor patient outcome. Slower gastric emptying leading to larger gastric residual volume appears to be associated with increased secretion of hormonal and neural mediators in response to nutrients and reduced capacity to absorb nutrients in the small bowel [10]. Prolonged gastric palsy may occur in surgical and trauma patients secondary to stress metabolism, the surgical procedure, or the use of opioids or sedatives, which often can be overcome by jejunal application.

The underlying mechanism of gastric motility disorders are not fully understood and the pharmacological options are limited. A relevant upper GI motility disorder can be defined in case of gastric reflux exceeding more than 2 L/d. The most simple and pragmatic approach during gastrointestinal dysmotility is to withhold any enteral supply of nutrients. A locally tailored feeding protocol is recommended.

The impact of the measurement of gastric residual volume has been assessed controversial. In two controlled studies (one multicenter), non-monitoring gastric residual volume was without significant effect on the risk of ventilator-associated pneumonia in adults receiving mechanical ventilation and early enteral feeding [24, 25]. According to the experience of the working group in intensive care patients after abdominal surgery, a gastric residual volume of more than 500 mL/6 h may be considered critical [26]. According to the gastrointestinal dysfunction score (GIDS) [27], an increased risk has to be considered if:

- No oral intake
- Absent bowel sounds
- Vomiting
- GRV >200 mL
- GI paralysis/dynamic ileus
- Abdominal distension
- Diarrhea (not severe)
- GI bleeding without transfusion
- Intraabdominal pressure (IAP) 12–20 mmHg.

7.5 Practical Considerations

Many studies have shown the benefits and feasibility of enteral feeding in the critically ill [17].

The presence of bowel sounds is not a necessary condition for the start of enteral feeding. A clearly defined feeding protocol has shown to decrease the rate of patients who cannot be enterally fed at all [28–30]. Heyland et al. [28] could demonstrate that an enhanced protein-energy provision via the enteral route feeding protocol will increase the delivery of calories. Protocols should be locally tailored according to expertise, local barriers, facilities, and patient subpopulation in the ICU [31].

In a lot of patients, interruption of enteral nutrition may be avoidable to prevent a cumulative caloric deficit [29]. According to a meta-analysis of 13 randomized trials comparing intermittent and continuous enteral feeding, continuous feeding may be more favorable regarding the mortality rate bearing a higher risk of constipation [32].

A locally tailored feeding protocol has proven benefits and is recommended [28]. In anecdotal reports, too rapid administration of feed may lead to the development of small bowel ischemia [33–35].

> Tolerance of tube feeding has to be monitored closely in patients with impaired gastrointestinal function. [36]

7.6 Enteral Feeding and Prone Position

Early enteral nutrition should be performed in patients managed in prone position [19].

7.7 Enteral Feeding and an Open Abdomen

Based on expert consensus, the ASPEN guidelines suggest early EN (24–48 h postinjury) in patients treated with an open abdomen in the absence of a bowel injury [37]. An algorithm was proposed by Friese [38] and Moore and Burlew [39].

7.8 Early Enteral Nutrition Is Feasible And May Be Performed in Patients [19]

- Receiving ECMO
- With traumatic brain injury
- With stroke (ischemic or hemorrhagic)
- With spinal cord injury
- With severe acute pancreatitis
- After GI surgery
- After abdominal aortic surgery
- With abdominal trauma when the continuity of the GI tract is confirmed/restored
- Receiving neuromuscular blocking agents
- Managed in prone position
- With open abdomen
- Regardless of the presence of bowel sounds unless bowel ischemia or obstruction is suspected in patients with diarrhea.

7.9 Enteral Nutrition During Hemodynamic Instability

Cautious enteral feeding in patients with the need for catecholamines or vasopressors may be considered feasible and tolerated [40]. A retrospective propensity score-matched study in patients with hemodynamic instability ($n = 357$ in each group) revealed a significantly improved survival in the group with early enteral feeding [41].

However, in a prospective observational study in 60 critically ill patients receiving catecholamines, plasma intestinal fatty-acid-binding protein, which is a marker of enterocyte damage, was higher than in controls not receiving catecholamines [42]. Nevertheless, the need for vasopressors and low cardiac output requiring dobutamine are risk factors for acute mesenteric ischemia [43].

There is still a risk for nonocclusive bowel disease and a lack of data from controlled randomized trials [44].

A prospective observational study from Spain investigated the feasibility and safety of early enteral nutrition in a high-risk group of feeding intolerance with multiple organ dysfunction and a high risk for mortality. There were 37 patients after cardiac surgery with hemodynamic failure (two or more vasoactive drugs and/ or mechanical circulatory support) requiring more than 24 h of mechanical ventilation [45]. In total, 25 patients (68.0%) had multiple organ dysfunction with a resulting mortality of 13.5%. Mean duration of enteral nutrition was 12.3 days. The energy target was achieved in 15 patients (40.4%). Most gastrointestinal complications seen were constipation (46%). No case of mesenteric bowel necrosis occurred. This study clearly pointed out the feasibility of enteral nutrition in hemodynamically compromised patients taking into account that careful clinical examination of the abdomen is required and the caloric target cannot be achieved in such patients via the enteral route in the majority of cases. In a retrospective study, 339 critically ill children receiving vasoactive agents were categorized whether they had received any enteral nutrition or not during any of the first 4 days in the pediatric ICU. No significant difference was observed in the frequency of adverse gastrointestinal outcomes with a tendency to lower mortality in the enterally fed group [46]. Regarding the effect of enterally administered caloric intake, Tian et al. [47] performed a meta-analysis of eight randomized controlled trials with 1895 patients. In a subgroup of patients with low energy intake of 33.3–66.6% of goal energy, a significantly decreased lower rate of mortality (relative risk 0.68; 95% CI, 0.51–0.92; $Pp< 0.01$) and gastrointestinal intolerance (relative risk 0.65; 95% CI 0.43–0.99; $Pp<0.05$) was observed. However, gastrointestinal intolerance was only reported in three studies, including 452 patients. One of these studies was a recent Australian multicenter double-blind randomized trial, which showed that the substitution of a 1.0 compared to a 1.5 kcal/mL enteral nutrition with fiber resulted in a 46% greater calorie delivery without adverse effects regarding gastric residual volume and diarrhea [48]. One hundred and twelve patients were critically ill with Acute Physiology and Chronic Health Evaluation Score more than 20 in both groups. The volume of enteral nutrition was 1221 mL/d (95% CI: 1120, 1322 mL/d) vs. 1259 mL/d (95% CI: 1143, 1374 mL/d), the increase of daily calories 1832 kcal/d (95% CI: 1681, 1984) vs. 1259 kcal (95% CI: 1143, 1374 kcal/d) ($Pp < 0.001$). However, concerns about the higher delivery by energy-dense formulae arise from a retrospective comparison in 40 patients (energy-dense vs. standard). In comparison with the standard, this study showed significantly slower gastric emptying in the group of patients with the energy-dense diet [49].

Therefore, it is recommended to start tube feeding with a low flow rate (e.g., 10–max. 20 mL/h) according to intestinal tolerance. It may therefore take 5–7 days before nutritional requirements can be achieved by the enteral route. In case of hemodynamic instability and the administration of catecholamines, limited enteral tolerance should be anticipated, and the flow rate may be reduced even to 5 mL/h. Close observation of the abdomen is mandatory. In the concept of "minimal trophic nutrition," complete stop of enteral supply should be avoided whenever possible [50].

Enteral nutrition should be administered very cautiously (5–10 mL/h) in case of clinical signs of compromised enteral tolerance:

- Abdominal pain, distension
- Increased reflux, increased GRV, persistent emesis
- Diminished bowel sounds, flatus, stool
- Metabolic acidosis and/or deficit
- X-ray with distended bowel loops.

Enteral nutrition should even be stopped in case of new onset of increased serum lactate and/or procalcitonin as a warning for threatening bowel ischemia.

If CT scan shows bowel loops with intramural air accumulation ("Pneumatosis intestinalis"), bowel ischemia has to be considered.

See also proposed algorithm according to [51]—Fig. 7.2.

7.10 Enteral-Feeding Monitor

The so-called enteral-feeding monitor was developed by the American surgeon Gerald Moss [52]. The concept is a special tube device combining enteral feeding with intermittent suction in order to avoid any bowel distension at the tip of the tube by accumulation of enteral diet, bowel secretion, and gas. Decompression is achieved by a double lumen tube with a thin feeding lumen which has a distal opening separate from the suction lumen. After filtration and degassing of the aspirate, cyclic refeeding can be performed according to intestinal tolerance. A large lumen feeding tube and good flow properties of the enteral diet are essential requirements. While this device may provide additional safety in the early phase of enterally fed critically ill patients it has not been established in clinical routine. Furthermore, an appropriate jejunal feeding device is not available on the European market.

7.11 Energy-Dense Versus Standard Formula

Taking into account impaired gastrointestinal tolerance, the question arises whether more energy-dense enteral nutrition may achieve an increase in calorie intake.

A multicenter double-blind randomized trial has shown that the substitution of a 1.0 with 1.5 kcal/mL enteral nutrition with fiber resulted in a 46% greater calorie delivery without adverse effects regarding gastric residual volume and diarrhea [48]. Slowed gastric emptying should be taken into account [49]. In a single-center PRCT, volume-based feeding has been proven to be safe and to meet caloric requirements better than the standard hourly based rate strategy [30].

In order to investigate the impact of an energy-dense enteral diet on outcome, a recent multicenter double-blind randomized trial was performed in critically ill ventilated patients with the majority from internal medicine [53]. Enteral nutrition was started within 12 h after admission and continued up to 28 days. Three thousand nine hundred and fifty seven patients could be analyzed on an intention-to-treat basis. The use of the high-density enteral nutrition (1.5 kcal/mL) led to higher energy supply (1863 ± 478 kcal/d vs. 1262 ± 313 kcal/d) without an increased rate of adverse gastrointestinal events. However, the need for insulin was higher in the 1.5 kcal group (55.8 vs. 49.0%) (RR 1.14; 95% CI, 1.07–1.21). Finally, the rate of survival at 90 days was not significantly different in the group with the energy-dense formulation (26.8% vs. 25.7%; relative risk, 1.05: 95% CI, 0.94–1.16; $p = 0.41$). It has to be discussed critically that on admission to the ICU, only 2% were malnourished according to BMI <18.5 kg/m^2. Therefore, potential benefits of an energy-dense formula in primarily malnourished patients remain a matter of discussion. Because adverse gastrointestinal events had not been observed, the results may serve as an argument for the use of an energy-dense diet in primarily malnourished patients taking into account the need for an intensified blood sugar monitoring.

In severely malnourished patients, the start and increase of nutritional support have to be performed very carefully under close monitoring of potassium, phosphate, and magnesium in order to avoid Refeeding Syndrome (see guidelines monitoring).

7.12 Enteral Tube Access

7.12.1 Gastric Tubes

According to the number of lumens, gastric tubes can be divided into one- or two-lumen tubes, whereas the second lumen acts as a vent. There are different sizes classified into the outer diameter in Charrière (Ch). Whereas 14–18Ch are used in adults, smaller sizes (8–14Ch) are predominately used in children. One lumen tubes are used during short interventions (e.g., operating theatre), they should have a great diameter, as their main function is draining of gastric content. These (often) low-priced tubes are usually made of polyvinylchloride (PVC), losing their elasticity after 24–72 h, depending on the manufacturer. A longer use could lead to mucosal lesions going from superficial ulcerations to bleedings or even perforations, hence these tubes should be removed as soon as possible.

If a gastric tube is applied for a longer period as it is required for enteral nutrition, it should be made of silicone or polyurethane. Due to the softener "phthalate," these tubes can be utilized over a period of several weeks. Gastric tubes with a small diameter are eligible for enteral nutrition and are usually well (or better) tolerated although the risk of occlusion is much higher in a thinner tube. If the gastric residual volume has to be measured, the diameter should be greater. The type of tube should be chosen according to the clinical indication.

Placement of a gastric tube is a routine procedure. Holding the tube against the patient's chest and measuring the distance between mandibular angle and epigastrium offers a good estimation of the tube's length needed for insertion. Even if the patient is not awake, topical anaesthesia is needed. Topical anaesthesia like lidocaine spray or gel are often used because of the anaesthetic and vasoconstrictive effects. Inclination of the head or active swallowing when the tip of the tube touches the posterior pharyngeal wall are appropriate methods that ease application of the tube in the awake patient. If anesthetised, tube application can be challenging, as the voluntary act of swallow is missing. Sometimes a laryngoscope and/or a Magill forceps can be helpful for placement at sight.

There are different bedside methods to monitor the tube placement: throat inspection and palpation of the tube on the posterior pharyngeal wall, instillation of 30–50 mL air through the tube with consequent auscultation of the epigastrium or aspiration of gastric contents with subsequent pH measurement. However, these methods are not very accurate concerning gastric localisation, although they are very common. Misplaced tubes can build up loops in the laryngopharyngeal area, or in the oesophagus, which may lead to pain, ulcers, or bleeding. Placement of the tube inside the lung is associated with high morbidity and mortality if it remains undetected and enteral nutrition is delivered endotracheal. The gold standard for checking the tube position, and the only method that is recommended, is a chest x-ray, deep enough so that the tube can be followed along its entire length. However, such radiographs are associated with x-ray exposure, so it is advisable to perform them as part of a routine radiological workup of the chest. For daily practice, if instillation of air fails to produce an audible sound above the epigastrium, one should always double check tube placement by an x-ray before starting enteral nutrition.

> IRIS-technology ("integrated realtime imaging system") is a fairly innovative technique which uses a single lumen tube with an integrated 3 mm-camera attached to a monitor, following the placement in real time. While guided placement is associated with lower complications it still requires some expertise [54].

In case of anticipated long-lasting enteral nutrition (>4 weeks), e.g., brain injury, percutaneous endoscopic gastrostomy should be considered.

7.12.2 Nasojejunal (Postpyloric) Tubes

Certain clinical scenarios—for example, severe gastroparesis due to complicating pancreatitis or shock states, or just the need to put a new intestinal anastomosis at rest—require postpyloric feeding. These tubes are made mostly of polyurethane and have one to three lumen. One lumen tubes do not allow aspiration of the stomach content, an additional gastric tube being required, inducing extra discomfort to the patient. Two lumen tubes solved this problem and the three lumen ones have an extra vent. As the calibre is smaller than in gastric tubes (8–9Ch), they are at higher risk of occlusion. Tube nursing is extremely important, a flush with 30–50 mL non-carbonated water is recommended after usage of the tube for medication, nutrition etc. The most common way to insert such tubes is endoscopically or guided by ultrasound.

If the patient has to undergo surgery, e.g., in case of severe acute pancreatitis, placement of a jejunal tube should be considered intraoperatively. In order to create safe enteral access, (fine) needle catheter jejunostomy (FNCJ) has proven to be most appropriate [52], feasible, and safe in those patients, as it is advisable to avoid later manipulations in the anastomotic area.

Other bedside modalities for insertion include magnet tracking tubes (a small magnet attached permanently to the tip of the tube, so that its placement can be visualised in real time using an external sensor array connected to a computer) or the so-called self-advancing tubes (they are placed in the stomach, then left to advance by themselves through the pylorus using the gastric motility). All these methods are time-consuming and sometimes require patient sedation. Thus, once in place, a good fixation of the tube is recommended, and a high degree of alertness against possible tube displacements should be taken (see also Fig. 7.1).

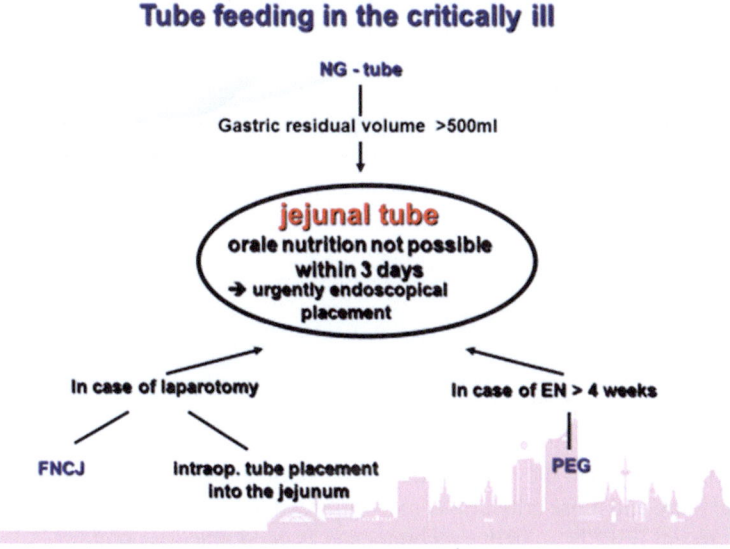

Fig. 7.1 Tube feeding in the critically ill

7.12.3 Prokinetics

The pharmacological options to treat gastrointestinal dysmotility are still limited [56]. In critically ill patients receiving gastric feeding, prokinetic agents may reduce the ICU length of stay (MD −2.03, 95% CI −3.96, −0.10; $Pp = 0.04$; low certainty) and the hospital length of stay [57]. During the past few years, the number of available prokinetic drugs has not increased. In our own daily practice, metoclopramide, erythromycin, and pyridostigmin, a cholinesterase inhibitor, are routinely used. Erythromycin is the medication of choice in case of persisting gastric paralysis. Comparing metoclopramide and erythromycin in a prospective RCT, MacLaren et al. [58] had proven that erythromycin is more effective on gastric motility. Continuing administration (>3 days) does not provide additional benefit. Furthermore, the risk to promote bacterial resistance has to be taken into account. In a meta-analysis, the effect of erythromycin in feeding intolerance remained inconclusive [59], while other authors more recently recommended the combination of erythromycin with metoclopramide [60]. To avoid adverse neurological reactions like dyskinesia and convulsions, warnings about the use of metoclopramide have been brought up by the regulatory agencies, and a restricted use was recommended by the European Medicines Agency in December 2013: short-term use up to 5 days only with a reduced dosage for adults up to 30 mg/d or 0.5 mg/kg body weight/day unrelated to the route of administration, no long-term use for patients with chronic disease like gastroparesis. An expert group reviewed the evidence for safety, effectiveness, and dosing of metoclopramide in critically ill patients as well as for alternatives. Some promising substances like the opioid antagonist alvimopan or the motilin agonist mitemcinal have not been sufficiently studied in critically ill patients [32]. Rhubarb derives from Chinese herbal medicine and has proven its feasibility as a prokinetic agent in comparison with metoclopramide and erythromycin for the successful placement of nasojejunal tubes in the critically ill [61]. Summarizing the recent data, van der Meer et al. [62] recommended not to abandon the use of metoclopramide in ICU patients, because metoclopramide is considered effective in enhancing gastric emptying and facilitating early enteral nutrition. This opinion is shared by the experts in the American Society for Parenteral and Enteral Nutrition guidelines [37].

7.13 Parenteral Nutrition

During the past years, the indication for parenteral nutrition in the critically ill has become more and more critical and individualized [63].
The recent ESPEN guideline recommends as good practice point.

> *Parenteral nutrition should not be started until all strategies to maximize enteral nutrition tolerance have been attempted* and
> *In patients who do not tolerate full dose enteral nutrition during the first week in the ICU, the safety and benefits of initiating should be weighed on a case-by-case basis.* [19]

The optimal amount of calories in the critically ill has been an ongoing matter of debate [2, 64–66]. To avoid a cumulative caloric deficit with negative impact on hospital outcome and rate of discharge to home, an improved energy and protein supply [67, 68] are the main objectives for combining enteral and parenteral nutrition.

In a meta-analysis [69] of these studies, no advantage was found of combined nutrition regarding mortality, infection, LOS, and length of artificial ventilation. Therefore, Heyland et al. [70] traditionally recommended not to begin with combined enteral and parental nutrition in critically ill patients without signs of malnutrition. They further recommended to decide on parenteral substrate intake on an individual basis in case of poor tolerance to enteral nutrition [70]. This should include consideration of the underlying pathology and the expected length of stay in the ICU.

The definition of enteral feeding intolerance may be a matter of debate. A recent meta-analysis has shown that the combination of GRV >250 mL combined with any other gastrointestinal symptom may be highly predictive for mortality, the incidence of pneumonia, and prolonged hospital length of stay [71].

In order to provide more evidence, during the past years, three large-scale multicenter studies investigated whether, in the case of impaired enteral tolerance, parenteral nutrition should be supplemented "early" (within 4 days) or "late" (after 7 days) [72–74]. The results were intensively discussed regarding a start of parenteral nutrition in malnourished patients and those with special risks on day 4 latest [73, 75]. So far, according to a recent meta-analysis, combination of EN with PN may improve nutrition intake in the acute phase. There is no clear evidence regarding benefits for patient outcomes [76].

The ESPEN guideline surgery recommendation states:

> If the energy and nutrient requirements cannot be met by oral and enteral intake alone (>50% of caloric requirement) for more than seven days, a combination of enteral and parenteral nutrition is recommended. [50]

See also proposed algorithm Fig. 7.2.

In most patients, individualized parenteral nutrition compounding is unnecessary. Special attention has to be attributed to patients with serious comorbidity (see chapters). Standardization may follow a protocol, and "All-In-One solutions" (AIO) (two-chamber bag with glucose and amino acids and an additional lipid emulsion, or three-chamber bag with glucose, amino acids, and lipids) may be used. The advantages of AIO solutions had been shown with regard to feasibility, time and cost saving, and the lower risk of contamination [77, 78].

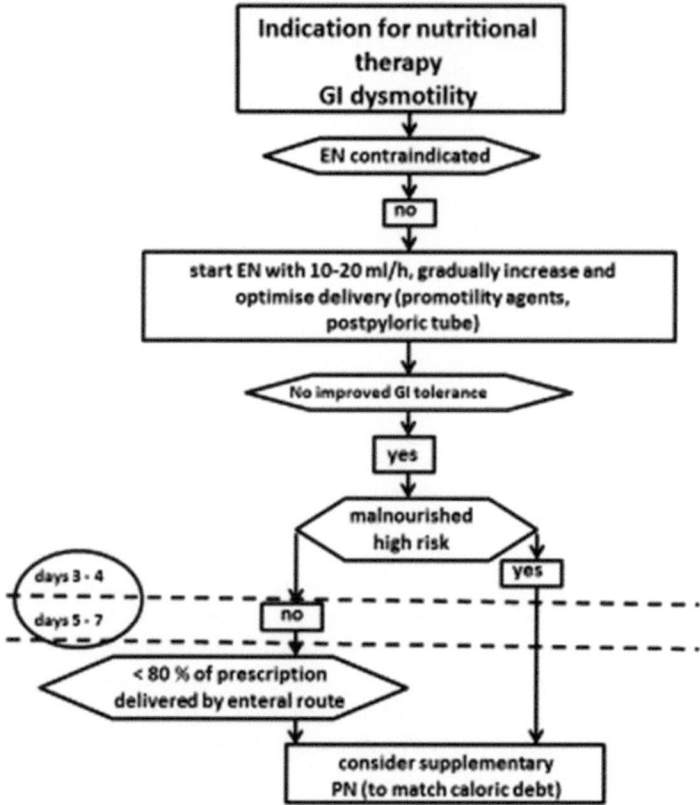

Fig. 7.2 Medical nutrition therapy in GI dysmotility [50]

7.14 Complications

Due to the fact that parenteral nutrition is applied very easily compared to the enteral route, there is always a great risk of *hyperalimentation* which could lead to a deleterious worsening of the clinical course with an increase of morbidity and mortality [2, 66, 72].

Related to central venous access, *catheter-related complications* with special regard to blood stream infections and thrombosis are the most frequent complications and a traditional argument against parenteral nutrition [79].

In severely malnourished patients, and with special regard to those with a long starving period, *refeeding syndrome* may occur within the first few days after starting nutritional therapy. Parenteral but also enteral (or oral) supply of carbohydrates and fluid will stimulate insulin secretion and intracellular shift of glucose and electrolytes. The decrease of serum potassium, magnesium, and phosphate levels will lead to impaired neuromuscular transmission causing life-threatening arrhythmias and convulsions. The ASPEN experts (2020) [80] propose that RS diagnostic criteria be stratified as follows: a decrease in any 1, 2, or 3 of serum phosphorus, potassium, and/or magnesium levels by 10–20% (mild), 20–30% (moderate), or >30% and/or organ dysfunction resulting from a decrease in any of these and/or due to thiamin deficiency (severe), occurring within 5 days of reintroduction of calories. There is a special risk in the frail elderly [81]. In high-risk patients, thiamine should be administered before the first feeding and continued with 200 mg once daily for 2 days. Calories and fluid administration should be started very carefully increasing slowly for several days.

Critically low levels which may be considered for parenteral supplementation are potassium 2.5, phosphate 0.35, and magnesium 0.4 mmol/L (CNSG East Cheshire NHS Trust Guidelines). In the author's own unit in high-risk patients, medical nutrition therapy will be initiated with intermediate care setting including ECG monitoring.

7.14.1 Refeeding Syndrome: Risk Patients According to NICE 2006 [82]

Moderate:
- Very little or no nutrition for over 5 days

High—have one of the following

- BMI less than 16 kg/m^2
- Unintentional weight loss greater than 15% in last 3–6 months
- Very little or no nutritional intake for more than 10 days
- Low levels potassium, phosphate or magnesium prior to feeding

Or two or more of the following:
- BMI less than 18.5 kg/m^2

Unintentional weight loss more than 10% in the last 3–6 months

- Very little or no nutritional intake for more than 5 days
- History of alcohol abuse, or drugs including chemotherapy, antacids, and diuretics.

Extremely High
- BMI under 14 kg/m^2

Or negligible intake for greater than 15 days
Septic blood stream infection

Hyperglycemia may be due either to hyperalimentation in a phase of insulin resistance or to underlying subclinical diabetes. Hyperglycemia is associated with increased mortality which has been the rationale for intensified insulin therapy [83]. In order to avoid any life-threatening hypoglycaemia, nowadays, glucose levels up to 180 mg/dL (10 mmol/L) are well tolerated. Reduction of glucose calories should be considered first, before insulin may be administered in nondiabetic patients with moderate dosages of 0–4 IU/h. Otherwise, reversible liver steatosis will develop within a few days.

7.14.2 Hypertriglyceridemia

Bolus application of lipids should be avoided. During continuous lipid infusion, serum triglyceride levels should not exceed 400 mg/dL [26]. Otherwise, hypertriglyceridemia is associated with low-grade inflammation and higher risk of acute pancreatitis [84].

7.14.3 Monitoring

Consensus exists that early full feeding may be harmful during the first few days [85]. Using clinical features on day 1–2, machine learning has shown predictive for enteral nutrition failure a large GRV on day 2, after BMI, followed by SOFA on day 1 [86]. Higher enteral calorie supply has been shown in a meta-analysis to be associated with higher GRV and use of prokinetics but not vomiting/regurgitation, diarrhea, or abdominal distension [87].

A new ICU care platform (smARTt+) has recently proven value to guide clinical nutrition in the critically ill in order to achieve caloric targets derived from calorimetry and to reduce GRV, length of stay, and mechanical ventilation [87]. Therefore, clinical observation of the patient's abdomen, bowel motility, and gastric reflux is mandatory. Gastric residual volume (GRV) measurement may be critically discussed [89]. It is not standardized, and the optimal threshold (<500 mL) is uncertain [16], the impact of the measurement of gastric residual volume has been controversial. In an important multicentric study in critically ill medical patients receiving mechanical ventilation and early enteral feeding, residual gastric volume had no significant effect on the risk of ventilator-associated pneumonia [24]. In the conclusion of a review of the literature [20] the monitoring of GRV may be still relevant in surgical ICU patients and severely critically ill patients with a high risk for gastrointestinal dysfunction. This has been emphasized in those patients with goal-directed enteral nutrition and volume-based feeding strategy.

For monitoring substrate supply, blood chemistry includes serum glucose, triglycerides, lactate, and procalcitonin [90], as well as phosphate levels to avoid a refeeding syndrome.

In order to avoid measurement of nitrogen balance, urea excretion rate per 24 h will help to estimate the extent of catabolism. Intramucosal pHi tonometry as a tool for the measurement of splanchnic perfusion has not been used frequently in clinical practice. It is the problem that sensitivity of the jejunal blood perfusion is not well represented by the more robust gastric perfusion [91].

7.15 Post-acute Phase: Post-extubation and Rehabilitation

It has been shown that after extubation, many patients will receive no more than 700 kcal/d [92]. Reasons to be discussed may be: in favour of oral feeding, medical nutrition therapy is stopped too early, especially in case of discharge from the ICU to the normal ward. Frequently, in many patients, oral intake from the normal hospital diet is rather limited due to post-critical weakness and fatigue. These patients have to be intensively encouraged and observed for oral food intake. Documentation of the amount of oral intake is mandatory. Supplementation with oral nutritional supplements may be reasonable; in some cases, enteral or even parenteral support has to be reconsidered.

During this phase of recovery from catabolic critical illness, substrate tolerance has been normalized with a metabolic shift to anabolism. From a nutritional point of view, insufficient caloric supply in this period has to be considered a "catastrophe." The amount of administered calories should be 1.2–1.5 fold higher than the calculated energy requirement. Because these patients are weaned from ventilation and able to eat, it will be frequently assumed that they will manage to cover these requirements by the oral route. It has been recently shown that this may be achieved only by a combination of oral and enteral feeding [93].

After critical illness, the anabolic energy requirements will be covered most likely by a combination of oral and enteral or even parenteral nutrition.

Keeping in mind post-intensive care syndrome (PICS), these patients should be monitored for adequate caloric intake and nutritional status even after hospital discharge in an integrated and holistic approach [94, 95].

7.16 Conclusion

Due to very low-quality evidence, there is still uncertainty whether early enteral nutrition, compared with delayed enteral nutrition, affects the risk of mortality within 30 days, feed intolerance or gastrointestinal complications, or pneumonia. There is currently also insufficient evidence regarding parenteral supplementation. There is still need for large, multicentric studies with rigorous methodology, which measure important clinical outcomes [96].

From a practical point for nutritional therapy, start of enteral nutrition is recommended within the first days of critical illness. In primarily malnourished patients and those with severe illness bearing the risk for an accumulating caloric and protein debt, parenteral supplementation should be considered in case of inappropriate enteral intake on day 4 at the latest. Taking into account local process-related barriers, a standard operative procedure (SOP) or feeding protocol is recommended.

References

1. Lambell KJ, King SJ, Forsyth AK, Tierney AC. Association of Energy and Protein Delivery on skeletal muscle mass changes in critically ill adults: a systematic review. JPEN J Parenter Enteral Nutr. 2018;42:1112–22. https://doi.org/10.1002/jpen.1151. Epub 2018 Mar 30
2. Matejovic M, Huet O, Dams K, Elke G, Vaquerizo Alonso C, Csomos A, Krzych ŁJ, Tetamo R, Puthucheary Z, Rooyackers O, Tjäder I, Kuechenhoff H, Hartl WH, Hiesmayr M. Medical nutrition therapy and clinical outcomes in critically ill adults: a European multinational, pro-

spective observational cohort study (EuroPN). Crit Care. 2022;26:143. https://doi.org/10.1186/s13054-022-03997-z. PMID: 35585554; PMCID: PMC9115983
3. Moore FA, Moore EE. The evolving rationale for early enteral nutrition based on paradigms of multiple organ failure: a personal journey. Nutr Clin Pract. 2009;24:297–304.
4. Alverdy JC, Krezalek MA. Collapse of the microbiome, emergence of the pathobiome, and the immunopathology of sepsis. Crit Care Med. 2017;45:337–47.
5. Krezalek MA, DeFazio J, Zaborina O, et al. The shift of an intestinal 'microbiome' to a 'pathobiome' governs the course and outcome of sepsis following surgical injury. Shock. 2016;45:475–82.
6. Alverdy JC, Luo JN. The influence of host stress on the mechanism of infection: lost microbiomes, emergent pathobiomes, and the role of interkingdom signaling. Front Microbiol. 2017;8:322.
7. Marik PE, Pinsky M. Death by TPN – the final chapter. Crit Care Med. 2008;36:1964–5.
8. Harvey SE, Parrott F, Harrison DA, Bear DE, Segaran E, Beale R, Bellingan G, Leonard R, Mythen MG, Rowan KM, Calories Trial Investigators. Trial of the route of early nutritional support in critically adults. N Engl J Med. 2014;371:1673–84.
9. Elke G, Wang M, Weiler N, et al. Close to recommended caloric and protein intake by enteral nutrition is associated with better clinical outcome of critically ill septic patients: a secondary analysis of a large international nutrition database. Crit Care. 2014;18:R29.
10. Elke G, van Zanten AR, Lermieux M, McCall M, Jeejeebhoy KN, Kott M, Jiang X, Day AG, Heyland DK. Enteral versus parenteral nutrition in critically ill patients: an updated systematic review and meta-analysis of randomized controlled trials. Crit Care. 2016;20:117. https://doi.org/10.1186/s13054-016-1298-1l.
11. Lewis SR, Schofield-Robinson OJ, Alderspn P, Smith AF. Enteral versus parenteral nutrition and enteral versus a combination of enteral and parenteral nutrition for adults in the intensive care unit. Cochrane Database Syst Rev. 2018;6:CDO12278. https://doi.org/10.1002/14651858.CD012276.pub2.
12. Tian F, Heighes PT, Allingstrup MJ, Doig GS. Early enteral nutrition provided within 24 hours of ICU admission: a meta-analysis of randomized controlled trials. Crit Care Med. 2018;46:1049–56. Epub ahead of print
13. Zhang G, Zhang K, Cui W, Hong Y, Zhang Z. The effect of enteral versus parenteral nutrition for critically ill patients: a systematic review and metaanalysis. J Clin Anesth. 2018;51:62–92.
14. Reignier J, Boisramé-Helms J, Brisard L, Lascarrou JB, Ait Hssain A, Anguel N, Argaud L, Asehnoune K, Asfar P, Bellec F, Botoc V, Bretagnol A, Bui HN, Canet E, Da Silva D, Darmon M, Das V, Devaquet J, Djibre M, Ganster F, Garrouste-Orgeas M, Gaudry S, Gontier O, Guérin C, Guidet B, Guitton C, Herbrecht JE, Lacherade JC, Letocart P, Martino F, Maxime V, Mercier E, Mira JP, Nseir S, Piton G, Quenot JP, Richecoeur J, Rigaud JP, Robert R, Rolin N, Schwebel C, Sirodot M, Tinturier F, Thévenin D, Giraudeau B, Le Gouge A. Enteral versus parenteral early nutrition in ventilated adults with shock: a randomised, controlled, multicentre, open-label, parallel-group study (NUTRIREA-2). NUTRIREA-2 Trial Investigators; Clinical Research in Intensive Care and Sepsis (CRICS) group. Lancet. 2018;391:133–43. https://doi.org/10.1016/S0140-6736(17)32146-3. Epub 2017 Nov 8
15. Compher C, Bingham AL, McCall M, Patel J, Rice TW, Braunschweig C, McKeever L. Guidelines for the provision of nutrition support therapy in the adult critically ill patient: the American Society for Parenteral and Enteral Nutrition. JPEN J Parenter Enteral Nutr. 2022;46:12–41. https://doi.org/10.1002/jpen.2267. Epub 2022 Jan 3. Erratum in: JPEN J Parenter Enteral Nutr. 2022;46(6):1458–9. https://doi.org/10.1002/jpen.2419. PMID: 34784064
16. Preiser JC, van Zanten AR, Berger MM, Biolo G, Casaer MP, Oig GS, Griffiths RD, Heyland DK, Hiesnayr M, Iapichino G, Laviano A, Pichard C, Singer P, Van den Berghe G, Wernerman J, Wischmeyer P, Vincent JL. Metabolic and nutritional support of critically ill patients: consensus and controversies. Crit Care. 2015;19:35.
17. Reintam Blaser A, Starkopf J, Alhazzani W, Berger MM, Casaer MP, Deane AM, Fruhwald S, Hiesmayr M, Ichai C, Jakob SM, Loudet CI, Malbran ML, Montejo-Gonzalez JC, Paugam-

Burtz C, Poeze M, Preiser JC, Singer P, van Zanten AR, De Waele J, Wendon J, Wernerman J, Whitehouse T, Wilmer A, Oudemans-van-Straten HM. ESCIM Working Group on gastrointestinal function early enteral nutrition in critically ill patients: ESCIM clinical practice guidelines. Intensive Care Med. 2017;43:380–98.
18. Elke G, Hartl WH, Kreymann KG, Adolph M, Felbinger TW, Graf T, de Heer G, Heller AR, Kampa U, Mayer K, Muhl E, Niemann B, Rümelin A, Steiner S, Stoppe C, Weimann A, Bischoff SC. DGEM Leitlinie Klinische Ernährung in der Intensivmedizin. Aktuel Ernahrungsmed. 2018;43:341–408.
19. Singer P, Reintam Blaser A, Berger MM, Alhazzani W, Calder P, Casaer M, Hiesmayr M, Mayer K, Montejo JC, Pichard C, Preiser JC, van Zanten ARH, Oczkowski S, Szczeklik W, Bischoff SC. ESPEN Guideline Clinical nutrition in the intensive care unit. Clin Nutr. 2019;38:48–79.
20. Elke G, Felbinger TW, Heyland D. Gastric residual volume in critically ill patients: a dead marker or still alive? Nutr Clin Pract. 2015;30:59–71.
21. Reintam Blaser A, Starkopf L, Deane AM, Poeze M, Starkopf J. Comparison of different definitions of feeding intolerance: a retrospective observational study. Clin Nutr. 2015;34:956–61.
22. Pironi L, Corcos O, Forbes A, Holst M, Joly F, Jonkers C, Klek S, Lal S, Blaser AR, Rollins KE, Sasdelli AS, Shaffer J, Van Gossum A, Wanten G, Zanfi C, Lobo DN. ESPEN Acute and Chronic Intestinal Failure Special Interest Groups intestinal failure in adults: recommendations from the ESPEN expert groups. Clin Nutr. 2018;37:1798–809.
23. Martinez EE, Douglas K, Nurko S, Mehta NM. Gastric dysmotility in critically ill children: pathophysiology, diagnosis, and management. Pediatr Crit Care Med. 2015;16:828–36.
24. Reignier J, Mercier E, le Gouge A, Boulain T, Desachy A, Bellec F, Clavel M, Frat J-P, Plantefeve G, Quenot J-P, Lasarrou J-B, Clinical Research in Intensive Care and Sepsis (CRICS) Group. Effect of non monitoring residual gastric volume on risk of ventilator-associated pneumonia in adults receiving mechanical ventilation and early enteral feeding: a randomized controlled trial. JAMA. 2013;309:249–56.
25. Poulard F, Dimet J, Martin-Lefevre L, Bontemps F, Fiancette M, Clementi E, Lebert C, Renard B, Reignier J. Impact of not measuring residual gastric volume in mechanically ventilated patients receiving enteral feeding: a prospective before-after study. JPEN. 2010;34:125–30.
26. Hartl WH, Parhofer KG, Kuppinger D, Rittler P. und das DGEM Steering Committee. S3 Leitlinie der Deutschen Gesellschaft für Ernährungsmedizin (DGEM) in Zusammenarbeit mit der GESKES und der AKE: Besonderheiten der Überwachung bei künstlicher Ernährung. Aktuel Ernahrungsmed. 2013;38:e90–100.
27. Reintam Blaser A, Padar M, Mändul M, Elke G, Engel C, Fischer K, Giabicani M, Gold T, Hess B, Hiesmayr M, Jakob SM, Loudet CI, Meesters DM, Mongkolpun W, Paugam-Burtz C, Poeze M, Preiser JC, Renberg M, Rooijackers O, Tamme K, Wernerman J, Starkopf J. Development of the Gastrointestinal Dysfunction Score (GIDS) for critically ill patients – a prospective multicenter observational study (iSOFA study). Clin Nutr. 2021;40:4932–40. https://doi.org/10.1016/j.clnu.2021.07.015. Epub 2021 Jul 18
28. Heyland DK, Dhaliwal R, Lemieux M, et al. Implementing the PEP uP protocol in critical care units in Canada: results of a multicenter, quality improvement study. JPEN J Parenter Enteral Nutr. 2015;39:98–706.
29. Peev MP, Yeh DD, Quraishi SA, et al. Causes and consequences of interrupted enteral nutrition: a prospective observational study in critically ill surgical patients. JPEN J Parenter Enteral Nutr. 2015;39:21–7.
30. McClave SA, Martindale RG, Rice TW, Heyland DK. Feeding the critically ill patient. Crit Care Med. 2014;42:2600–10.
31. Kozeniecki M, McAndrew N, Patel JJ. Process-related barriers to optimizing enteral nutrition in a tertiary medical intensive care unit. Nutr Clin Pract. 2016;31:80–5.
32. Wu JY, Liu MY, Liu TH, Kuo CY, Hung KC, Tsai YW, Lai CC, Hsu WH, Chuang MH, Huang PY, Tay HT. Clinical efficacy of enteral nutrition feeding modalities in critically ill

patients: a systematic review and meta-analysis of randomized controlled trials. Eur J Clin Nutr. 2023;77:1026–33. https://doi.org/10.1038/s41430-023-01313-8. Epub ahead of print
33. Jorba R, Fabregat J, Borobia FG, Torras J, Poves I, Jaurrieta E. Small bowel necrosis in association with early postoperative enteral feeding after pancreatic resection. Surgery. 2000;128:111–2.
34. Scaife CL, Saffle JR, Morris SE. Intestinal obstruction secondary to enteral feedings in burn trauma patients. J Trauma. 1999;47:859–63.
35. Schloerb PR, Wood JG, Casillan AJ, Tawfik O, Udobi K. Bowel necrosis caused by water in jejunal feeding. JPEN. 2004;28:27–9.
36. Durham CM, Frankenfield D, Belzberg H, Wiles C, Cushing B, Grant Z. Gut failure–predictor of or contributor to mortality in mechanically ventilated blunt trauma patients? J Trauma. 1994;37:30–4.
37. McClave SA, Taylor BE, Martindale RG, et al. Society of Critical Care Medicine, American Society for Parenteral and Enteral Nutrition. Guidelines for the provision and assessment of nutrition support therapy in the adult critically ill patient: Society of Critical Care Medicine (SCCM) and American Society for Parenteral and Enteral Nutrition (A.S.P.E.N.). JPEN J Parenter Enteral Nutr. 2016;40:159–211.
38. Friese RS. The open abdomen: definitions, management principles, and nutrition support considerations. Nutr Clin Pract. 2012;27:492–8.
39. Moore SM, Burlew CC. Nutrition support in the open abdomen. Nutr Clin Pract. 2016;31:9–13.
40. Zaloga GP, Roberts PR, Marik P. Feeding the hemodynamically unstable patient: a critical evaluation of the evidence. Nutr Clin Pract. 2003;18:285–93.
41. Khalid I, Doshi P, DiGiovine B. Early enteral nutrition and outcomes of critically ill patients treated with vasopressors and mechanical ventilation. Am J Crit Care. 2010;18:281–8.
42. Piton G, Cypriani B, Regnard J, et al. Catecholamine use is associated with enterocyte damage in critically ill patients. Shock. 2015;43:437–42.
43. Piton G, Le Gouge A, Boisramé-Helms J, Anguel N, Argaud L, Asfar P, Botoc V, Bretagnol A, Brisard L, Bui HN, Canet E, Chatelier D, Chauvelot L, Darmon M, Das V, Devaquet J, Djibré M, Ganster F, Garrouste-Orgeas M, Gaudry S, Gontier O, Groyer S, Guidet B, Herbrecht JE, Hourmant Y, Lacherade JC, Letocart P, Martino F, Maxime V, Mercier E, Mira JP, Nseir S, Quenot JP, Richecoeur J, Rigaud JP, Roux D, Schnell D, Schwebel C, Silva D, Sirodot M, Souweine B, Thieulot-Rolin N, Tinturier F, Tirot P, Thévenin D, Thiéry G, Lascarrou JB, Reignier J, Clinical Research in Intensive Care and Sepsis (CRICS) Group. Factors associated with acute mesenteric ischemia among critically ill ventilated patients with shock: a post hoc analysis of the NUTRIREA2 trial. Intensive Care Med. 2022;48:458–66. https://doi.org/10.1007/s00134-022-06637-w. Epub 2022 Feb 22. PMID: 35190840
44. Bruns BR, Kozar RA. Feeding the postoperative patient on vasopressor support. Nutr Clin Pract. 2016;31:14–7.
45. Flordelis Lasierra JL, Perez-Vela JL, Umezawa Makikado LD, et al. Early enteral nutrition with hemodynamic failure following cardiac surgery. JPEN J Parenter Enteral Nutr. 2015;39:154–62.
46. Panchal AK, Manzi J, Connolly S, et al. Safety of enteral feedings in critically ill children receiving vasoactive agents. JPEN J Parenter Enteral Nutr. 2016;40:236–41.
47. Tian F, Wang X, Gao X, et al. Effect of initial caloric intake via enteral nutrition in critical illness: a meta-analysis of randomised controlled trials. Crit Care. 2015;19:180.
48. Peake SL, Davies AR, Deane AM, et al. Use of concentrated enteral nutrition solution to increase calorie delivery to critically ill patients: a randomized double-blind clinical trial. Am J Clin Nutr. 2014;100:616–25.
49. Kar P, Plummer MP, Chapman MJ, et al. Energy-dense formulae may slow gastric emptying in the critically ill. J Parenter Enter Nutr. 2008;32:412–9.

50. Weimann A, Braga M, Carli F, Higashiguchi T, Hübner M, Klek S, Laviano A, Lobo DN, Ljungqvist O, Martindale R, Waitzberg D, Bischoff SC, Singer P. ESPEN guideline clinical nutrition in surgery. Clin Nutr. 2017;36:623–50.
51. Weimann A, Felbinger T. Gastrointestinal dysfunction in the critically ill—a role for nutrition. Curr Opin Clin Nutr Metab Care. 2016;19:353–9.
52. Moss G. Development of automated postoperative enteral nutrition: restricting feeding site inflow to match peristaltic outflow. Ann Surg Innov Res. 2015;9:12.
53. The TARGET Investigators, for the ANZICS Clinical Trials Group, Chapman M, Peake SL, Bellomo R, Davies A, Deane A, Horowitz M, Hurford S, Lange K, Little L, Mackle D, O'Connor S, Presneill J, Ridley E, Williams P, Young P. Energy-dense versus routine enteral nutrition in the critically ill. N Engl J Med. 2018;379:1823–34.
54. Taylor SJ, Karpasiti T, Milne D. Safety of blind versus guided feeding tube placement: misplacement and pneumothorax risk. Intensive Crit Care Nurs. 2023;76:103387. https://doi.org/10.1016/j.iccn.2023.103387. Epub 2023 Jan 17. PMID: 36657250
55. Weimann A, Braunert M, Müller T, Bley T, Wiedemann B. Feasibility and safety of needle catheter jejunostomy for enteral nutrition in surgically treated severe acute pancreatitis. JPEN J Parenter Enteral Nutr. 2004;28:324–7.
56. Herbert MK, Holzer P. Standardized concept for the treatment of gastrointestinal dysmotility in critically ill patients—current status and future options. Clin Nutr. 2008;27:25–41.
57. Peng R, Li H, Yang L, Zeng L, Yi Q, Xu P, Pan X, Zhang L. The efficacy and safety of prokinetics in critically ill adults receiving gastric feeding tubes: a systematic review and meta-analysis. PLoS One. 2021;16:e0245317. https://doi.org/10.1371/journal.pone.0245317. PMID: 33428672; PMCID: PMC7799841
58. MacLaren R, Kiser TH, Fish DN, Wischmeyer PE. Erythromycin vs metoclopramide for facilitating gastric emptying and tolerance to intragastric nutrition in critically ill patients. JPEN J Parenter Enteral Nutr. 2008;32:412–9.
59. Chen YT, Tai KY, Lai PC, Huang YT. Should we believe the benefit of intravenous erythromycin in critically ill adults with gastric feeding intolerance? Reinspecting the pieces of evidence from a series of meta-analyses. JPEN J Parenter Enteral Nutr. 2022;46:1449–54. https://doi.org/10.1002/jpen.2352. Epub 2022 Mar 15
60. Szczupak M, Jankowska M, Jankowski B, Wierzchowska J, Kobak J, Szczupak P, Kosydar-Bochenek J, Krupa-Nurcek S. Prokinetic effect of erythromycin in the management of gastroparesis in critically ill patients-our experience and literature review. Front Med (Lausanne). 2024;9:1440992. https://doi.org/10.3389/fmed.2024.1440992. PMID: 39314225; PMCID: PMC11416996
61. Li J, Gu Y, Zhou R. Rhubarb to facilitate placement of nasojejunal feeding tubes in patients in the intensive care unit. Nutr Clin Pract. 2016;31:105–10.
62. van der Meer YG, Venhuizen WA, Heyland DK, van Zanten AR. Should we stop prescribing metoclopramide as a prokinetic drug in critically ill patients. Crit Care. 2014;18:502.
63. Hill A, Elke G, Weimann A. Nutrition in the intensive care unit-a narrative review. Nutrients. 2021;13(8):2851. https://doi.org/10.3390/nu13082851. PMID: 34445010; PMCID: PMC8400249
64. Arabi YM, Aldawood AS, Hadddad SH, et al. PermiT Trial Group. Permissive underfeeding or standard enteral feeding in critically ill adults. N Engl J Med. 2015;372:2398–408.
65. Petros S, Horbach M, Seidel F, Weidhase L. Hypocaloric vs. normocaloric nutrition in critically ill patients: a prospective randomized pilot trial. JPEN J Parenter Enteral Nutr. 2016;40:242–9.
66. Braunschweig CA, Sheean PM, Petersen SJ, Perez SG, Freels S, Lateef O, Gurka D, Fantuzz G. Intensive nutrition in acute lung injury: a clinical trial (INTACT). JPEN J Parenter Enteral Nutr. 2015;39:13–20.

67. Yeh DD, Fuentes E, Quraishi SA, et al. Adequate nutrition may get you home effect of caloric/protein deficits on the discharge destination of critically ill surgical patients. JPEN J Parenter Enteral Nutr. 2016;40:37–44.
68. Compher C, Chittams J, Sammero T, Nicolo M, Heyland DK. Greater protein and energy intake may be associated with improved mortality in higher risk critically ill patients: a multicenter multinational observational study. Crit Care Med. 2017;41:104–12.
69. Dhaliwal R, Jurewitsch B, Harrietha D, Heyland DK. Combination enteral and parenteral nutrition in critically ill patients: harmful or beneficial? A systematic review of the evidence. Intensive Care Med. 2004;30:1666–771.
70. Heyland DK, Dhaliwal R, Drover JW, Gramlich L, Dodek P, Canadian Critical Care Clinical Practice Guidelines Committee. Canadian clinical practice guidelines for nutrition support in mechanically ventilated, critically ill adult patients. JPEN J Parenter Enteral Nutr. 2003;27:355–73.
71. Li J, Wang L, Zhang H, Zou T, Kang Y, He W, Xu Y, Yin W. Different definitions of feeding intolerance and their associations with outcomes of critically ill adults receiving enteral nutrition: a systematic review and meta-analysis. J Intensive Care. 2023;11:29. https://doi.org/10.1186/s40560-023-00674-3. PMID: 37408020; PMCID: PMC10320932
72. Casaer MP, Mesotten D, Hermans G, Wouters PJ, Schetz M, Meyfroidt G, Van Cromphaut S, Ingels C, Meersseman P, Muller J, Vlasselaers D, Debaveye Y, Desmet L, Dubois J, Van Assche A, Vanderheyden S, Wilmer A, Van den Berghe G. Early versus late parenteral nutrition in critically ill adults. N Engl J Med. 2011;365:506–17.
73. Heidegger CP, Berger MM, Graf S, Zingg W, Darmon P, Costanza MC, Thibault R, Pichard C. Optimisation of energy provision with supplemental parenteral nutrition in critically ill patients: a randomised controlled clinical trial. Lancet. 2013;381:385–93.
74. Doig GS, Simpson F, Sweetman EA, Finfer SR, Cooper DJ, Heighes PT, Davies AR, O'Leary M, Solano T, Peake S, Early PN, Investigators of the ANZICS Clinical Trial Group. Early parenteral nutrition in critically ill patients with short term relative contraindications to early enteral nutrition: a randomized controlled trial. JAMA. 2013;22:2130–8.
75. Oshima T, Hiesmayer M, Pichard C. Parenteral nutrition in the ICU setting: need for a shift in utilization. Curr Opin Clin Nutr Metab Care. 2016;19:144–50.
76. Hill A, Heyland DK, Ortiz Reyes LA, Laaf E, Wendt S, Elke G, Stoppe C. Combination of enteral and parenteral nutrition in the acute phase of critical illness: an updated systematic review and meta-analysis. JPEN J Parenter Enteral Nutr. 2022;46:395–410. https://doi.org/10.1002/jpen.2125. Epub 2021 Jun 8
77. Pichard C, Schwarz G, Frei A, Kyle U, Romand JA, Sierro C. Economic investigation of the use of three-compartment total parenteral nutrition bag: prospective randomized unblended controlled study. Clin Nutr. 2000;19:245–51.
78. Menne R, Adolph M, Brock E, Schneider H, Senkal M. Cost analysis of parenteral nutrition regimens in the intensive care unit: three-compartment bag system vs. multibottle system. JPEN J Parenter Enteral Nutr. 2008;32:506–12.
79. Teja B, Bosch NA, Diep C, Pereira TV, Mauricio P, Sklar MC, Sankar A, Wijeysundera HC, Saskin R, Walkey A, Wijeysundera DN, Wunsch H. Complication rates of central venous catheters: a systematic review and meta-analysis. JAMA Intern Med. 2024;184(5):474–82. https://doi.org/10.1001/jamainternmed.2023.8232. Erratum in: JAMA Intern Med. 2024;184(6):707. doi: 10.1001/jamainternmed.2024.2175. PMID: 38436976; PMCID: PMC12285596
80. da Silva JSV, Seres DS, Sabino K, Adams SC, Berdahl GJ, Citty SW, Cober MP, Evans DC, Greaves JR, Gura KM, Michalski A, Plogsted S, Sacks GS, Tucker AM, Worthington P, Walker RN, Ayers P, Parenteral Nutrition Safety and Clinical Practice Committees, American Society for Parenteral and Enteral Nutrition. ASPEN consensus recommendations for refeeding syndrome. Nutr Clin Pract. 2020;35:178–95. https://doi.org/10.1002/ncp.10474. Epub 2020 Mar 2. Erratum in: Nutr Clin Pract 2020 Jun;35(3):584–585
81. Aubry E, Friedli N, Schuetz P, Stanga Z. Refeeding syndrome in the frail elderly population: prevention, diagnosis and management. Clin Exp Gastroenterol. 2018;11:255–64.

82. https://www.bapen.org.uk/nutrition-support/assessment-and-planning/nutritional-assessment?start=2 (letzter Aufruf: 5.8.23).
83. Van den Berghe G, Wouters P, Weekers F, Verwaest C, Bruyninckx F, Schetz M, et al. Intensive insulin therapy in the critically ill patients. N Engl J Med. 2001;345:1359–67.
84. Hansen SEJ, Madsen CM, Varbo A, Nordestgaard BG. Low-grade inflammation in the association between mild-to-moderate hypertriglyceridemia and risk of acute pancreatitis: a study of more than 115000 individuals from the general population. Clin Chem. 2019;65:321–32. https://doi.org/10.1373/clinchem.2018.294926. Epub 2018 Dec 5
85. Reintam Blaser A, Rooyackers O, Bear DE. How to avoid harm with feeding critically ill patients: a synthesis of viewpoints of a basic scientist, dietitian and intensivist. Crit Care. 2023;27:258. https://doi.org/10.1186/s13054-023-04543-1. PMID: 37393289; PMCID: PMC10314407
86. Raphaeli O, Statlender L, Hajaj C, Bendavid I, Goldstein A, Robinson E, Singer P. Using machine-learning to assess the prognostic value of early enteral feeding intolerance in critically ill patients: a retrospective study. Nutrients. 2023;15:2705. https://doi.org/10.3390/nu15122705. PMID: 37375609; PMCID: PMC10305247
87. Murthy TA, Plummer MP, Tan E, Chapman MJ, Chapple LS. Higher versus lower enteral calorie delivery and gastrointestinal dysfunction in critical illness: a systematic review and meta-analysis. Clin Nutr. 2022;41:2185–94. https://doi.org/10.1016/j.clnu.2022.08.011. Epub 2022 Aug 19
88. Kagan I, Hellerman-Itzhaki M, Bendavid I, Statlender L, Fishman G, Wischmeyer PE, de Waele E, Singer P. Controlled enteral nutrition in critical care patients – a randomized clinical trial of a novel management system. Clin Nutr. 2023;42:1602–9. https://doi.org/10.1016/j.clnu.2023.06.018. Epub ahead of print. PMID: 37480797
89. Feng L, Chen J, Xu Q. Is monitoring of gastric residual volume for critically ill patients with enteral nutrition necessary? A meta-analysis and systematic review. Int J Nurs Pract. 2023;29:e13124. https://doi.org/10.1111/ijn.13124. Epub ahead of print. PMID: 36540042
90. Markogiannakis H, Memos N, Messaris E, et al. Predictive value of procalcitonin for bowel ischemia and necrosis in bowel obstruction. Surgery. 2011;149:394–403.
91. Zhang X, Xuan W, Yin P, Wang L, Wu X, Wu Q. Gastric tonometry guided therapy in critical care patients: a systematic review and meta-analysis. Crit Care. 2015;19:22. https://doi.org/10.1186/s13054-015-0739-6. PMID: 25622724; PMCID: PMC4350856
92. Peterson SJ, Tsai AA, Scala CM, Sowa DC, Sheean PM, Braunschweig CL. Adequacy of oral intake in critically ill patients 1 week after extubation. J Am Diet Assoc. 2010;110:427–33.
93. Ridley E, Parke RL, Davies AR, Bailey M, Hodgson C, Deane AM, McGuinness S, Coopper DJ. What happens to nutrition intake in the post-intensive care unit hospitalization period? An observational cohort study in critically ill adults. J Parenter Enteral Nutr JPEN. 2019;43:88–95.
94. Moisey LL, Merriweather JL, Drover JW. The role of nutrition rehabilitation in the recovery of survivors of critical illness: underrecognized and underappreciated. Crit Care. 2022;26:270. https://doi.org/10.1186/s13054-022-04143-5. PMID: 36076215; PMCID: PMC9461151
95. Renner C, Jeitziner MM, Albert M, Brinkmann S, Diserens K, Dzialowski I, Heidler MD, Lück M, Nusser-Müller-Busch R, Sandor PS, Schäfer A, Scheffler B, Wallesch C, Zimmermann G, Nydahl P. Guideline on multimodal rehabilitation for patients with post-intensive care syndrome. Crit Care. 2023;27:301. https://doi.org/10.1186/s13054-023-04569-5. PMID: 37525219; PMCID: PMC10392009
96. Padilla FP, Martínez G, Vernooij RW, Urrútia G, Figuls MRI, Cosp XB. Early enteral nutrition (within 48 hours) versus delayed enteral nutrition (after 48 hours) with or without supplemental parenteral nutrition in critically ill adults. Cochrane Database Syst Rev. 2019;2019:CD012340. https://doi.org/10.1002/14651858.CD012340.pub2. PMID: 31684690; PMCID: PMC6820694

Immunonutrition and Pharmaconutrition

Aileen Hill and Christian Stoppe

8.1 Introduction

Micronutrients have numerous essential functions in the human biology, such as support of metabolism, maintenance of an adequate immune activity, defence against oxidative stress, for DNA synthesis and diverse cell signalling processes. For these reasons, micronutrients should be considered as an integral part of the daily medical nutrition therapy in critically ill patients.

Several observational studies demonstrated a significant deficiency of micronutrients during critical illness, which correlated with severity of illness in concerning patients [1–3]. Besides, a prolonged use of technical assist devices such as extracorporeal life support (ECLS, ECMO) or dialysis can trigger or aggravate pre-existing micronutrient deficiencies [4]. Given their role as essential cofactors of many antioxidant or anti-inflammatory enzymes (e.g., glutathione peroxidase (GPX) or superoxide dismutase (SOD)), the need to compensate a significant deficiency of micronutrients to maintain an adequate immune response is urgent, especially in critically ill patients. Furthermore, it becomes obvious *why* in the past, clinicians repeatedly attempted to substitute micronutrients to further optimize the critically ill patients' antioxidant and anti-inflammatory defence mechanisms.

In fact, several experimental studies demonstrated that an application of, for example, antioxidant trace elements result in a significant increase of the dependent anti-oxidant enzyme activity [5]. Yet, based on heterogeneous data received from adequately designed multicentre trials, the resulting meta-analyses could not demonstrate clinically relevant effects of micronutrients, which questions the role of their supplementation during the daily routine in the clinical practice. The available evidence for the most relevant micronutrients will be outlined in the following chapter.

8.2 Targeting the Inflammatory Response

Patients with critical illness frequently experience a complex systemic inflammatory response syndrome (SIRS). As part of this, reactive oxidative and nitrogen species, as well as pro-inflammatory cytokines such as TNFα, IL-1-β, IL-6 and IL-8, are repeatedly released, triggering leukocyte extravasation, intravascular leukostasis, lipid peroxidation, cell death, vasodilation, capillary fluid leakage in the tissues. To mitigate the effects of the pro-inflammatory mechanisms, a compensatory anti-inflammatory response syndrome (CARS) is activated in parallel [6]. The balance within the organism between enough inflammation to heal and defend against secondary infection on the one side, and too much damage to the body through the inflammation cascades on the other hand, is crucial for the outcome of the patient. The consequences of these mechanisms include mild adverse effects, such as fever and tissue edema, moderate adverse effects, for example, hemodynamic instability and coagulopathy, as well severe complications, such as acute organ injury requiring mechanical support and death [7].

The antioxidant micronutrients copper, selenium, zinc, and vitamins A, E and C belong to the body' first line of antioxidant defences mechanisms. Several observational clinical studies demonstrated that blood levels of these antioxidants frequently decrease below reference ranges during critical illness, which may further aggravate the inflammatory response [8–10], which illuminates a clinical scenario to compensate the occurring deficiencies to enable an optimal immune response. In fact, based on these studies, several interventional trials followed, which investigated if supplementation with antioxidant trace elements or vitamins may influence the outcomes of critically ill patients. The aggregated data of 34 studies including 4678 patients were meta-analysed [11] and indicated that a supplementation of combined antioxidants may reduce the mortality relative risk [RR], 0.89 [95% CI 0.79–0.99], whereas the certainty of the received evidence remained questionable, as eight studies with low risk of bias (RR, 1.08; 95% CI 0.95–1.23; TSA CI, 0.64–1.82; moderate QOE) did not show mortality reduction with antioxidants supplementation.

8.3 Supplementation Recommendations

While general ICU patients receiving full enteral nutrition support might not need an additional supplementation of micronutrients, these should be given daily in patients receiving parenteral nutrition (PN) exclusively or as combined or supplemental PN, as commercial PN solutions do not contain micronutrients for stability reasons. Therefore, micronutrients should be added to the PN shortly before it is administered to the patient.

Based on the existing heterogeneous evidence and conflicting studies, until today neither the European nor American Society of Parenteral and Enteral Nutrition (ESPEN or ASPEN) can give recommendations above the compensation of deficiencies for when regarding the supplementation of selenium, zinc or vitamins in critically ill patients [12, 13]. Until now, guideline recommendations are limited to the supplementation of these micronutrients in case of supposed, ideally measured deficiencies, whereas the latter is known to be cumbersome. Therefore, efforts should be increased to establish a monitoring of these micronutrients, which should be integrated into the clinical routine in critically ill patients on medical nutrition therapy to avoid deficiency as well as overdosage.

The recent ESPEN micronutrient guidelines provide a clear guidance for all micronutrients [14].

8.4 Micronutrients of Special Interest

8.4.1 Selenium

Selenium belongs to the most studied micronutrient in the field of critical care medicine. A significant decrease of circulating selenium levels has repeatedly been shown in several observational studies in different settings of critical illness, whereas the extend of decrease was closely related to the severity of illness and demonstrated to be independently associated with the development of organ dysfunctions [15–18]. An increase of selenium was shown to correlate with an increase of the powerful antioxidant glutathione peroxidase activity [15, 19], which itself may neutralize either reactive oxygen or nitrogen species. Clinicians and researchers followed this exciting idea to further optimize the patient's antioxidant defence by an exogenous supplementation with selenium.

Notably, a meta-analysis of 9 trials by Huang et al. found a significant reduction in mortality (RR = 0.83; 95% CI, 0.70–0.099; $P = 0.04$) with the use of higher doses of selenium in critical illness [20]. Yet, two recent large-scale studies could not confirm clinically significant effects of selenium on the mortality in general critically ill patients, regardless of whether it was given as combination therapy or monotherapy [21, 22], while a previous study demonstrated a significant reduction in mortality in severely ill ICU patients receiving a high-dose selenium monotherapy [23]. Based on the two most recent studies about selenium supplementation in critically ill patients, a following meta-analysis could not anymore demonstrate a clinically meaningful effect of selenium in these patients [24].

Recently, a large-scale RCT evaluated the potential clinical significance of a high-dose selenium supplementation, which was given perioperatively in patients scheduled to undergo cardiac surgery with increased risk for postoperative complications. Despite the demonstrated efficacy to compensate the well-known preoperative selenium deficiencies and the frequently observed significant decrease of intraoperative selenium levels, no difference could be detected between the treatment groups with respect to the development of postoperative organ dysfunctions. Yet, based on an embedded lab study, it could be demonstrated that potential confounding factors, such as the patients' comorbidities and co-medications inhibited the translation of high selenium levels in an increase of the antioxidant acting glutathione peroxidase, so that more investigations are needed to further carefully observe such factors. Based on the currently existing evidence, the dietary-recommended intake (DRI) of 55 μg/day [20–90 μg/day] should be considered, but no recommendations can be given for dosages beyond these. In situation of acute inflammation or sepsis, alone or associated with increased intake of copper and zinc according to previous European and American nutrition society recommendations, however, higher doses might be worth to be considered [25].

8.4.2 Zinc

In a comparable manner, observational studies demonstrated a significant decrease of the essential trace element zinc, whereas the extend of inflammation inversely correlated with the measured blood levels of this mineral. Furthermore, previous studies demonstrated that circulating zinc levels were closely related to markers of inflammation, and low zinc levels were associated with the development of organ dysfunctions and ultimately mortality [26, 27]. Yet, it still remains controversial whether a decrease of zinc levels results from the acute-phase response, or if the zinc is bound to the endothelium, transporter enzymes or simply re-distributed into different body components. Although a compensation of such deficiency would obviously be desirable to prevent a further suppression of the immune competence and prevent the development of secondary infections, current guidelines cannot give recommendations about zinc supplementation in septic patients due to absence of adequately designed interventional studies.

An RCT of 100 patients with severe head trauma demonstrated a remarkable increase in zinc plasma concentrations and urinary excretion [28], which was in accordance with another RCT of 68 patients with severe head trauma, where no statistically relevant differences could be demonstrated between both groups with respect to the clinical outcomes [29].

A recent meta-analysis reported no difference in mortality with zinc supplementation when combining these trials with limited confidence in the results ($n = 168$, relative risk 0.73 (95% confidence intervals 0.41-1.28)) [30]. In a meta-analysis of four RCTs and four non-randomized studies of patients with severe burn injury ($n = 398$), intravenous combined zinc, selenium and copper after burn injury decrease infectious complications (95% CI: -1.70, -0.80, $P < 0.00001$). There was no evidence to support an effect of combined supplementation on overall mortality or LOS in patients with severe burn injury [31].

8.4.3 Vitamin C

Vitamin C is an essential, water-soluble micronutrient, which acts as electron donor in multiple reactions and thus exerts many crucial functions in the human body. Vitamin C is required for more than 60 enzymatic reactions, restores vascular responsiveness to vasoconstrictors, ameliorates microcirculatory blood flow, preserves endothelial barriers, prevents apoptosis and augments the bacterial defence [32–34]. Based on its redox-potential and powerful antioxidant capacity, vitamin C has been called the most important antioxidant, scavenging free radicals and thereby preventing damage to macromolecules, such as lipids or DNA [35]. Vitamin C showed organo-protective effects in the nervous, cardiovascular, respiratory, gastrointestinal, coagulation and immune systems in preclinical and clinical trials [36].

Vitamin C concentrations are lowered in severe illness, in patients recovering from surgery, in patients after cardiac surgery and in patients developing multiorgan failure as shown by observational studies. Supplementation of vitamin C in the general ICU population was not associated with an overall reduced risk of mortality, infection, or hospital length-of-stay, but a different meta-analysis showed decrease in duration of mechanical ventilation and ICU stay [37–40].

Notably, Marik et al. introduced the concept that an adjuvant treatment with corticosteroids alone [41], or in combination with intravenous vitamin C and thiamine, may improve outcomes of critically ill patients with septic shock [42]. These so-called metabolic resuscitation strategies therefore may expand the current management of sepsis by a combined application of hydrocortisone, ascorbate, and thiamine, which should be started timely together with early initiation of antibiotics, fluids and norepinephrine. A published retrospective before-after study provided the first evidence of the beneficial effects of this concept by a significantly reduced SOFA score and mortality in this group [42]. However, following systematic reviews could not confirm any significant effects of combined vitamin C strategies, whereas strong beneficial effects were detected when vitamin C was given as high-dose single strategy [43].

Building up on the following vitamin C pioneer trial, which demonstrated a survival benefit of high-dose vitamin C in patients with ARDS [44], the so-called LOVIT trial was conducted to evaluate the clinical significance of high-dose vitamin C in patients with sepsis. The primary endpoint of this study was a composite endpoint of death or persistent organ dysfunction, which was significantly higher in patients who received high-dose vitamin C at 50 mg/kg/6 h [45]. Potential explanations for this surprising finding were discussed extensively and could be due to the imbalances in the baseline characteristics (sicker patients in treatment group) or heterogeneity in the application strategy [46] and fact that a high number of patients were transferred from other ICUs, so that the treatment might have been initiated too late to translate into a clinically meaningful difference [47]. Furthermore, a recently published study highlighted the importance of a prolonged treatment duration, so the used treatment period (mostly 4 days) may have been too short to translate into clinically meaningful results. Importantly, the most recent SRMA including the LOVIT trial still demonstrated a significant reduction of 30-day or hospital mortality in the intravenous vitamin C monotherapy subgroup [48], whereas a high statistical heterogeneity reduces the certainty of this finding.

Overall, given the unique pleiotropic functions of vitamin C, it still has to be evaluated if other risk patient populations who are exposed to inflammation, ischemia/reperfusion or oxidative stress, such as patients after cardiac arrest, cardiac surgery, polytrauma and burn trauma, ischemic stroke, or undergoing major surgical procedures, benefit from this intervention [49–52].

8.4.4 Vitamin D

Vitamin D3 (cholecalciferol), a precursor of a potent steroid hormone, is absorbed from food sources or produced by the skin in the presence of sunlight. Vitamin D insufficiency defined as 25-hydroxy-vitamin-D [25(OH)D] serum levels ≤20 ng/mL (equals 50 nmol/L) is reported in 40–70% of all ICU patients and is associated with an increased risk of mortality, organ dysfunctions, infections, prolonged ICU and hospital stay as well as expanded duration of mechanical ventilation [53]. While the largest prospective interventional trial including 492 critically ill patients failed to show beneficial effects of high-dose (540.000 IU) oral cholecalciferol supplementation in the general ICU population, a significantly reduced risk of 28-day mortality has been observed in a subgroup of patients with severe 25(OH)D deficit <12 ng/mL (equals 30 nmol/L) [54]. An earlier meta-analysis showed incongruent results regarding the effect of vitamin D supplementation on mortality in ICU patients [53, 55] possibly due to small sample sizes (less than 750 patients analysed) and a heterogeneous study procedure with respect to vitamin D deficiency, study drug (active vs. inactive vitamin D), dosage (200.000–540.000 IU) and timing (up to 72 h after ICU admission). In contrast, patients receiving prehospital vitamin D supplements had significantly shorter ICU stay, days of mechanical ventilation and rates of mortality [56], supporting the importance of the availability of biological active vitamin D at the time of acute illness.

A recent multicentre, randomized, double-blind, placebo-controlled phase III trial of 1360 patients at high risk for ARDS and mortality showed no benefit from high-dose vitamin D3 supplementation [57]. A following meta-analysis aggregated currently available evidence and included 16 RCTs with 2449 patients [58]. The received data demonstrated that vitamin D administration was associated with lower overall mortality rates, reduced intensive care unit length of stay and shorter duration of mechanical ventilation. Notably, it was further demonstrated that the parenteral administration of vitamin D was associated with a greater effect on overall mortality than enteral administration [58]. Another large ongoing vitamin D trial in ICU patients (NCT 03188796) will provide more evidence in this field.

Therefore, although being inexpensive, but effective to raise 25(OH)D serum levels, it still needs to be clarified if supplementation leads to improved clinical outcomes in vitamin D deficient ICU patients [53]. The evidence to date does not support the use of single high-dose vitamin D in all critically ill patients, whereas a deficit should be treated with daily doses.

8.4.5 Glutamine

The several potent immune modulating properties of glutamine resulted in many clinical studies, testing its relevance in different clinical settings. Plasma glutamine levels have repeatedly been shown to be low during critical illness, and low values were associated with poor outcome. In fact, older studies demonstrated the clinical significance of glutamine supplementations if given enterally or parenterally in smaller groups of critically ill patients [59–61].

Yet, based on current evidence, influenced by the REDOX study that demonstrated significantly higher mortality in those patients who received glutamine compared with those who did not [22], led to meta-analysis demonstrating no overall significant benefits on mortality, infections or hospital length of stay in patients suffering from burn, trauma, and in mixed ICU populations [12]. Therefore, the additional application of glutamine is not anymore recommended in the routine of critically ill patients.

Notably, based on the results received from few smaller studies, indicating significant benefits of glutamine in patients with burn injuries and trauma [62], current guidelines still emphasized the potential role of glutamine for these patients if given enterally as low dose [13]. Yet, most recent data could not provide evidence for its use: the Re-Energize study was a double-blind, randomized, placebo-controlled trial, which assigned patients with deep second- or third-degree burns to receive enterally delivered glutamine or placebo to evaluate its clinical significance [63]. No effect on the primary endpoint, the time to discharge alive from the hospital or any secondary endpoint could be demonstrated. A following meta-analysis, which included the data received from the Re-Energize study, showed that glutamine supplementation, regardless of administration, does not appear to improve clinical outcomes in patients with severe burn injuries, so that actual recommendations for its use have to be adapted to consider this evidence [64].

8.5 Special Groups of Critically Ill Patients

While most interventional studies were conducted in ICU-patients with sepsis or septic shock, the hitherto received results cannot be easily transferred to other groups of critically ill patients. For example, although recent meta-analyses could not demonstrate a positive effect of selenium supplementation in patients with sepsis, a subgroup analysis revealed that there was a positive effect of parenteral selenium supplementation on the reduction of infectious complications in RCTS of non-septic patients [24]. Based on these results, further studies in specific subgroups of critical illness need to evaluate if a high-dose micronutrient supplementation may lead to clinically meaningful effects. In this context, Berger et al. reported earlier that this strategy might be of special relevance in patients with trauma or burn injuries [18]. In this context, the recent ASPEN guidelines further noted that, based on their own meta-analysis, the administration of antioxidants and trace elements can be considered in critically ill patients with burns and trauma requiring mechanical ventilation, as it was demonstrated to be associated with a significant reduction in overall mortality (RR = 0.8; 95% CI 0.7–0.92; $P = 0.001$), whereas infectious complications, ICU or hospital length of stay, and duration of mechanical ventilation were not significantly different between patients groups. Based on these results, further studies in critically ill patients, others than septic patients, are still required.

8.6 Why Did Several Studies in the Past Fail to Demonstrate Beneficial Effects?

Although inflammation and oxidative stress represent attractive therapeutic targets in critical illness so that antioxidants have been tested in critically ill patients for decades, overall results remain inconsistent without clear clinical meaningful effects. The reasons for this are matter of ongoing debates and remain speculative. Some might argue, the heterogeneity in trials regarding patients, diseases and supplementation makes it difficult to aggregate the resulting evidence. Attempts to carefully identify these patients who may benefit most from pharmaconutrient supplementation are still missing. Further, the heterogeneity in dosing, timing, combination, or delivery of antioxidants remains problematic. Last, the timing of initiating an anti-inflammatory and anti-oxidant strategy seems of high importance, as it often may simply be too late for a specific intervention to translate into clinically meaningful effects. This might be of special relevance in patients with sepsis, as the time point of onset of sepsis often occurred several hours to day before admission to an ICU, so that the accompanying inflammatory response in such patients might be too advanced to be a target for an inflammatory strategy. Further, Jain et al. speculated that adverse off-target effects may have contributed to their failure, as ROS are critical signalling molecules for cell homeostasis and adaptation to stress (e.g., hypoxia) processes and that their positive effects may be neutralized with antioxidants [65]. Patients with sepsis commonly show a period of relative immunosuppression after the initial cytokine storm, during which they are at increased risk of nosocomial infection or viral reactivation. Regarding the important role of ROS in activating lymphocytes and monocytes, it remains speculative if the ROS production contributes to the variability in inflammatory responses and immune competence. Therefore, the timing of pharmaconutrient-supplementation seems to play a crucial role and may have been too late in recent studies performed in critically ill patients. Here, the use of antioxidants may be beneficial during the initial acute phase of exaggerated inflammatory responses but may be detrimental during periods of relative immunosuppression [6]. In contrast, patients undergoing major surgical procedures are known to be exposed to an intense inflammatory response as part of the perioperative inflammatory response. The scheduled setting of some surgeries may thus open the chance for a preoperative optimization strategy to restore endogenous antioxidants by supplementing vitamins or trace elements alone or in various combinations in these patients.

References

1. Knoell DL, Julian MW, Bao S, et al. Zinc deficiency increases organ damage and mortality in a murine model of polymicrobial sepsis*. Crit Care Med. 2009;37:1380–8. https://doi.org/10.1097/CCM.0b013e31819cefe4.
2. Forceville X, Vitoux D, Gauzit R, et al. Selenium, systemic immune response syndrome, sepsis, and outcome in critically ill patients. Crit Care Med. 1998;26:1536–44.
3. Heyland DK, Dhaliwal R, Suchner U, Berger MM. Antioxidant nutrients: a systematic review of trace elements and vitamins in the critically ill patient. Intensive Care Med. 2004;31:327–37. https://doi.org/10.1007/s00134-004-2522-z.
4. Stoppe C, Nesterova E, Elke G. Nutritional support in patients with extracorporeal life support and ventricular assist devices. Curr Opin Crit Care. 2018;24:269–76. https://doi.org/10.1097/MCC.0000000000000512.
5. Manzanares W, Biestro A, Torre MH, et al. High-dose selenium reduces ventilator-associated pneumonia and illness severity in critically ill patients with systemic inflammation. Intensive Care Med. 2011;37:1120–7. https://doi.org/10.1007/s00134-011-2212-6.
6. Hotchkiss RS, Monneret G, Payen D. Sepsis-induced immunosuppression: from cellular dysfunctions to immunotherapy. Nat Rev Immunol. 2013;13:862–74. https://doi.org/10.1038/nri3552.
7. Fry DE. Sepsis, systemic inflammatory response, and multiple organ dysfunction: the mystery continues. Am Surg. 2012;78:1–8.
8. Berger MM, Chiolro RL. Antioxidant supplementation in sepsis and systemic inflammatory response syndrome. Crit Care Med. 2007;35:S584–90. https://doi.org/10.1097/01.CCM.0000279189.81529.C4.
9. Mertens K, Lowes DA, Webster NR, et al. Low zinc and selenium concentrations in sepsis are associated with oxidative damage and inflammation. Br J Anaesth. 2015;114:990–9. https://doi.org/10.1093/bja/aev073.
10. Preiser J-C. Oxidative stress. J Parenter Enter Nutr. 2012;36:147–54. https://doi.org/10.1177/0148607111434963.
11. Gudivada KK, Kumar A, Shariff M, Sampath S, Varma MM, Sivakoti S, Krishna B. Antioxidant micronutrient supplementation in critically ill adults: a systematic review with meta-analysis and trial sequential analysis. Clin Nutr. 2021;40:740–50. https://doi.org/10.1016/j.clnu.2020.06.033. Epub 2020 Jul 14. PMID: 32723509. Manzanares W, Dhaliwal R, Jiang X, et al. Antioxidant micronutrients in the critically ill: a systematic review and meta-analysis. Crit Care. 2012;16:R66. https://doi.org/10.1186/cc11316
12. McClave SA, Taylor BE, Martindale RG, et al. Guidelines for the provision and assessment of nutrition support therapy in the adult critically ill patient: Society of Critical Care Medicine (SCCM) and American Society for Parenteral and Enteral Nutrition (A.S.P.E.N.). J Parenter Enter Nutr. 2016;40:159–211. https://doi.org/10.1177/0148607115621863.
13. Singer P, Blaser AR, Berger MM, et al. ESPEN guideline on clinical nutrition in the intensive care unit. Clin Nutr. 2019;38:48–79. https://doi.org/10.1016/j.clnu.2018.08.037.
14. Berger MM, Shenkin A, Schweinlin A, Amrein K, Augsburger M, Biesalski HK, Bischoff SC, Casaer MP, Gundogan K, Lepp HL, de Man AME, Muscogiuri G, Pietka M, Pironi L, Rezzi S, Cuerda C. ESPEN micronutrient guideline. Clin Nutr. 2022;41:1357–424. https://doi.org/10.1016/j.clnu.2022.02.015. Epub 2022 Feb 26. PMID: 35365361
15. Manzanares W, Biestro A, Galusso F, et al. Serum selenium and glutathione peroxidase-3 activity: biomarkers of systemic inflammation in the critically ill? Intensive Care Med. 2008;35:882–9. https://doi.org/10.1007/s00134-008-1356-5.
16. Benstoem C, Goetzenich A, Kraemer S, et al. Selenium and its supplementation in cardiovascular disease-what do we know? Nutrients. 2015;7:3094–118. https://doi.org/10.3390/nu7053094.

17. Stoppe C, Schälte G, Rossaint R, et al. The intraoperative decrease of selenium is associated with the postoperative development of multiorgan dysfunction in cardiac surgical patients. Crit Care Med. 2011;39:1879–85. https://doi.org/10.1097/CCM.0b013e3182190d48.
18. Berger MM, Soguel L, Shenkin A, et al. Influence of early antioxidant supplements on clinical evolution and organ function in critically ill cardiac surgery, major trauma, and subarachnoid hemorrhage patients. Crit Care. 2008;12:R101. https://doi.org/10.1186/cc6981.
19. Stoppe C, Spillner J, Rossaint R, et al. Selenium blood concentrations in patients undergoing elective cardiac surgery and receiving perioperative sodium selenite administration. Nutrition. 2013;29:158–65. https://doi.org/10.1016/j.nut.2012.05.013.
20. Huang T-S, Shyu Y-C, Chen H-Y, et al. Effect of parenteral selenium supplementation in critically ill patients: a systematic review and meta-analysis. PLoS One. 2013;8:e54431. https://doi.org/10.1371/journal.pone.0054431.
21. Bloos F, Trips E, Nierhaus A, et al. Effect of sodium selenite administration and procalcitonin-guided therapy on mortality in patients with severe sepsis or septic shock: a randomized clinical trial. JAMA Intern Med. 2016;176:1266–76. https://doi.org/10.1001/jamainternmed.2016.2514.
22. Heyland D, Muscedere J, Wischmeyer PE, et al. A randomized trial of glutamine and antioxidants in critically ill patients. N Engl J Med. 2013;368:1489–97. https://doi.org/10.1056/NEJMoa1212722.
23. Angstwurm MWA, Engelmann L, Zimmermann T, et al. Selenium in Intensive Care (SIC): results of a prospective randomized, placebo-controlled, multiple-center study in patients with severe systemic inflammatory response syndrome, sepsis, and septic shock*. Crit Care Med. 2007;35:118–26. https://doi.org/10.1097/01.CCM.0000251124.83436.0E.
24. Manzanares W, Lemieux M, Elke G, et al. High-dose intravenous selenium does not improve clinical outcomes in the critically ill: a systematic review and meta-analysis. Crit Care. 2016;20:356. https://doi.org/10.1186/s13054-016-1529-5.
25. Stoppe C, McDonald B, Meybohm P, Christopher KB, Fremes S, Whitlock R, Mohammadi S, Kalavrouziotis D, Elke G, Rossaint R, Helmer P, Zacharowski K, Günther U, Parotto M, Niemann B, Böning A, Mazer CD, Jones PM, Ferner M, Lamarche Y, Lamontagne F, Liakopoulos OJ, Cameron M, Müller M, Zarbock A, Wittmann M, Goetzenich A, Kilger E, Schomburg L, Day AG, Heyland DK, SUSTAIN CSX Study Collaborators. Effect of high-dose selenium on postoperative organ dysfunction and mortality in cardiac surgery patients: the SUSTAIN CSX Randomized Clinical Trial. JAMA Surg. 2023;158:235–44. https://doi.org/10.1001/jamasurg.2022.6855. PMID: 36630120; PMCID: PMC9857635
26. Shanley TP, Cvijanovich N, Lin R, et al. Genome-level longitudinal expression of signaling pathways and gene networks in pediatric septic shock. Mol Med. 2007;13:495–508. https://doi.org/10.2119/2007-00065.Shanley.
27. Besecker BY, Exline MC, Hollyfield J, et al. A comparison of zinc metabolism, inflammation, and disease severity in critically ill infected and noninfected adults early after intensive care unit admission. Am J Clin Nutr. 2011;93:1356–64. https://doi.org/10.3945/ajcn.110.008417.
28. Khazdouz M, Mazidi M, Ehsaei MR, Ferns G, Kengne AP, Norouzy AR. Impact of zinc supplementation on the clinical outcomes of patients with severe head trauma: a double-blind randomized clinical trial. J Diet Suppl. 2018;15:1–10.
29. Young B, Ott L, Kasarskis E, Rapp R, Moles K, Dempsey RJ, et al. Zinc supplementation is associated with improved neurologic recovery rate and visceral protein levels of patients with severe closed head injury. J Neurotrauma. 1996;13:25–34.
30. Vesterlund GK, Jensen TS, Ellekjaer KL, Moller MH, Thomsen T, Perner A. Effects of magnesium, phosphate, or zinc supplementation in intensive care unit patients-a systematic review and meta-analysis. Acta Anaesthesiol Scand. 2023;67:264–76.
31. Kurmis R, Greenwood J, Aromataris E. Trace element supplementation following severe burn injury: A systematic review and meta-analysis. J Burn Care Res. 2016;37:143–59. https://doi.org/10.1097/BCR.0000000000000259. PMID: 26056754
32. Tyml K. Vitamin C and microvascular dysfunction in systemic inflammation. Antioxidants (Basel). 2017;6:49. https://doi.org/10.3390/antiox6030049.

33. Oudemans-van Straaten HM, Spoelstra-de Man AM, de Waard MC. Vitamin C revisited. Crit Care. 2014;18:460. https://doi.org/10.1186/s13054-014-0460-x.
34. Yamamoto T, Kinoshita M, Shinomiya N, et al. Pretreatment with ascorbic acid prevents lethal gastrointestinal syndrome in mice receiving a massive amount of radiation. J Radiat Res. 2010;51:145–56.
35. Berger MM, Oudemans-van Straaten HM. Vitamin C supplementation in the critically ill patient. Curr Opin Clin Nutr Metab Care. 2015;18:193–201. https://doi.org/10.1097/MCO.0000000000000148.
36. Hill A, Wendt S, Benstoem C, et al. Vitamin C to improve organ dysfunction in cardiac surgery patients-review and pragmatic approach. Nutrients. 2018;10:974. https://doi.org/10.3390/nu10080974.
37. Spoelstra-de Man AME, Elbers PWG, Oudemans-van Straaten HM. Making sense of early high-dose intravenous vitamin C in ischemia/reperfusion injury. Crit Care. 2018;22:70. https://doi.org/10.1186/s13054-018-1996-y.
38. Borrelli E, Roux-Lombard P, Grau GE, et al. Plasma concentrations of cytokines, their soluble receptors, and antioxidant vitamins can predict the development of multiple organ failure in patients at risk. Crit Care Med. 1996;24:392–7.
39. Langlois PL, Manzanares W, Adhikari NKJ, et al. Vitamin C administration to the critically ill: a systematic review and meta-analysis. JPEN J Parenter Enteral Nutr. 2019;43:335–46. https://doi.org/10.1002/jpen.1471.
40. Hemilä H, Chalker E. Vitamin C can shorten the length of stay in the ICU: a meta-analysis. Nutrients. 2019;11:708. https://doi.org/10.3390/nu11040708.
41. Annane D, Renault A, Brun-Buisson C, et al. Hydrocortisone plus fludrocortisone for adults with septic shock. N Engl J Med. 2018;378:809–18. https://doi.org/10.1056/NEJMoa1705716.
42. Marik PE, Khangoora V, Rivera R, et al. Hydrocortisone, vitamin C, and thiamine for the treatment of severe sepsis and septic shock: a retrospective before-after study. Chest. 2017;151:1229–38. https://doi.org/10.1016/j.chest.2016.11.036.
43. Stoppe C, Lee ZY, Ortiz L, Heyland DK, Patel JJ. The potential role of intravenous vitamin C monotherapy in critical illness. JPEN J Parenter Enteral Nutr. 2022;46:972–6. https://doi.org/10.1002/jpen.2338. Epub 2022 Feb 13. PMID: 35088422
44. Fowler AA 3rd, Truwit JD, Hite RD, Morris PE, DeWilde C, Priday A, Fisher B, Thacker LR 2nd, Natarajan R, Brophy DF, Sculthorpe R, Nanchal R, Syed A, Sturgill J, Martin GS, Sevransky J, Kashiouris M, Hamman S, Egan KF, Hastings A, Spencer W, Tench S, Mehkri O, Bindas J, Duggal A, Graf J, Zellner S, Yanny L, McPolin C, Hollrith T, Kramer D, Ojielo C, Damm T, Cassity E, Wieliczko A, Halquist M. Effect of vitamin C infusion on organ failure and biomarkers of inflammation and vascular injury in patients with sepsis and severe acute respiratory failure: the CITRIS-ALI randomized clinical trial. JAMA. 2019;322:1261–70. https://doi.org/10.1001/jama.2019.11825. Erratum in: JAMA 2020 Jan 28;323(4):379. PMID: 31573637; PMCID: PMC6777268
45. Lamontagne F, Masse MH, Menard J, Sprague S, Pinto R, Heyland DK, Cook DJ, Battista MC, Day AG, Guyatt GH, Kanji S, Parke R, McGuinness SP, Tirupakuzhi Vijayaraghavan BK, Annane D, Cohen D, Arabi YM, Bolduc B, Marinoff N, Rochwerg B, Millen T, Meade MO, Hand L, Watpool I, Porteous R, Young PJ, D'Aragon F, Belley-Cote EP, Carbonneau E, Clarke F, Maslove DM, Hunt M, Chassé M, Lebrasseur M, Lauzier F, Mehta S, Quiroz-Martinez H, Rewa OG, Charbonney E, Seely AJE, Kutsogiannis DJ, LeBlanc R, Mekontso-Dessap A, Mele TS, Turgeon AF, Wood G, Kohli SS, Shahin J, Twardowski P, Adhikari NKJ, LOVIT Investigators and the Canadian Critical Care Trials Group. Intravenous vitamin C in adults with sepsis in the intensive care unit. N Engl J Med. 2022;386:2387–98. https://doi.org/10.1056/NEJMoa2200644. Epub 2022 Jun 15. PMID: 35704292
46. Stoppe C, Hill A, Christopher KB, Kristof AS. Toward Precision in Nutrition Therapy. Crit Care Med. 2025;53(2):e429–e440. https://doi.org/10.1097/CCM.0000000000006537. Epub 2024 Dec 17. PMID: 39688452; PMCID: PMC11801434.

47. Stoppe C, Preiser JC, de Backer D, Elke G. Intravenous vitamin C in adults with sepsis in the intensive care unit: still LOV'IT? Crit Care. 2022;26:230. https://doi.org/10.1186/s13054-022-04106-w. PMID: 35908003; PMCID: PMC9339181
48. Lee ZY, Ortiz-Reyes L, Lew CCH, Hasan MS, Ke L, Patel JJ, et al. Intravenous vitamin C monotherapy in critically ill patients: a systematic review and meta-analysis of randomized controlled trials with trial sequential analysis. Ann Intensive Care. 2023;13:14.
49. Rozemeijer S, de Grooth HJ, Elbers PWG, Girbes ARJ, den Uil CA, Dubois EA, et al. Early high-dose vitamin C in post-cardiac arrest syndrome (VITaCCA): study protocol for a randomized, double-blind, multi-center, placebo-controlled trial. Trials. 2021;22:546.
50. Hill A, Clasen KC, Wendt S, Majoros AG, Stoppe C, Adhikari NK, et al. Correction: Hill, A.; et al. Effects of vitamin C on organ function in cardiac surgery patients: a systematic review and meta-analysis. *Nutrients*. 2019, 11, 2103. Nutrients. 2020;12:3910.
51. Berger MM. Antioxidant micronutrients in major trauma and burns: evidence and practice. Nutr Clin Pract. 2006;21:438–49.
52. Sanchez-Moreno C, Dashe JF, Scott T, Thaler D, Folstein MF, Martin A. Decreased levels of plasma vitamin C and increased concentrations of inflammatory and oxidative stress markers after stroke. Stroke. 2004;35:163–8.
53. Amrein K, Papinutti A, Mathew E, et al. Vitamin D and critical illness: what endocrinology can learn from intensive care and vice versa. Endocr Connect. 2018;7:R304–15. https://doi.org/10.1530/EC-18-0184.
54. Amrein K, Schnedl C, Holl A, et al. Effect of high-dose vitamin D3 on hospital length of stay in critically ill patients with vitamin D deficiency: the VITdAL-ICU randomized clinical trial. JAMA. 2014;312:1520–30. https://doi.org/10.1001/jama.2014.13204.
55. Langlois PL, Szwec C, D'Aragon F, et al. Vitamin D supplementation in the critically ill: a systematic review and meta-analysis. Clin Nutr. 2018;37:1238–46. https://doi.org/10.1016/j.clnu.2017.05.006.
56. Leclair TR, Zakai N, Bunn JY, et al. Vitamin D supplementation in mechanically ventilated patients in the medical intensive care unit. JPEN J Parenter Enteral Nutr. 2019;144:74. https://doi.org/10.1002/jpen.1520.
57. Ginde AA, Brower RG, Caterino JM, Finck L, Banner-Goodspeed VM, Grissom CK, Hayden D, Hough CL, Hyzy RC, Khan A, et al. Early high-dose vitamin D3 for critically ill, vitamin D-deficient patients. N Engl J Med. 2019;381:2529–40. https://doi.org/10.1056/NEJMoa1911124.
58. Menger J, Lee ZY, Notz Q, Wallqvist J, Hasan MS, Elke G, Dworschak M, Meybohm P, Heyland DK, Stoppe C. Administration of vitamin D and its metabolites in critically ill adult patients: an updated systematic review with meta-analysis of randomized controlled trials. Crit Care. 2022;26:268. https://doi.org/10.1186/s13054-022-04139-1. PMID: 36068584; PMCID: PMC9446655
59. Pasin L, Landoni G, Zangrillo A. Glutamine and antioxidants in critically ill patients. N Engl J Med. 2013;369:482–4. https://doi.org/10.1056/NEJMc1306658.
60. Fadda V, Maratea D, Trippoli S, Messori A. Temporal trend of short-term mortality in severely ill patients receiving parenteral glutamine supplementation. Clin Nutr. 2013;32:492–3. https://doi.org/10.1016/j.clnu.2013.01.017.
61. Stehle P, Ellger B, Kojic D, et al. Glutamine dipeptide-supplemented parenteral nutrition improves the clinical outcomes of critically ill patients: a systematic evaluation of randomised controlled trials. Clin Nutr ESPEN. 2017;17:75–85. https://doi.org/10.1016/j.clnesp.2016.09.007.
62. van Zanten ARH, Dhaliwal R, Garrel D, Heyland DK. Enteral glutamine supplementation in critically ill patients: a systematic review and meta-analysis. Crit Care. 2015;19:294. https://doi.org/10.1186/s13054-015-1002-x.

63. Heyland DK, Wibbenmeyer L, Pollack JA, Friedman B, Turgeon AF, Eshraghi N, Jeschke MG, Bélisle S, Grau D, Mandell S, Velamuri SR, Hundeshagen G, Moiemen N, Shokrollahi K, Foster K, Huss F, Collins D, Savetamal A, Gurney JM, Depetris N, Stoppe C, Ortiz-Reyes L, Garrel D, Day AG, RE-ENERGIZE Trial Team. A randomized trial of enteral glutamine for treatment of burn injuries. N Engl J Med. 2022;387:1001–10. https://doi.org/10.1056/NEJMoa2203364. Epub 2022 Sep 9. PMID: 36082909

64. Ortiz-Reyes L, Lee ZY, Lew CH, Hill A, Jeschke MG, Turgeon AF, Cancio L, Stoppe C, Patel JJ, Day AG, Heyland DK. The efficacy of glutamine supplementation in severe adult burn patients: a systematic review with trial sequential meta-analysis. Crit Care Med. 2023;51:1086–95. https://doi.org/10.1097/CCM.0000000000005887. Epub 2023 Apr 28. PMID: 37114912

65. Jain M, Chandel NS. Rethinking antioxidants in the intensive care unit. Am J Respir Crit Care Med. 2013;188:1283–5. https://doi.org/10.1164/rccm.201307-1380CP.

Excel Worksheet for Calculating an Adapted Nutrition Plan

9

Ulrich Fauth

9.1 Properties of the Excel Worksheet

In generally, an Excel worksheet enables a quick calculation of the dosage of enteral and parenteral solutions in the context of artificial nutrition. The user is supported in determining the requirements for water, carbohydrates, amino acids, and fat, and the infusion volumes are calculated after selecting the solutions to be used. Mixed enteral/parenteral nutrition is taken into account, as is the supply of fat-containing medication via syringe pumps.

Discontinuous regimes with night breaks can be taken into account when calculating the infusion rates. Calculated requirements and intake via the determined nutritional regime are shown in tabular form for the main ingredients. The names and compositions of the solutions used can be freely selected. The structure of the calculations is open so that the functionality of the file can be changed and extended by the user if required.

9.2 Structure and Functional Principle of the File

The calculations are simple and easy to understand based on the shapes visible in the file. They are carried out in the following steps:

U. Fauth (Retired) (✉)
Kassel, Germany
e-mail: ulrichfauth@ulrichfauth.de

© The Author(s), under exclusive license to Springer Nature
Switzerland AG 2025
A. Rümelin et al. (eds.), *Nutrition in ICU Patients*,
https://doi.org/10.1007/978-3-032-00818-3_9

Steps for Calculating the Dosage of Enteral and Parenteral Solutions

- Input of anthropometric data (user).
- Determination of the need for water and energy-supplying substances.
- Determining the proportion of enteral intake (user).
- Determining the supply of other relevant solutions (electrolyte solutions, syringe pumps, fat-containing medication, e.g., propofol; hemofiltration with citrate-buffered replacement solution) (user).
- Calculation of the ingredients to be supplemented by parenteral means until required.
- Calculation of the dosage of infusion solutions to cover the parenteral portion.
- Rounding the calculated infusion volumes to the desired values.
- Calculation of the infusion rates for the parenteral solutions.

Before use on the patient, the names and compositions of the solutions must be defined in the "Solutions" sheet. Like the other spreadsheets, the sheet is protected without a password when the file is delivered. The Excel function "Unprotect sheet" removes the write protection of the sheet. After entering the data, it is essential to set write protection with a password again to prevent accidental changes by the user. All entries, calculations, and outputs in the context of the nutrition calculation are made in the "Plan" worksheet. The required steps are processed in the table from top to bottom. Only fields that require or allow an entry can be changed (after setting the sheet protection). All other fields are locked. Selectable fields have the colors green and blue. The fields for selecting solutions and some infusion rates can alternatively be set via slide switches positioned to the right of the input field. Some fields have a comment (red triangle at the top right of the field), which is displayed when the cursor is moved over the field. The locked fields can also be selected so that the stored formulas are visible.

9.3 Possibilities and Limitations of the Procedure, Practical Experience

The file should enable simple calculation of water and nutrient requirements as well as dosing of the enteral and parenteral solutions required to cover requirements.

In principle, all calculations can also be carried out on a pocket calculator. However, the time required would not be feasible in the routine operation of an averagely staffed intensive care unit.

Despite these limitations, the Excel sheet has been in use in various intensive care units for many years and has proven to be a simple, time-saving, and sufficiently accurate tool to support the creation of nutrition plans. In particular, the routine use of the method avoids overly crude artificial feeding based solely on bottles and bag volumes, as can occasionally be observed when staffing levels are tight.

9.4 Further Development of the Method

The procedure is based on simple balancing calculations and the functions provided in Excel. With the version presented, the possibilities of this methodological approach are largely exhausted. The consideration of further parenteral components of the patient's therapy (e.g., citrate solution for hemofiltration) may appear desirable. However, it must be remembered that the approach presented here for planning artificial nutrition can only ever be a relatively rough estimate. We do not know the actual requirements of the individual patient, nor the metabolic utilization of the solutions that we administer. In the author's opinion, the consideration of further special cases (beyond propofol sedation) feigns a "pseudo-accuracy" of the calculated nutritional regime that does not stand up to critical assessment.

AI-based approaches are conceivable in principle, but they would require a bidirectional interface between Excel and the AI software used.

It should also be considered to what extent extended functionalities overlap with the functions of patient data management systems (PDMS). These systems cover the majority of conceivable time-dependent functions and process the data within a single system. An Excel-based program can only ever represent a stand-alone solution for special applications, and creating interfaces to the database of a PDMS is unlikely to be trivial.

Children and Adolescents 10

Frank Jochum, Antonia Nomayo, Harry Nomayo, and Hanna Petersen

10.1 Introduction

> Clinical nutrition strategies in children and adolescents differ significantly from those used in adults. This is due to the specific physiology of the maturing body, whose organs and body structures are subject to dynamic development of both functionality and growth.

Pediatric patients are also very different physically: body weight alone ranges from less than 500 g in extremely premature babies to more than 100 kg in obese adolescents. Healthcare professionals must be aware that children have less developed compensatory mechanisms than adults due to lower body reserves and functionally immature metabolic processes. A qualified prescribing practice for an age-adapted diet is required, based on the current individual nutritional needs, with components calculated within narrow margins. Energy and nutrient demands change greatly from birth to late adolescence and can largely fluctuate depending on life situation.

Harry Nomayo died before publication of this work was completed.

F. Jochum (✉)
Ev. Waldkrankenhaus Spandau, Klinik für Kinder- und Jugendmedizin,
Institut für Ernährungsforschung, Berlin, Germany

Medizinische Hochschule Brandenburg, Theodor Fontane (MHB), Neuruppin, Germany
e-mail: frank.jochum@jsd.de

A. Nomayo · H. Petersen
Ev. Waldkrankenhaus Spandau, Klinik für Kinder- und Jugendmedizin,
Institut für Ernährungsforschung, Berlin, Germany

H. Nomayo (Deceased)
Parkstein, Deutschland

The nutritional supply to children should not only provide the energy needed to maintain body functions, but also the quality and quantity of nutrients needed for age-appropriate growth and proper organ development must also be met. An unbalanced diet can compromise the maturation and differentiation of organs and cause irreversible functional impairments (e.g., of the central nervous system). Consequently, fluid, energy, and nutrient intake must be adjusted to the age-specific needs in all developmental stages from early childhood to adolescence. And as in any treatment strategy in pediatric intensive care, nutrition therapy should be tailored to the individual patient.

Physiological principles, nutritional needs for children of various age groups, and practical implementation will be briefly addressed below.

10.2 Physiological Principles

10.2.1 Fluid Balance

Body water content varies with age, decreasing from about 90% in a premature infant born at 24 weeks gestation to about 55–60% in adolescents or adults. Fluid turnover is higher in neonates than in older children due to renal immaturity, higher energy expenditure, greater body surface area as compared to body volume, immature epidermal layer resulting in high insensible perspiration, and rapid body growth (see Fig. 10.1). Likewise, compared to adults, children exhibit reduced water and electrolyte balance regulation mechanisms with lower concentration capacity, lower glomerular filtration capacity, decreased tubular reabsorption, and H+ ion excretion.

In the newborn infant, the very dynamic postnatal adaptation processes pose particular challenges for an adequate fluid and nutrients supply, especially in premature infants. Due to the activation of metabolic and renal functions, the fluid requirement initially increases day by day after birth. Therefore, daily adjustments and specific intake recommendations are crucial during the immediate postnatal period (see Table 10.1).

10.2.2 Energy and Nutrient Requirements

> In relation to body weight, children have higher energy and nutrient requirements than older patients. These increased needs are due to higher (metabolic) activity and body growth. Childhood is characterized by recurring periods of accelerated growth (e.g., the pubertal growth spurt), during which exceptionally high substrate requirements must be met to ensure unimpaired growth and development.

It should also be noted that, unlike adults, premature infants and newborns are unable to synthesize various nutrient substrates from precursors in sufficient

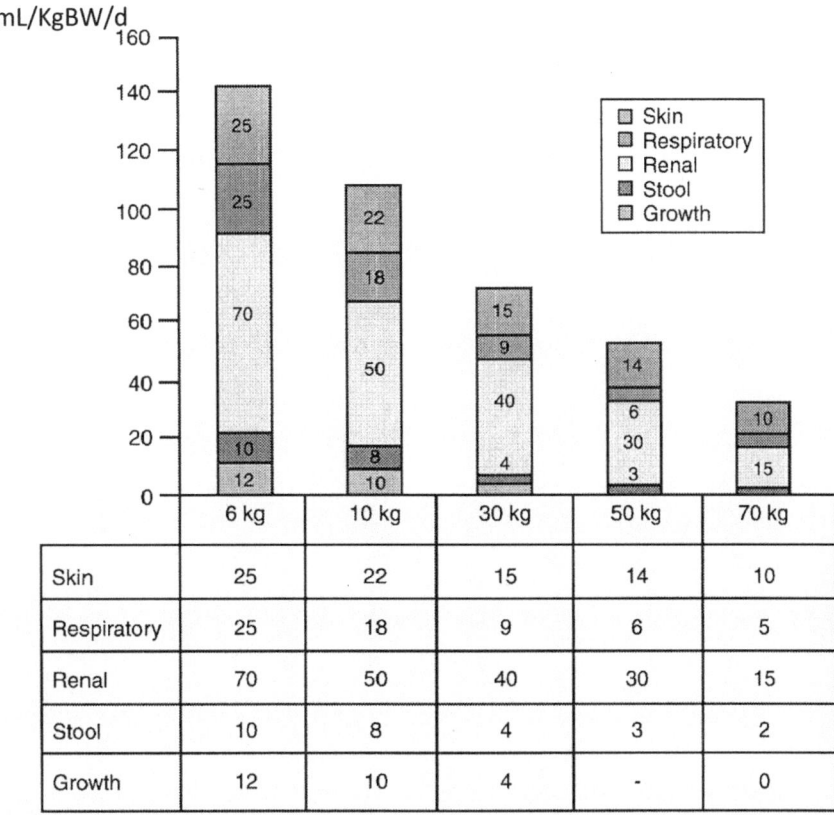

Fig. 10.1 Fluid losses in infants, young children, adolescents, and adults. (Modified after Fusch and Jochum [1])

quantities due to the immaturity of certain enzyme systems. In this specific patient group, these substrates become "conditionally essential" and therefore must be externally supplemented, until a sufficient intrinsic production is ensured upon reaching metabolic maturity.

10.2.3 Food Programming

In addition to the well-known short-term nutritional effects of food intake, there is clear evidence of long-term nutrition-induced metabolic changes during early childhood ("food programming"/Koletzko et al. [2]). During the period from fetal life to late infancy, there appears to be a particular vulnerability to nutrition-related adverse long-term effects, which are not observed in other phases of life, in older children or adults. To prevent unfavorable metabolic imprinting due to imbalanced nutrient intake in early life, which may subsequently increase disease risk in adulthood,

Table 10.1 Recommended fluid supply (in mL/KGBW/d) in preterm and term born neonates during the first days of life

	First day of life	Second day of life	Third day of life	Fourth day of life	Fifth day of life	Intermediate phase of adaptation	Phase of stable growth
Preterm neonates birth weight <1000 g	80–100	100–120	120–140	140–160	160–180	140–160	140–160
Preterm neonates birth weight <1500 g	70–90	90–110	110–130	130–150	160–180	140–160	140–160
Preterm neonates birth weight >1500 g	60–80	80–100	100–120	120–140	140–160	140–160	140–160
Term newborns	40–60	50–70	60–80	60–100	100–140	140–170	140–160

Adapted from Jochum et al. [14]
mL/KGBW/d milliliter per kilogram bodyweight and per day

clinical nutrition strategies should focus on an age-appropriate nutrient composition and quantity to avoid both malnutrition and overfeeding.

10.3 Practical Approach to Nutritional Therapy in Pediatric Patients

> For the reasons mentioned above, a need-oriented nutrient supply is even more important for the younger pediatric patient. With increasing age, improved compensatory and regulatory mechanisms are available to maintain body homeostasis.

Therefore, nutritional recommendations intended for older patient groups, with mere interpolation based on the body weight or body surface, are insufficient to meet the fundamentally differing nutritional needs of the pediatric patient (see above). If available, nutritional products with age-adapted composition (e.g., pediatric infusion solutions) should be used.

> In pediatric patients the choice of the preferred nutritional route (oral, enteral, partially parenteral, or totally parenteral) should always be based on the medical indication and guided by the principle of "as minimally invasive as possible."

This strategic approach is associated with the lowest complication rate. Therefore, oral feeding should be preferred to the greatest possible extent, and whenever possible, the enteral route should be chosen over parenteral access. Total or partial parenteral nutrition should be implemented if the first two options are considered inadequate and should be accompanied by (minimal) enteral nutrition whenever there are no contraindications.

However, in preterm infants below 35 weeks of gestation, full enteral nutrient supply cannot be established immediately after birth due to immaturity of the gastrointestinal system. For these children, (partial) parenteral nutrition will be necessary at least during the first days of life while enteral feeding is introduced gradually.

Standardized formulations and structured prescription processes in (partial) parenteral nutrition therapy have the potential to minimize errors in everyday clinical practice and improve patient safety, especially when feeding premature babies. It is more and more common to use specialized nutrition-calculating software for prescription of (parenteral) nutrition, e.g., in the neonatal intensive care setting. Standardized prescription sheets or nutrient calculators should consider both parenteral and enteral nutrient supply, and respective absorption rates of different nutrients.

10.3.1 Short- or Long-Term Parenteral Nutrition

If sufficient nutrient intake via the natural enteral route cannot be established, parenteral nutrient supply must be initiated to prevent catabolic metabolism. Depending on the current nutritional status, to some extent, the body's electrolyte and micronutrient reserves can be considered, when determining the type of nutritional support. A basic distinction can be made between short- and long-term parenteral nutrition.

> In practice, the infusion of a glucose solution with an adapted potassium and sodium supplementation is sufficient for short-term parenteral nutrition in children with adequate nutritional status and with a low risk of malnutrition. However, if parenteral nutrition is expected to be required for more than 3–7 days, total parenteral nutrition should be provided, including adequate amounts of all macronutrients, electrolytes, minerals (including magnesium, calcium, and phosphate), trace elements, and vitamins. This approach should be considered whenever parenteral nutrition provides >50% of the age-appropriate energy requirements.

10.3.2 Nutritional Support in Critically Ill Children

Although high-level evidence on optimal nutrition practice in pediatric intensive care medicine is scarce, guideline recommendations on basis of expert consensus methodology are available [3, 4]. There is evidence that it may be beneficial to withhold total parenteral nutrition in critically ill children during the early-acute phase of intensive care (approx. first 1–3 days after admission) to prevent a "nutri-trauma," which can be caused by excessive macronutrient intake in the situation of an impaired post-aggression metabolism. On the other hand, malnourishment and macronutrient deficiencies during critical illness have been shown to increase patient morbidity and mortality [5, 6].

In critically ill term neonates and children, it is therefore suggested to initiate nutritional support at (N)ICU admission carefully, starting at the range of or just below predicted resting energy expenditure, while providing micronutrients (trace elements, vitamins, minerals, and electrolytes)—withholding total parenteral nutrition (including the provision of amino acids) can be considered in critically ill children for up to 7 days—while accepting the risk of temporary undernutrition [4].

> In order to avoid growth faltering, loss of body mass, and functional impairments, premature babies on parenteral nutrition should receive at least the basic requirements of macronutrients (protein, carbohydrates, and fat). The clinical phase of critical illness should be carefully monitored and nutrient supply adjusted accordingly depending on the stage of the disease (e.g., increased nutrient supply for tissue repair in the late-acute or convalescence phase may be considered) [7].

10 Children and Adolescents

Enteral nutrition is also the preferred form of nutrient intake for critically ill children. In the absence of any contraindications, early enteral nutrition should be commenced within 24–48 h of admission to the (N)ICU and be gradually increased according to institutional policy, if necessary accompanied by (partial) parenteral nutrient supply [4, 7].

10.3.3 Monitoring

In principle, assessment of the nutritional status is recommended in all pediatric patients, e.g., by routinely performing and evaluating anthropometric measurements, both on admission to the NICU or PICU, and throughout the clinical course [4].

Close monitoring of fluid balance is particularly important in pediatric patients, as their high fluid turnover is accompanied by immature regulatory mechanisms and a higher risk for clinically relevant imbalances (see above). Regular (if necessary, several times a day) clinical assessments, including measurement of body weight and urine output, fluid balance, as well as acid–base status, serum electrolytes, and blood glucose monitoring, are required, especially when starting parenteral nutrition.

In the case of medium- and long-term enteral or parenteral nutrition therapy, in addition to routine clinical examinations, weight, length, and head circumference gain should be documented in growth charts.

Moreover, the following laboratory parameters should be measured at regular intervals (e.g., initially weekly) in adaptation to the clinical situation: acid–base status, blood glucose, electrolytes, hematocrit, blood count with mean corpuscular volume (MCV) and mean corpuscular hemoglobin (MCH), urea, creatinine, transaminases, γ-GT, alkaline phosphatase (AP), urine osmolarity, or specific weight. Once stable conditions have been achieved, the control intervals can be extended. To monitor adequacy in long-term parenteral nutrition therapy for substrates outside of routine diagnostics, relevant surrogate parameters rather than actual serum levels can be determined: low body stores of vitamin B12, folic acid, vitamin B6, copper, or iron may be indicated by deviations in MCV, and serum levels of AP might be an indicator for insufficient calcium intake (elevated AP), or severe zinc deficiency (decreased AP), low vitamin K uptake manifests in abnormal clotting tests, etc. Those routine parameters can be included into regular monitoring in order to avoid specialized laboratory testing, which may require high blood volumes, are expensive, and are often more difficult to interpret. Diagnostics should be expanded to include specific testing (e.g., plasma concentration of vitamins, trace elements, etc.), if clinical signs of deficiencies or excessive intakes are suspected and the use of the above-mentioned indicator tests fails to clarify the clinical situation.

Cave The following information should be considered when monitoring newborn infants:

- In neonates during the first few weeks of life, urine specific weight or osmolarity is of diagnostic significance only if the results show elevated values. Due to renal immaturity, low (or normal) values may be caused by low renal concentrating ability in preterm and term neonates and do not provide reliable information about the fluid balance.
- When treating preterm and term neonates as well as young infants, healthcare professionals must have access to laboratory testing that is equipped with micro-blood volume methods, having in mind that only small sample quantities are attainable.

10.3.4 Methods of Venous Access

The type of access for parenteral nutrition should be chosen individually, taking into account the feasibility, underlying disease, osmolarity of the nutritional solution used, as well as the expected duration of parenteral nutrition. In neonates, the use of peripheral intravenous catheters (PIVCs) is associated with fewer serious complications (e.g., central line–associated bloodstream infections, thrombosis, etc.) in comparison to central venous catheters (CVCs). This advantage must be weighed against various limitations in the use of peripheral venous access: restrictions in the osmolarity of the nutrition solutions used, higher risk of extravasations with possible tissue necrosis, and the need for repetitive venipunctures. In newborns and children on prolonged parenteral nutrition, peripherally inserted central venous catheters (PICCs) or tunneled CVCs should be used. However, in older pediatric patients, and in children requiring long-term parenteral nutrition or home parenteral nutrition, a tunneled CVC is recommended for PN access.

Implanted central venous access devices for long-term parenteral nutrition (e.g., Broviac catheters) must be handled with particular caution to prevent infection and thrombosis. Blood samplings and unnecessary manipulations should, if possible, be avoided with this type of access. A catheter with the minimum number of lumens and ports required for individualized treatment should be selected. Preferable materials for catheters in long-term PN are silicone and polyurethane, whereas antimicrobial coating for CVCs does not seem to provide any benefit and is therefore not recommended. In the absence of any signs for catheter-related complications, CVCs and PICCs should not be replaced routinely [8].

For enteral nutrition in preterm infants, gastric tube feeding is common practice until adequate nutritional intake is achieved through oral feeding. In this setting, enteral nutrition is provided via nasogastric or orogastric tubes. It should be noted that nasogastric tubes, especially in the case of a large tube diameter and low body weight, may impair airflow and thus lead to respiratory distress [9], whereas orogastric tubes may be associated with an increased risk of displacement. Currently, there are no clinical guidelines for the choice of the feeding tube access, and the practice of feeding tube placement is largely based on the subjective experience and preference of the different neonatal centers.

Long-term oro- or nasogastric tube feeding is not recommended in older children for reasons of comfort and due to the risk of tube displacement. Should there be a foreseeable need for long-term enteral nutrition therapy, the option of a percutaneous endoscopic gastro- or jejunostomy should be considered.

10.4 Clinical Nutrition in Preterm and Term Neonates

From a physiological point of view, and in line with the gradual development of the digestive capacity of the gastrointestinal tract, the newborn baby goes through a period of considerable fasting from birth until the start of adequate breast milk secretion of the mother. This is approximately during the first 3–4 days after birth. However, postnatal fasting does not usually result in a nutritional gap, as the healthy newborn uses its existing energy reserves from glycogen and fat stores, together with the small amounts of colostrum ingested during the first few days of life. Furthermore, energy requirements are low in the immediate postnatal period because energy metabolism is reduced at the initial stages. This balanced situation predisposes that the newborn has adequate body stores with neither a decrease in available body reserves nor additional pathologies preventing the proper mobilization of required energy reserves.

Preterm infants <35 completed weeks of gestation and sick term infants are unlikely to be able to mobilize the required energy either from sufficient enteral nutrition or body reserves due to various reasons (e.g., immaturity of the gastrointestinal tract, muscular and neurological functional limitations, or reduced adipose tissue mass). In this group of patients, total or partial parenteral nutrition is generally required to meet the generally higher nutrient requirements for accelerated growth and the possibly increased disease-related energy needs.

Despite concerns that an early exposure to enteral feedings in very immature newborns may lead to complications due to food intolerance and an increased risk of necrotizing enterocolitis (NEC), the early initiation of trophic feeds (small nonnutritive feeding volumes) and a gradual increase in milk volumes soon after birth instead of enteral fasting did not result in these adverse effects [10]. Similarly, earlier and faster progression in enteral feeding volumes did not lead to higher incidence of NEC or mortality, whereas a faster increment of enteral feedings had the potential to reduce the time on parenteral nutrition, length of hospital stay, and possibly the incidence of invasive infections [11, 12]. Therefore, an early enteral nutrition management strategy should also be implemented in small preterm infants in order to achieve full enteral nutrition as quickly as possible while carefully monitoring possible feeding-related complications, such as regurgitation, reflux, and NEC.

Taking into account the different nutritional requirements, it is generally useful to distinguish between recommendations for the first 5–7 days of life and recommendations for the subsequent period of stable growth (beginning from the second week of life), as well as to differentiate between the fluid and nutrient requirements of preterm infants and term newborns, based on their body weight.

A subdivision based on birth weight and gestational age is therefore advisable, resulting in the following frequently used classification:

- Preterm infants birth weight <1000 g (extremely low birth weight, ELBW).
- Preterm infants birth weight between 1000 and 1500 g (very low birth weight, VLBW).
- Preterm infants birth weight >1500 g.
- Term infants ≥37 + 0 weeks of gestation at birth.

10.4.1 Nutrition in Newborns During the Phase of Postnatal Adaptation

The transition from intrauterine to extrauterine life involves major changes, particularly in the metabolism of water and electrolytes. During the early postnatal period, various adaptation phases can be distinguished. The highly dynamic initial "transition phase," which lasts the first hours to days after birth, defines a period of oliguria followed by a phase of increased urine production, as well as relatively high sodium excretion, leading to a redistribution of body fluid compartments. This transitional phase usually ends when the nadir of postnatal weight loss has been reached and the high insensitive water losses then gradually decrease again with increasing renal function and progressive epidermal cornification processes. The early adaptation phase is followed by a period of stabilization ("intermediate" adaptation phase) of fluid and electrolyte balance, until the newborn enters the phase of continuous and stable growth.

In preterm infants, a "restrictive" fluid management from the beginning of life has been shown to favorably impact clinical outcome by decreasing the risk for persistent ductus arteriosus (PDA) and NEC [13].

An overview of the recommended fluid supply during the first days of life, according to birth weight, is provided in Table 10.1.

Despite the importance of a strict fluid management, an optimal energy supply should be ensured from the first day of life to prevent energy deficiency and to meet the requirements for an appropriate growth trajectory according to birth percentiles.

It is suggested that the level of energy and protein provided even in the first week of life may have a significant impact on later neurological outcome in very immature preterm infants, with each additional gram of nutrients and energy sources provided having a beneficial effect on later neurological development [15].

Early life nutrition therapy in preterm or sick infants usually involves parenteral nutrition. The initiation of parenteral nutrition with target nutrient doses in the sense of an "aggressive" parenteral nutrition regimen has been shown to be well tolerated in stable infants [16]. However, it is common practice to initiate parenteral nutrition more cautiously with macronutrient doses that initially meet basal requirements and then gradually increase nutrient delivery while monitoring metabolic tolerance.

In VLBW preterm infants, the initiation of parenteral lipid and protein supplementation from the first day of life has proven to enable a positive nitrogen balance and an increased protein synthesis from the onset, which improves short-term growth and is recommended. A positive nitrogen balance can be achieved with an intake of at least 1.5 g protein per kilogram bodyweight from the first day of life on, and maintained by a promptly increased protein supply up to a maximum of 2.5–3.5 g/KGBW/d within 2–3 days after birth, thus preventing a net loss of body mass or growth faltering during the early postnatal period. Moreover, early parenteral protein substitution may result in a lower incidence of hyperkalemia in preterm infants and possibly in improved insulin sensitivity (with fewer episodes of neonatal hyperglycemia).

Higher overall energy supply, with low fluid volumes, can be achieved using parenteral lipids from the first days of life. In VLBW infants, it is recommended that intravenous lipid supply be started as soon as possible after birth (no later than the second day of life) with a lipid emulsion dosage at least providing an adequate intake of essential fatty acids (e.g., minimum intake of 0.25 g/KGBW/d of linoleic acid). Lipid supply should not exceed amounts of 4 g/KGBW/d in neonates.

With carbohydrates being the main energy source in parenteral nutrition, the amount of parenteral carbohydrate intake should be balanced between the effort to meet the high energy needs and the prevention of excessive glucose load resulting in hyperglycemia and hepatic steatosis. Blood glucose levels repeatedly exceeding 145 mg/dL (180 mg/dL in preterm infants) or falling below 45 mg/dL are associated with increased morbidity and mortality, as well as poorer outcome, and should be avoided. In principle, the only appropriate carbohydrate-containing basic infusion solutions are glucose solutions, with the possibility of using high-concentrated (10–15% glucose solution) or low-concentrated (7.5% or 5% glucose solution) glucose solutions depending on metabolic monitoring (blood glucose control). The recommended parenteral glucose supply for neonates is based on intrinsic rates for gluconeogenesis and glucose oxidation and should also take into account the age (postnatal days), actual metabolic situation, and phase of illness, starting with 5.8–11.5 g/KGBW/d in stable preterm infants on the first day of life (3.6–7.2 g/KGBW/d in term infants) and gradually increasing to a target intake of around 11.5–14.4 g/KGBW/d (term infants 7.2–14.4 g/KGBW/d) [17, 18, 19].

It should be noted that mineral and electrolytes homeostasis must be closely monitored and sufficient supplies of sodium, potassium, and phosphate must be provided under the currently recommended high macronutrient (e.g., protein) intakes, especially in very immature and growth-retarded preterm infants. This is to prevent the occurrence of a "refeeding-like syndrome," a potentially life-threatening condition caused by severe micronutrient imbalances [20, 21]!

In critically ill neonates with an impaired metabolic regulation, e.g., due to severe infection or surgical stress, the tolerance of parenteral nutrition therapy must be monitored, and the intakes adjusted accordingly [7]. In this situation, it is common practice to reduce the macronutrient intake to basic requirements and an energy supply in the area of resting energy expenditure, similar to the conditions on the first day of life.

10.4.2 Initiating Enteral Nutrition in Very Premature Neonates

Studies in both animals and humans have shown that enteral nutrition is essential to facilitate intestinal maturation [22], while providing energy and nutrients to intestinal cells from the intraluminal space. Early enteral administration of nutrient-rich solutions is thus advisable in extremely premature infants. The fear that early enteral nutrition might increase the risk of NEC, a dreaded complication associated with nutrition therapy in preterm infants, was not supported by recent research. On the contrary, an earlier start with progressive enteral feeds seemed to be advantageously associated with a lower risk of invasive infections, probably due to a shorter duration on PN with fewer (central) venous catheter-days [10, 11]. Initiating enteral nutrition with very low nutrition volumes ("minimal" or "trophic feeding") soon after birth followed by a gradual increase of enteral feeding volumes under continuous monitoring of gastrointestinal tolerance ("progressive enteral feeding") is now common practice in most neonatal centers.

To ensure safe and effective practice, it should be mandatory to prescribe enteral and parenteral nutrition therapy for preterm and term neonates on the basis of standardized, well-informed prescription guidelines. Through implementation of a standardized feeding regimen alone, the risk for severe complications, e.g., NEC, can be decreased [23].

Meta-analysis data suggest that the incidence of NEC can be further reduced through prophylactic enteral administration of specific probiotic bacteria [24]. Depending on the prevalence of NEC in the respective perinatal center, routine prophylactic administration of a probiotic strain (combination) with proven effectiveness in NEC prevention should be considered for infants at risk. However, certainty about the optimal strains, doses, and timing of this preventive strategy still remains to be determined.

10.4.3 Nutrition in Newborns After the Adaptation Phase

Implementing enteral nutrition is usually completed in the phase of stable growth (from the second week of life) in premature neonates and sick term infants. Should parenteral nutrition still be required in this phase, treatable reasons for the delayed implementation of enteral feeding should be sought. In most cases, nutrient supply via the enteral route is provided by administration of mothers' own milk, donor breast milk, infant formula, or specialized preterm formula.

Daily fluid requirements vary widely in neonates and infants, depending on age, maturity, and activity. Generally, enteral fluid requirements around 150–180 mL/KGBW, or around 140–160 mL/KGBW parenterally supplied fluid volumes can be considered adequate in most stable term and preterm newborns during the phase of stable growth [14, 25]. Yet, in order to provide adequate amounts of nutrients in preterm infants' fluid, demands may increase to up to 200 mL/KGBW/d. In addition, special circumstances associated with altered fluid requirements must be considered, such as the increased fluid requirements associated with fever, increased gastrointestinal losses or tachypnea, as well as decreased fluid requirements due to respiratory therapy with humidified breathing gas.

Protein requirements in relation to body weight, which depend on growth rate and body stores, are significantly higher in growth-restricted preterm infants and very premature infants with catch-up growth than in eutrophic term neonates. Recommendations for enteral protein intake for preterm infants, classified by birth weight, are in the range of 3.5–4.5 g/KGBW/d (see Table 10.2; Embleton et al. [25], s.o.). Recommendations for lower protein intake apply to term infants and should principally mimic those of healthy, breastfed newborns. These are estimated at approximately 2.5 g/KGBW/d (website DGE [26]) for term-born neonates by means of enteral nutrition, and at approximately 1.5–3.0 g/KGBW/d via parenteral nutrition [17]. After the neonatal period, the enteral protein requirement in healthy infants decreases from approximately 2.5–1.3 g/KGBW/d throughout the first year of life [26], and a minimum amino acid intake of 1.0 g/KGBW should be provided via parenteral nutrition to infants and children from 1 month to 3 years of age [17].

A separate supplementation of individual amino acids, such as glutamine, arginine, or taurine to reduce neonatal morbidities (e.g., reduce the incidence of NEC), is not recommended for routine clinical practice because there is insufficient evidence for clinical benefit.

Energy requirements in this phase of life also vary widely, ranging from approximately 115–160 kcal/KGBW/d for VLBW preterm infants on enteral nutrition [25], while the parenteral energy supply in principal may be somewhat lower (approx. 90–120 kcal/KGBW/d) due to the lack of gastrointestinal losses [27]. In clinical practice, however, individual energy and nutrient requirements can be estimated by relating the weight gain achieved to the targeted (intrauterine) growth curves.

If other etiologies for failure to achieve "percentile-parallel growth" can be ruled out, insufficient energy supply results in a drop, whereas excessive energy supply results in a recovery of weight in comparison to intrauterine percentiles. The optimal growth rate for premature infants is still a matter of debate. There is some evidence indicating that growth exceeding the intrauterine development could lead to obesity at adult age [28]. In addition to the quantity of nutrient intake, the effect of nutrient quality is also the subject of ongoing research. For example, it is suggested that the quality and composition of lipid emulsions used for PN, such as solutions rich in long-chained-polyunsaturated fatty acids, may be beneficial in the prevention or resolution of parenteral nutrition–associated cholestasis.

Table 10.2 Recommendations for enteral protein intake in neonates with different birth weight (on basis of Embleton et al. [25] and DGE [26])

Birth weight (g)	<1000 g	1000–1800 g	>1800 g
Daily protein requirements (g)	4.0–4.5	3.5–4.0(–4.5)	ca. 2.5

10.4.4 Preferred Food for Newborns

Breast milk is the best form of physiological nutrition for premature and term neonates and is thus considered the gold standard. For very small preterm infants, specific substrate and energy requirements are indicated due to their higher energy and nutrient needs. Milk fortification, e.g., with protein, and energy or specific preterm formula is generally prescribed for this population. To avoid typical diseases of the preterm infant and because of the immaturity of various metabolic systems, a separate supplementation of vitamins, calcium, phosphorus, and iron is also often advisable.

10.5 Clinical Nutrition in Older Infants, School Children, and Adolescents

The principles of nutritional therapy for older children are similar to those described for neonates. It is easier to make recommendations for this population because there is no adaptation or stabilization phase and the metabolic and regulatory mechanisms are more mature than in neonates. However, nutrient requirements should be assessed in relation to body weight and age, particularly in relation to total energy, protein, and fluid requirements.

An age-matched nutritional substrate intake is also required for older pediatric patients (see Table 10.3); however, with increasing age, better compensation mechanisms for balancing fluctuations in nutrient intake are more readily available. In general, a short-term phase of reduced nutrient intake, which is associated with depletion of body stores, can be tolerated for a maximum of 1 week in children beyond infancy, depending on the preexisting nutritional status. During this period, partial parenteral nutrition may be sufficient, while mobilizing available body stores. If requirement- and age-adequate enteral nutrition intake cannot be guaranteed, thereafter, the implementation of complete parenteral nutrition therapy must be considered (see above).

Certain specific metabolic functions in childhood and adolescence differ from those in adulthood. For this reason, clinical nutrition therapy requires specific and age-appropriate sources of nutrition. Both enteral and parenteral nutrition therapies should always be performed, relying on products tailored to the specific needs of

Table 10.3 Approximated daily energy, protein, and fluid intake for children at different ages (per kilogram of body weight and day) (on basis of ESPGHAN/ESPEN Guidelines 2018) and DGE 2024 [14, 17, 26, 27]

	Unit	Age				
Substrate	Years	2nd month to >1 year	1–3	3–7	7–12	12–18
Energy	kcal/KGBW/d	90–100	75–90	75–90	60–75	30–60
Protein	g/KGBW/d	1.0–2.5	1.0–2.0	0.9–2.0	0.9–2.0	0.9–2.0
Fluid	mL/KGBW/d	120–150	80–120	80–100	60–80	50–70

KGBW/d Kilogram body weight per day

either children or adolescents, such as pediatric amino acid solutions and tube feeding formulas for children of different ages, containing different amounts of protein and energy. The use of fiber-rich nutrition must also be considered in children, if there are no contraindications.

10.6 Perioperative Nutrition in Children and Adolescents

The risk of catabolism from prolonged perioperative fasting periods is higher in children and adolescents than in adults. Patients with preexisting nutritional deficiencies, toddlers, and infants are at particular risk. Establishing a structured perioperative nutritional approach when planning surgery can help to prevent the development of deficits and improve the postoperative outcome. If possible, an age-appropriate nutritional status should be attained prior to (elective) surgery to reduce the risk of postoperative complications.

10.6.1 Preoperative Planning

The scheduled preoperative fasting period should be as short as possible, and the time limits should be strictly adhered to. Children should, for example, be requested to eat and drink until the mandatory fasting period. If adequate enteral nutrition until that time is not possible, partial parenteral fluid and nutrient supply appear indicated, with the aim of limiting catabolism while providing energy and basic structural elements. Should there be a state of malnutrition prior to performing surgery, preoperative nutrition therapy should be implemented. While this strategy aims to improve nutritional status, it has also been shown to improve postoperative outcome.

Examples of recommended fasting periods for elective surgery are as follows [29]:

- Age <12 months: 4 h of formula milk fasting, 3 h of breast milk fasting, 1 h of clear fluid fasting.
- Age >12 months: 6-h fasting for solid food, 4 h for nonclear fluids.

10.6.2 Intraoperative Infusion Therapy

Intraoperative infusion requirements include preoperative deficits (such as fasting periods, enhanced losses, as well as nutritional deficits on account of prior medical history), basic water and electrolyte requirements for the operative period, along with intraoperative correction requirement that are dependent on the duration of the intervention as well as on the severity of surgical trauma. In principle, when choosing perioperative infusion solutions for children, it must be taken into account that large amounts of hypotonic infusion solutions reduce serum osmolality and can cause unforeseen electrolyte and fluid shifts. Intraoperative hyponatremia, which has been shown to be associated with poor postoperative outcome, increases the risk of cerebral edema and encephalopathy occurrence, particularly in critically ill children [30]. Isotonic and physiological infusion solutions must be administered perioperatively whenever possible. Intraoperative parenteral glucose administration must be considered in specific settings only, when the risk of hypoglycemia is particularly increased, as in any condition leading to an impaired fasting tolerance. This includes neonates, as well as critically ill children with sepsis or SIRS, children with preoperative malnutrition, preexisting parenteral nutrition therapy, diabetes mellitus or other metabolic disorders, and children with an impaired liver function. In otherwise healthy children, the risk of intraoperative hypoglycemia occurrence remains low, whereas severe hyperglycemia may be associated with numerous adverse complications, such as osmotic diuresis, increased infection rate, or wound healing disorders [31]. In critically ill children or patients with enhanced cerebral vulnerability, hyperglycemia can result in increased perioperative mortality. The occurrence of intraoperative hypo- and hyperglycemia episodes must therefore be prevented with utmost attention.

Using balanced electrolyte solutions with minimal glucose and additional metabolic anions designed to prevent hyperchloremic acidosis (for example, Ringer-Lactate with 1–2.5% glucose) represents a potential compromise [32].

10.6.3 Postoperative Planning

In the absence of contraindications, early initiation of enteral nutrition following surgery appears to be the optimal solution for children ("fast track" concept). Rapid physiological re-alimentation, whenever possible, was shown to promote recovery while enhancing the child's satisfaction, decreasing infection rates, and shortening hospital stay. Healthy children may already be able to start drinking in the recovery room, after minor surgery without intestinal involvement, after protective reflexes have been restored. The indication for partial parenteral or enteral nutrition therapy following surgery depends on the preexisting nutritional status and feeding ability that must be individually assessed. Catabolism should be avoided so as not to impair the healing process. If from a surgical perspective, the postoperative fasting period exceeds 2–3 days (below 50% of the age-related energy needs), parenteral nutrition therapy should be applied.

References

1. Fusch C, Jochum F. In: Tsang RC, Uauy R, Koletzko B, Zlotkin S, editors. Nutrition in the preterm infant. Cincinnati, OH: Digital Educational Publishing, Inc.; 2005. p. 201–45.
2. Koletzko B, Schiess S, Brands B, et al. Infant feeding practice and later obesity risk. Indications for early metabolic programming. Bundesgesundheitsblatt Gesundheitsforschung Gesundheitsschutz. 2010;53:666–73.

3. Mehta NM, Skillman HE, Irving SY, et al. Guidelines for the provision and assessment of nutrition support therapy in the Pediatric critically ill patient: Society of Critical Care Medicine and American Society for Parenteral and Enteral Nutrition. JPEN J Parenter Enteral Nutr. 2017;41:706–42. https://doi.org/10.1177/0148607117711387. Epub 2017 Jun 2. PMID: 28686844
4. Tume LN, Valla FV, Joosten K, et al. Nutritional support for children during critical illness: European Society of Pediatric and Neonatal Intensive Care (ESPNIC) metabolism, endocrine and nutrition section position statement and clinical recommendations. Intensive Care Med. 2020;46:411–25. https://doi.org/10.1007/s00134-019-05922-5. Epub 2020 Feb 20. PMID: 32077997; PMCID: PMC7067708
5. de Souza Menezes F, Leite HP, Koch Nogueira PC. Malnutrition as an independent predictor of clinical outcome in critically ill children. Nutrition. 2012;28:267–70. https://doi.org/10.1016/j.nut.2011.05.015. Epub 2011 Aug 27. PMID: 21872433
6. Bechard LJ, Duggan C, Touger-Decker R, et al. Nutritional status based on body mass index is associated with morbidity and mortality in mechanically ventilated critically ill children in the PICU. Crit Care Med. 2016;44:1530–7. https://doi.org/10.1097/CCM.0000000000001713. PMID: 26985636; PMCID: PMC4949117
7. Moltu SJ, Bronsky J, Embleton N, et al. ESPGHAN Committee on Nutrition. Nutritional management of the critically ill neonate: a position paper of the ESPGHAN committee on nutrition. J Pediatr Gastroenterol Nutr. 2021;73:274–89. https://doi.org/10.1097/MPG.0000000000003076. PMID: 33605663
8. Kolaček S, Puntis JWL, Hojsak I. ESPGHAN/ESPEN/ESPR/CSPEN working group on pediatric parenteral nutrition. ESPGHAN/ESPEN/ESPR/CSPEN guidelines on pediatric parenteral nutrition: venous access. Clin Nutr. 2018;37:2379–91. https://doi.org/10.1016/j.clnu.2018.06.952. Epub 2018 Jun 18. PMID: 30055869
9. Greenspan JS, Wolfson MR, Holt WJ, Shaffer TH. Neonatal gastric tube intubation: differential respiratory effects between nasogastric and orogastric tubes. Pediatr Pulmonol. 1990;8:254–8.
10. Morgan J, Bombell S, McGuire W. Early trophic feeding versus enteral fasting for very preterm or very low birth weight infants. Cochrane Database Syst Rev. 2013;2013:CD000504. https://doi.org/10.1002/14651858.CD000504.pub4. PMID: 23543508
11. Young L, Oddie SJ, McGuire W. Delayed introduction of progressive enteral feeds to prevent necrotising enterocolitis in very low birth weight infants. Cochrane Database Syst Rev. 2022;1:CD001970. https://doi.org/10.1002/14651858.CD001970.pub6. PMID: 35049036; PMCID: PMC8771918
12. Oddie SJ, Young L, McGuire W. Slow advancement of enteral feed volumes to prevent necrotising enterocolitis in very low birth weight infants. Cochrane Database Syst Rev. 2017;8:CD001241. https://doi.org/10.1002/14651858.CD001241.pub7. Update in: Cochrane Database Syst Rev. 2021;8:CD001241. https://doi.org/10.1002/14651858.CD001241.pub8. PMID: 28854319; PMCID: PMC6483766.
13. Bell EF, Acarregui MJ. Restricted versus liberal water intake for preventing morbidity and mortality in preterm infants. Cochrane Database Syst Rev. 2014;2014:CD000503. https://doi.org/10.1002/14651858.CD000503.pub3. Epub 2014 Dec 4. PMID: 25473815; PMCID: PMC7038715
14. Jochum F, Moltu SJ, Senterre T, et al. ESPGHAN/ESPEN/ESPR/CSPEN working group on pediatric parenteral nutrition. ESPGHAN/ESPEN/ESPR/CSPEN guidelines on pediatric parenteral nutrition: fluid and electrolytes. Clin Nutr. 2018;37:2344–53. https://doi.org/10.1016/j.clnu.2018.06.948. Epub 2018 Jun 18. PMID: 30064846
15. Stephens BE, Walden RV, Gargus RA, et al. First-week protein and energy intakes are associated with 18-month developmental outcomes in extremely low birth weight infants. Pediatrics. 2009;123:1337–43.
16. Ibrahim HM, Jeroudi MA, Baier RJ, et al. Aggressive early total parenteral nutrition in low-birth-weight infants. J Perinatol. 2004;24:482–6.

17. van Goudoever JB, Carnielli V, Darmaun D, et al. ESPGHAN/ESPEN/ESPR/CSPEN working group on pediatric parenteral nutrition. ESPGHAN/ESPEN/ESPR/CSPEN guidelines on pediatric parenteral nutrition: amino acids. Clin Nutr. 2018;37:2315–23. https://doi.org/10.1016/j.clnu.2018.06.945. Epub 2018 Jun 18. PMID: 30100107
18. Lapillonne A, Fidler Mis N, Goulet O, et al. ESPGHAN/ESPEN/ESPR/CSPEN working group on pediatric parenteral nutrition. ESPGHAN/ESPEN/ESPR/CSPEN guidelines on pediatric parenteral nutrition: lipids. Clin Nutr. 2018;37:2324–36. https://doi.org/10.1016/j.clnu.2018.06.946. Epub 2018 Jun 18. PMID: 30143306
19. Mesotten D, Joosten K, van Kempen A, et al. ESPGHAN/ESPEN/ESPR/CSPEN working group on pediatric parenteral nutrition. ESPGHAN/ESPEN/ESPR/CSPEN guidelines on pediatric parenteral nutrition: carbohydrates. Clin Nutr. 2018;37:2337–43. https://doi.org/10.1016/j.clnu.2018.06.947. Epub 2018 Jun 18. PMID: 30037708
20. Sung SI, Chang YS, Choi JH, et al. Increased risk of refeeding syndrome-like hypophosphatemia with high initial amino acid intake in small-for-gestational-age, extremely-low-birthweight infants. PLoS One. 2019;14:e0221042. https://doi.org/10.1371/journal.pone.0221042. PMID: 31442245; PMCID: PMC6707589
21. Moltu SJ, Strømmen K, Blakstad EW, et al. Enhanced feeding in very-low-birth-weight infants may cause electrolyte disturbances and septicemia–a randomized, controlled trial. Clin Nutr. 2013;32:207–12. https://doi.org/10.1016/j.clnu.2012.09.004. Epub 2012 Sep 21. PMID: 23043722
22. Sangild PT. Minireview: gut responses to enteral nutrition in preterm infants and animals. Exp Biol Med. 2006;231:1695–711.
23. Patole SK, de Klerk N. Impact of standardised feeding regimens on incidence of neonatal necrotising enterocolitis: a systematic review and meta-analysis of observational studies. Arch Dis Child Fetal Neonatal Ed. 2005;90:F147–51. https://doi.org/10.1136/adc.2004.059741. PMID: 15724039; PMCID: PMC1721845
24. Sharif S, Meader N, Oddie SJ, Rojas-Reyes MX, McGuire W. Probiotics to prevent necrotising enterocolitis in very preterm or very low birth weight infants. Cochrane Database Syst Rev. 2023;7:CD005496. https://doi.org/10.1002/14651858.CD005496.pub6. PMID: 37493095; PMCID: PMC10370900
25. Embleton ND, Jennifer Moltu S, Lapillonne A, et al. Enteral nutrition in preterm infants (2022): a position paper from the ESPGHAN committee on nutrition and invited experts. J Pediatr Gastroenterol Nutr. 2023;76:248–68. https://doi.org/10.1097/MPG.0000000000003642. Epub 2022 Oct 28. PMID: 36705703
26. Website DGE (Deutsche Gesellschaft für Ernährung). http://www.dge.de/wissenschaft/referenzwerte/. Accessed 7 July 2024.
27. Joosten K, Embleton N, Yan W, et al. ESPGHAN/ESPEN/ESPR/CSPEN working group on pediatric parenteral nutrition. ESPGHAN/ESPEN/ESPR/CSPEN guidelines on pediatric parenteral nutrition: energy. Clin Nutr. 2018;37:2309–14. https://doi.org/10.1016/j.clnu.2018.06.944. Epub 2018 Jun 18. PMID: 30078715
28. Lucas A. Programming by early nutrition in man. Ciba Found Symp. 1991;156:38–50.
29. Frykholm P, Disma N, Andersson H, et al. Pre-operative fasting in children: a guideline from the European Society of Anaesthesiology and Intensive Care. Eur J Anaesthesiol. 2022;39:4–25. https://doi.org/10.1097/EJA.0000000000001599. PMID: 34857683
30. Duke T, Molyneux EM. Intravenous fluids for seriously ill children: time to reconsider. Lancet. 2003;362:1320–3.
31. Lönnqvist PA. Inappropriate perioperative fluid management in children: time for a solution?! Ped Anesthesia. 2007;17:203–5.
32. Sümpelmann R, Becke K, Crean P, et al. European consensus statement for intraoperative fluid therapy in children. Eur J Anaesthesiol. 2011;28:6.

Obesity and Cachexia

11

Matthias Pirlich

The nutritional status is a critical factor for the clinical course of the seriously ill. This holds for obesity as well as for cachexia. Both nutrition disorders may be accompanied by an unfavorable outcome regarding complication rate, wound healing, duration of mechanical ventilation, length of ICU stay, and mortality. Even though the predictive importance of the nutritional status is already well documented for many diseases, an adequate nutritional therapy receives most often only minor attention during daily routine. Therefore, the screening for malnutrition in hospitals is still an exemption in many countries. For intensive care patients, an especially high risk exists that an underlying nutritional problem may be unrecognized. They are often admitted as emergencies where the severity of disease forces a prioritization during which nutrition may easily be regarded circumstantial. The particularities of nutrition for obese and cachectic intensive care patients will be addressed in the following chapter.

11.1 Definitions

For intensive care patients, the same definitions of obesity and cachexia apply as for other patients (see also Chap. 4). Obesity is quantified by BMI according to the WHO criteria (Table 11.1).

M. Pirlich (✉)
Praxis Kaisereiche, Endocrinology, General Medicine, Clinical Nutrition, Berlin, Germany
e-mail: pirlich@kaisereiche.de

© The Author(s), under exclusive license to Springer Nature Switzerland AG 2025
A. Rümelin et al. (eds.), *Nutrition in ICU Patients*,
https://doi.org/10.1007/978-3-032-00818-3_11

Table 11.1 Classification of obesity according to WHO [22]

Obesity class I:	BMI 30–34.9 kg/m²
Obesity class II:	BMI 35–39.9 kg/m²
Obesity class III:	BMI ≥40 kg/m²

Table 11.2 Thresholds for severity grading of malnutrition into stage 1 (moderate) and stage 2 (severe) malnutrition according to the recent GLIM recommendations

	Phenotypic criteria		
	Weight loss (%)	Low body mass index (kg/m²)	Reduced muscle mass
Stage 1 moderate malnutrition (requires 1 phenotypic criterion that meets this grade)	5–10% within the past 6 mo, or 10–20% beyond 6 mo	<20 if <70 yr <22 if ≥70 yr	Mild to moderate deficit (per validated assessment methods, see EWGSOP2)
Stage 2 severe malnutrition (requires 1 phenotypic criterion that meets this grade)	>10% within the past 6 mo, or >20% beyond 6 mo	<18.5 if <70 yr <20 if ≥70 yr	Severe deficit (per validated assessment methods)

The term cachexia is synonymous to disease-related malnutrition with inflammation [4]. Modern cachexia definitions are based on the combination of weight loss and disease activity/inflammation. In 2011, an international consensus group gave the following definition for tumor cachexia [7], which is also applicable for other diseases:

- Weight loss >5% in the past 6 months (as long as no starving is present) or
- BMI <20 kg/m² and weight loss >2% or
- Diminished skeletal muscle mass (<5 percentile) and weight loss >2%

More recently, the Global Leadership Initiative on Malnutrition (GLIM), an international consensus group covering all major national and umbrella scientific societies in the field of clinical nutrition, has proposed a concept for diagnosing malnutrition based on three phenotypic (weight loss, low BMI, low muscle mass) and two etiologic (decreased food intake, disease burden/inflammation) criteria [5]. The grading of malnutrition into moderate and severe malnutrition is based on the three etiologic criteria (Table 11.2).

With intensive care patients, however, the sometimes-significant water deposits following, e.g., multi-organ failure, make all weight-related quantities hard to interpret. This adds further importance to an assessment of the nutritional status right at the beginning of a disease. A meticulous (third-party) history regarding earlier usual body weight, weight loss and recent nutrition intake, as well as a qualified physical examination, allows in most cases an evaluation of the nutritional status.

Independent from the above, validated screening instruments such as the NRS-2002 assume that the seriously ill are always in a catabolic situation and thus carry a high nutritional risk [9]. The 2023 ESPEN practical guidelines on clinical nutrition in the intensive care unit states: "Every critically ill patient staying for more than 48 h in the ICU should be considered at risk for malnutrition [19]."

11.2 Prevalence

In most countries, the prevalence of overweight and obesity is increasing in the general population. The German Health Interview and Examination Survey for Adults [13] demonstrated an increase of the prevalence of overweight (BMI >25 kg/m^2) with rising age in men up to 80% until the age of 60 (including 25–30% obese) with a stagnation until higher age. For women, the prevalence of overweight increases almost continually with rising age. The prevalence of obesity for women above 55 years was 25–35%. Regarding obesity in intensive care unit patients, the big database of the nutrition Day project allows a more global perspective and shows a large variability between continents (summary of these data in [18]): Prevalence rates of obesity (BMI >30 kg/m^2) in the ICU were 39% in the United States, 22% in Europe, 17% in South America, and 10% in the Asian/Pacific region.

The prevalence of cachexia/disease-related malnutrition differs between different regions and countries, but also according to the different screening or diagnostic instruments used. On admission to the hospital, about 25–30% of all adult patients show a clinically manifest malnutrition in European studies [14] with a higher prevalence in geriatric and cancer patients and in patients with gastrointestinal diseases [16]. A systematic review of 66 studies from 12 countries in Latin America, however, showed an even higher prevalence of 40–60% [6].

Cachexia is a risk factor for morbidity, complications, loss of functionality, prolonged hospital and ICU stay, and mortality. This has been impressively shown in a meta-analysis including 12 studies on malnutrition in adults with COVID-19 [3]: patients with malnutrition had a more than threefold higher in-hospital mortality compared to well-nourished subjects. Similar strong associations between malnutrition and mortality have also been observed in severely or critically ill COVID-19 patients [23].

11.3 Special Aspects in Obesity Class I and II

Obesity increases the risk for insulin resistance, diabetes mellitus, high blood pressure, cardiovascular diseases, hepatic cirrhosis, deep venous thrombosis, degenerative joint disorders, pulmonary dysfunctions, and several tumor entities. Therefore, obese intensive care patients commonly suffer from several chronic comorbidities with impact on the prognosis. The problem of insulin resistance deserves prior attention when dealing with the nutrition of the patient.

> Note: Beside glucose monitoring for manifested diabetes mellitus, patients with mild obesity do not seem to require special adaptations for the medical nutrition on the ICU.

The obese seriously ill patient is not protected by his excess of energy reserves from falling into an acute state of malnutrition via catabolism. Insulin resistance, reduced utilization of energy substrates, increased mobilization of fatty acids, and hyperlipidemia even produce an increased vulnerability for the reduction of fat-free mass through increasing protein degradation during insufficient nutrition intake. During the course of severe diseases, this may lead to sarcopenic obesity, which is associated with worsened outcome and increased mortality.

Therefore, the fundamental principles of nutrition for intensive care patients also apply for mild obesity. Alike lean patients, they benefit from an early low-dose enteral nutrition (avoiding overfeeding!) if there is no contraindication. The energy and protein goal (defined as >70% but not exceeding 100% of the resting energy expenditure) should be achieved progressively, but not before the first 48–72 h. According to the ESPEN guidelines [19], an iso-caloric high-protein diet can be administered. The energy intake should preferentially be guided by indirect calorimetry, and the protein intake by measurement of urinary nitrogen losses. If these measures are not available it is recommended to provide energy based on the calculation of ideal body weight (0.9 × (height in cm—100 (male) or -106 (female))). Under the assumption that about 10% of excess weight of obese individuals are muscle mass (with higher energy utilization than fat mass), it is recommended to add 20–25% of the excess weight (actual body weight − ideal body weight) to the ideal body weight (=adjusted body weight) for calculations of energy requirements [19].

The protein intake can be calculated as 1.3 g/kg adjusted body weight/d if estimation of nitrogen balance is not available.

11.4 Specific Recommendations for Nutrition in Class III Obesity

11.4.1 Access Route

Patients with class III obesity (BMI >40 kg/m^2) have an increased intra-abdominal pressure which fosters gastroesophageal reflux und aspiration. It is hence recommended to place enteral feeding tubes postpyloric, ideally behind the ligament of Treitz. The use of a PEG being quite rare is most often technically unproblematic with class III obesity but may, however, come along with a higher complication rate. The risk of a tube dislocation is increased as the massive fat storage thickens the large net [17]. Thus, it is recommended by some authors to additionally fix the stomach at the anterior abdominal wall through either surgically or endoscopically placed sutures.

11.4.2 Energy and Protein Demand

The ESPEN guideline on clinical nutrition in the intensive care unit does not specifically address the nutrition in the class III obese patient, but mention the concept of controlled undernutrition with relatively larger dose of protein in this patient group.

Some stratification of the energy and protein targets was suggested in the ASPEN guidelines with a high-protein and hypocaloric nutrition for class III obese intensive care patients in order to preserve the fat-free mass and to reduce the amount of fat mass and improve insulin sensitivity [11].

In accordance with the ESPEN guidelines, it is recommended to determine the energy demand by indirect calorimetry and the protein demand by nitrogen balance studies. Alternatively, if this is not available, it is proposed to use predictive equations, which, however, are considered as less accurate in patients with obesity. A simple approach is based on the actual or ideal body weight [11]:

Recommended caloric intake for obese:

- 65–70% of the calorimetric or calculated demand (all class of obesity) or
- 11–14 kcal/kg *actual body weight* for patients with BMI 30–50 kg/m^2 and
- 22–25 kcal/kg *ideal body weight* for patients with BMI >50 kg/m^2

The recommended protein intake is depending on the degree of obesity and is oriented at the ideal body weight (IBW):

Obesity degree I	>2 g/kg IBW/d
Obesity degree II	>2 g/kg IBW/d
Obesity degree III	>2.5 g/kg IBW/d

11.4.3 Types of Tube Feeding Formulae

The daily demand of liquid of class III obese patients is often increased. Therefore, it is recommended by some authors that the energy density of food should not exceed 1.0 kcal/mL [10]. However, tube feeding formulae closely adapted to the previously mentioned requirements of obese intensive care patients are not easy to find. While the protein calorie to total calorie ratio should be >30%, the standard tube feeding formulae available on the market contain 15–20% and the high-protein versions do not exceed 20–25% showing a calorie density >1 kcal/mL.

> Note: The proposed concept of high-protein, hypocaloric nutrition in class III obesity is therefore only feasible through a combination of industrial manufactured enteral formula and an enteral or parenteral addition of protein resp. amino acid solutions.

As obesity may come along with a chronic systemic inflammation, the importance of immune-modulating substrates resp. fatty acids with anti-inflammatory properties has been discussed. Because of the absence of specific studies, it is not possible to give recommendations, which exceeds the general statements for critically ill patients.

11.4.4 Monitoring of Nutrition Therapy for Obese

Obesity is associated with insulin resistance and alterations of metabolism, and thus, a close monitoring of glucose, triglyceride, and cholesterol levels is necessary. Also, the substrate and insulin supply must be adapted correspondingly. Insulin administration is recommended when glucose levels exceed 10 mmol/L [19]. Based on an increased risk for nonalcoholic steatohepatitis, a regular determination of the liver function tests is required twice weekly [2]. Ideally, the efficiency of protein intake is tested by the nitrogen balance [protein supply (g/d)/6.25 − (24 h urinary nitrogen excretion + 4 g)].

11.5 Specific Nutritional Recommendation for Cachexia

Advanced cachexia comes along with an increased mortality rate for critically ill patients with best survival for patients with BMI 30–39.9 kg/m^2 in this meta-analysis [1]. The existing deficits of macro- and micronutrients as well as the concept of an increased demand through stress metabolism lead to the concept of hyperalimentation which is nowadays regarded dangerous and obsolete. Especially during the early phase of severe illness, the decisive limitation of the nutrition supply lies in the limited nutrient utilization. Hence, a phase-adapted nutrient supply is required for cachexia (see Chap. 2). Furthermore, a deficiency of macronutrients is frequently associated with a deficiency of micronutrients, which promotes the potentially life-threatening refeeding-syndrome (see Sect. 11.6), and thus provides another reason for a hypocaloric nutrition.

11.5.1 Access Route

In general, the enteral route should be chosen whenever possible which is also true for cachexia. The same considerations as for other intensive care patients apply for the choice of the type of tube. The gastrointestinal tolerance is, however, often limited with extreme cachexia, and therefore, a combined enteral and parental nutrition might be needed in individual cases to cover the nutrient demand (see Chap. 12).

11.5.2 Energy and Protein Demand

The energy demand in preexisting cachexia varies between patients and during disease according to nutritional status, body composition, severity of disease, endogenous nutrient production, medical treatment, and several other factors. Therefore, the best way to assess the energy demand is indirect calorimetry. If this technique is not available, one might use the oxygen consumption (VO_2) from pulmonary catheter or carbon dioxide production (VCO_2) measured from the ventilator (e.g., calculation of resting energy expenditure = $VCO_2 \times 8.19$, according to [21]) with the limitation in patients treated with FiO_2 >0.6 (lower reliability).

Predictive equations are also commonly used, but they are considered as less accurate. As a very pragmatic approach, the calorie demand after the early phase of acute illness can be estimated based on body weight (20–25 kcal/kg body weight/d) [19]. During the recovery phase of the disease, however, an increased energy demand of >25 kcal/kg body weight/d must be assumed.

> Note: For cachectic intensive care patients, a hyperalimentation during early phase and a hypoalimentation in recovery phase must be avoided.

The normal protein demand of healthy subjects is about 0.8 g/kg body weight/d, but it is higher at higher age and in disease and malnutrition. The general recommendation regarding the protein intake of intensive care patients is 1.3 g/kg body weight/d according to the 2023 ESPEN guidelines [19]. Although no specific recommendations exist for preexisting cachexia, it can be assumed that this applies also for these patients.

It is important to mention that cachectic patients in the postacute or recovery phase require special attention and careful monitoring of their food intake to supply sufficient macronutrients [8]. Peterson et al. [15] demonstrated that 1 week after extubation many patients received no more than 700 kcal/d, probably because of the false assumption that patients who were able to eat will automatically manage to cover their energy and protein demands. In this situation, dietary advice, fortified food, the use of protein- and energy-rich oral nutritional supplements, and supplementary enteral or even parenteral nutrition might be necessary to achieve anabolism.

11.5.3 Types of Tube Feeding

> To cover the increased demand associated with cachexia, a high-protein formula with a protein contend of 20–25% of the total energy is recommended.

Concerning the use of immune modulating or other specific diets in cachexia, the same recommendations apply as for other intensive care patients.

11.6 The Refeeding Syndrome

The refeeding syndrome was observed for the first time in cachectic Japanese prisoners of war during the 1950s. After resuming normal nutrition intake, they surprisingly died from cardiac arrhythmia and cardiac insufficiency. By now it is well known that all diseases and clinical situations associated with a pronounced micronutrient deficiency, pose a risk for the refeeding syndrome (Table 11.3). This may also concern obese patients with malabsorption or severe weight loss, especially after bariatric surgery [12].

The cause is primarily a deficiency of thiamine, phosphate, and other micronutrients, which becomes evident through "physiological" substrate intake where especially the glucose-induced insulin release causes a shift of potassium, phosphate, and magnesium toward the intracellular compartment. This may cause severe neuromuscular dysfunctions. Typical findings are also hypomagnesemia, hypokalemia, lactic acidosis, and fluid retention. Clinically, the patients often demonstrate neuromuscular dysfunctions, Wernicke's encephalopathy, hypoventilation, cardiac arrhythmia, and cardiac and renal insufficiency. The prevention of the refeeding syndrome consists primarily of an extremely careful substrate intake of <50% of the calculated demand (Benchmark: initial 10 kcal/kg bodyweight/d), with a gradual increase closely monitored over 7–10 days. Additionally, to the normal intake of dietary minerals and trace elements, all patients who have an increased risk should receive 200–300 mg/d thiamine and 200% of RDI of other vitamins during the first

Table 11.3 Risk groups for refeeding syndrome

Chronic under- and malnutrition	Anorexia nervosa
	Chronic alcohol abuse
	Cachexia of any origin
	Severe weight loss in morbid obesity, after bariatric surgery
	High metabolic stress or fasting >7 days
Elderly patients	Comorbidities
	Reduced physiologic capacities
Malabsorption	Celiac disease, Whipple disease
	Chronic inflammatory bowel disease
	Chronic pancreatitis
	Short bowel syndrome

3–5 days [20]. Besides the normal monitoring, phosphate, calcium, potassium, sodium, chloride, magnesium, and the blood gas analysis have to be determined at least once daily, and if necessary substituted.

In patients with manifest hypophosphatemia (<0.65 mmol/L or drop of >0.16 mmol/L), electrolytes should be measured two to three times per day and supplemented [19].

> Note: The prevention of the refeeding syndrome is based mainly on a very careful increase of the amount of food given (initially 10 kcal/kg body weight/d) together with a careful monitoring and the supplementation of thiamine, phosphate, and other micronutrients.

References

1. Akinnusi ME, Pineda LA, Solh AA. Effect of obesity on intensive care morbidity and mortality: a meta-analysis. Crit Care Med. 2008;36:151–8.
2. Berger MM, Reintam-Blaser A, Calder PC, et al. Monitoring nutrition in the ICU. Clin Nutr. 2019;38:584–93.
3. Boaz M, Kaufman-Shriqui V. Systematic review and meta-analysis: malnutrition and in-hospital death in adults hospitalized with COVID-19. Nutrients. 2023;15:1298. https://doi.org/10.3390/nu15051298.
4. Cederholm T, Barazzoni R, Austin P, et al. ESPEN guidelines on definitions and terminology of clinical nutrition. Clin Nutr. 2017;36:49–64.
5. Cederholm T, Jensen G, Correia MITD, et al. GLIM criteria for the diagnosis of malnutrition—a consensus report from the global clinical nutrition community. Clin Nutr. 2019;38:1–9.
6. Correia MITD, Perman MI, Waitzberg DL. Hospital malnutrition in Latin America: a systematic review. Clin Nutr. 2017;36:958–67.
7. Fearon K, Strasser F, Anker SD, et al. Definition and classification of cancer cachexia: an international consensus. Lancet Oncol. 2011;12:489–95.
8. Hill A, Elke G, Weimann A. Nutrition in the intensive care unit—a narrative review. Nutrients. 2021;13:2851. https://doi.org/10.3390/nu13082851.
9. Kondrup J, Allison SP, Elia M, Vellas B, Plauth M. ESPEN guidelines for nutrition screening 2002. Clin Nutr. 2003;22:415–21.
10. McClave SA, Kushner R, Van Way CW, et al. Nutrition therapy of the severely obese, critically ill patient: summation of conclusions and recommendations. JPEN. 2011;35:88S–96S.
11. McClave SA, Taylor BE, Martindale RG, et al. Guidelines for the provision and assessment of nutrition support therapy in the adult critically ill patient: Society of Critical Care Medicine (SCCM) and American Society for Parenteral and Enteral Nutrition (ASPEN). JPEN. 2016;40:159–211.
12. Mehanna HM, Moledina J, Travis J. Refeeding syndrome: what it is, and how to prevent and treat it. BMJ. 2008;336:1495–8.
13. Mensink GBM, Schienkiewitz A, Haftenberger M, Lampert T, Ziese T, Scheidt-Nave C. Overweight and obesity in Germany. Results of the German health interview and examination survey for adults (DEGS1). Bundesgesundheitsbl. 2013;56:786–94.
14. Norman K, Pichard C, Lochs H, Pirlich M. Prognostic impact of disease-related malnutrition. Clin Nutr. 2008;27:5–15.
15. Peterson SJ, Tsai AA, Scala CM, et al. Adequacy of oral intake in critically ill patients 1 week after extubation. J Am Diet Assoc. 2010;110:427–33.

16. Pirlich M, Schütz T, Norman K, et al. The German hospital malnutrition study. Clin Nutr. 2006;25:563–72.
17. Port AM, Apovian C. Metabolic support of the obese intensive care unit patient: a current perspective. Curr Opin Clin Nutr Metab Care. 2010;13:184–91.
18. Singer P, Blaser AR, Berger MM, et al. ESPEN guideline on clinical nutrition in the intensive care unit. Clin Nutr. 2019;38:48–79.
19. Singer P, Blaser AR, Berger MM, et al. ESPEN practical and partially revised guideline: clinical nutrition in the intensive care unit. Clin Nutr. 2023;42:1671–89.
20. Stanga Z, Sobotka L, Schuetz P. Refeeding syndrome. In: Sobotka L, editor. Basics in clinical nutrition. Prague: Galen; 2019. p. 393–89.
21. Stapel SN, de Grooth HJ, Alimohamed H, et al. Ventilator derived carbon dioxide production to assess energy expenditure in critically ill patients: proof of concept. Crit Care. 2015;19:370.
22. WHO Expert Consultation. Appropriate body-mass index for Asian populations and its implications for policy and intervention strategies. Lancet. 2004;363:157–63.
23. Zhao X, Li Y, Ge Y, et al. Evaluation of nutrition risk and its association with mortality risk in severely and critically ill COVID-19 patients. JPEN. 2021;45:32–42.

Gastrointestinal Sonography in Nutritional Management: A Clinical Perspective

12

Nick Weidner

12.1 Introduction

When examining healthy individuals, gastric emptying is a complex process that varies significantly from person to person and is influenced by numerous factors such as food composition or comorbidities. Typically, the gastric emptying process is more pulsatile than continuous. The usual rate of emptying ranges between 1 and 4 kcal/min (4 and 17 kJ/min) [1].

Nutrition for critically ill patients is a constant challenge due to different phases of illness accompanied by varying metabolic changes, necessitating individual adjustments in nutrient intake. In this context, the caloric goal plays a crucial role, as both insufficient and excessive caloric intake can adversely affect mortality. Due to motility disorders, a purely enteral approach often leads to undernutrition, with the rate of emptying significantly delayed compared to healthy individuals.

To ensure adequate substrate supply, it may be necessary to initiate supplemental parenteral therapy in cases of inadequate enteral absorption but adequate utilization. In this context, measuring gastric clearance is of immense importance, as it serves as an indicator of nutrient transport and thus a predictor of adequate nutrient intake.

Scintigraphy is considered the gold standard for monitoring gastric emptying [2]. However, the method's drawbacks include the need for specific equipment and the radiation exposure to the patient. This technique is particularly impractical in an intensive care setting, as it cannot be seamlessly integrated into daily routines. Likewise, the alternative method of isotope breath testing, which involves administering carbon-13 labelled isotopes in food, is impractical for daily use in an intensive care unit due to the required equipment.

N. Weidner (✉)
Department of Interdisciplinary Intensive Care, Helios Clinics, Erfurt, Germany
e-mail: n.weidner@gmx.biz

In daily practice in intensive care units, gastric reflux testing has become established. However, this method is controversial, showing little correlation with the actual volume of gastric contents and is even considered obsolete by some [3].

In recent years, sonography has gained popularity in daily routines due to improvements in ultrasound devices and the introduction of handheld units. A variety of point-of-care methods have been established, offering the ability to make quick, reliable, bedside assessments with low interobserver variability, thus enabling ad hoc planning of further therapy.

While sonography has not yet been fully established in the nutritional therapy of intensive care patients, it has proven to be a valuable diagnostic tool for evaluating gastric residual volume with reliable predictability in perioperative medicine. For this reason, gastric sonography is viewed with high confidence for nutritional management.

12.2 Sonographic Evaluation of the Stomach

Sonography of the stomach is an essential skill that has been integrated into the educational curricula of various medical training programs across Europe, including Germany. This aspect of medical education emphasizes the importance of understanding and applying different transducer placements to obtain optimal imaging results for diagnostic purposes.

For standard sonographic examination of the stomach, two types of transducers are commonly used: the curved-array transducer and the sector transducer. Each of these transducers offers specific advantages in visualizing abdominal structures, allowing for detailed examination of the stomach and surrounding areas.

The stomach is anatomically located near the distal esophagus and the cardia, close to where the aorta passes through the diaphragm at the aortic hiatus, with the esophageal hiatus also in close proximity. By visualizing the descending aorta and following it to its passage below the diaphragm, sonographers can identify the cardia of the stomach. This area is crucial for evaluating various gastrointestinal (GI) conditions and assessing the stomach's anatomy and function (Fig. 12.1).

A significant aspect of gastric sonography is the ability to observe the typical five-layer structure of the intestinal wall, which is evident in sonographic imaging. This layered structure is crucial for diagnosing various gastrointestinal diseases and conditions, as alterations in the appearance of these layers can indicate pathology. The five layers, from the outermost to the innermost, include the serosa, muscularis, submucosa, mucosa, and the luminal interface, each with its distinctive sonographic appearance.

Incorporating sonography of the stomach into medical training programs is a critical step toward ensuring that future healthcare professionals are well prepared to conduct thorough abdominal examinations. This preparation is essential for the accurate diagnosis and effective management of patients with gastrointestinal conditions. Sonographic examination of the stomach, with its ability to provide

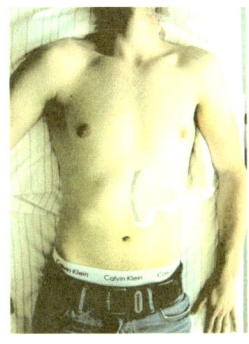
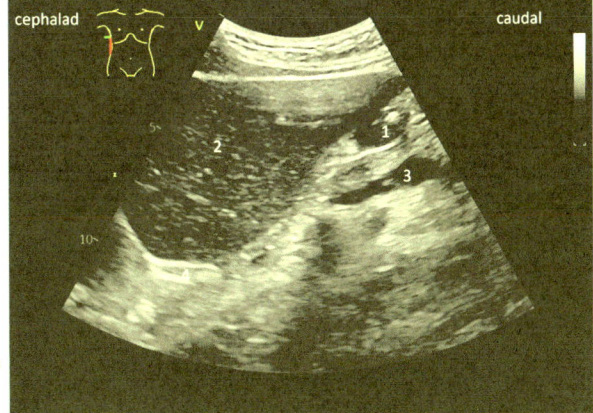

subcostal view – cranio-caudal orientation
numbers idicate
1 – stomach
2 – liver, left lobe
3 – portal vein, confluens
4 – kardia of stomach

Fig. 12.1 Subcostal view showing cardia and antral section of stomach

real-time imaging, offers a noninvasive and immediate method to assess various gastric and surrounding anatomical structures.

When performing a sonographic examination of the stomach, one of the techniques involves visualizing the stomach laterally, in relation to the spleen (Fig. 12.2). To achieve this, the sonographer locates the spleen along the middle to posterior axillary line. The transducer is then moved ventrally (toward the front of the body) until the fundus and corpus of the stomach become visible. This approach helps in assessing the upper portion of the stomach, providing valuable insights into its size, shape, and any pathological changes.

However, it's important to note that when the stomach is empty, its visualization might be challenging. The empty stomach may not display sufficiently in sonographic images and can be obscured by the left colic flexure (the bend of the colon near the spleen). This highlights the necessity for healthcare professionals to be adept at maneuvering the transducer and applying various imaging techniques to adequately visualize and assess the stomach (Figs. 12.1 and 12.2). Mastery of these skills allows for a more comprehensive examination, facilitating the identification of abnormalities and guiding appropriate patient management strategies.

The corpus can also be displayed in the middle clavicular line as a left upper abdomen cross-section. The lower edge of the rib cage can serve as a point of orientation for this. Visualization may be hindered by overlaps with gas-filled colon.

The visualization of the antrum has become the standard procedure. Due to its anatomical relationship to the left liver lobe, the antrum is easily identifiable and accessible for sonography (Fig. 12.1). Visualization is possible in both supine and right lateral decubitus positions. The right lateral decubitus position is ideal for assessment, as the stomach contents move toward the pylorus. To avoid confusion with the pylorus or duodenum, the sonographic window should display the abdominal aorta. The aorta is shown dorsal to the stomach. Depending on the anatomical

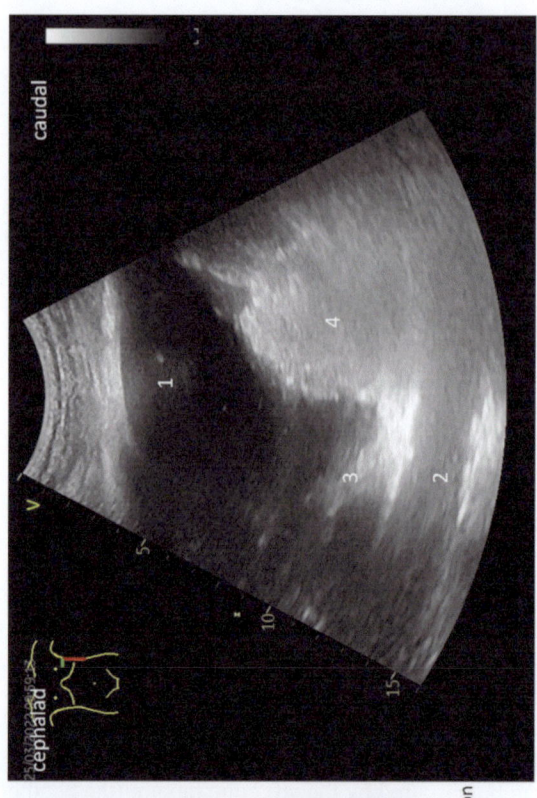

left lateral view – cranio-caudal orientation
numbers idicate
1 – stomach, fundus
2 – descending thoracic aorta
3 – diaphragm
4 – large bowel, left flexure

Fig. 12.2 Left lateral view of stomach filled with fluid, which can be misleading and interpreted as free intraabdominal fluid

position, the superior mesenteric artery may also be visible, appearing dorsal to the stomach (Fig. 12.1, no. 1).

The identification of the stomach via sonography is facilitated by its distinctive reflection pattern, characterized by a classical five-layer stratification. This stratification is a hallmark of gastrointestinal tract imaging and serves as a key diagnostic feature for sonographers. Understanding and recognizing these layers are crucial for assessing the integrity and pathology of the stomach wall. Here's a breakdown of these layers from the outermost to the innermost:

1. Serosa: This is the outermost layer of the stomach, appearing as a thin hyperechoic (bright on ultrasound) line. The serosa acts as a protective lining for the stomach.
2. Submucosa: Just beneath the serosa, this hyperechoic segment is slightly thicker and provides support to the mucosa. Its echogenicity is due to the presence of connective tissue and vessels within this layer.
3. Muscularis propria: Located between the submucosa and the muscularis mucosae, this structure appears hypoechoic (darker on ultrasound) and is composed of the smooth muscle layers of the stomach wall. It is responsible for the stomach's motility and mixing actions.
4. Muscularis mucosae: This thin hypoechoic layer follows the submucosa and serves as a boundary between the submucosa and the mucosa. It provides structural support to the mucosa and contributes to the stomach's flexibility.
5. Mucosa: The innermost layer, directly adjacent to the stomach lumen, appears as a very thin hyperechoic line. It becomes hyperechoic due to the transition from the solid tissue of the mucosa to the intraluminal air or fluid, creating a significant impedance mismatch, which results in a bright reflection.

This layered structure is not unique to the stomach and can be observed in various parts of the gastrointestinal tract, although the thickness and appearance of these layers can vary depending on the specific organ and its functional state. Accurate identification and assessment of these layers are essential in diagnosing conditions such as gastritis, tumors, and ulcers, making sonography an invaluable tool in gastrointestinal imaging.

12.3 Gastric Residual Volume

Determining the gastric residual volume is essential in clinical settings, especially for managing nutrition in critically ill or hospitalized patients. The cross-sectional area (CSA) in the antral region serves as a crucial measure for this purpose, with the area being calculated by measuring the transverse and longitudinal diameters around the antrum's outer edges.

Two primary methods have emerged for calculating gastric residual volume from the CSA: the Bouvet method and the Perlas method [4]. Each has its unique approach and considerations:

12.3.1 Bouvet Method [5]

This method is noted for its complexity, integrating multiple variables into its calculation, including patient height, ASA (American Society of Anesthesiologists) classification, body weight, and age. This comprehensive approach aims to account for various physiological factors that could influence gastric residual volume, making the Bouvet method thorough but also more complex to apply.

$$GV = -215 + 57\log CSA\left(mm^2\right) - 0.78 \times age(y) - 0.16 \times Größe(cm) - 0.25 \\ \times weight(kg) - 0.8 \times ASA + 16\,mL(emergency) + 10\,mL(PPI)$$

Calculation of GRV considering Bouvet

12.3.2 Perlas Method [6]

Designed for simplicity, the formula proposed by Perlas et al. focuses solely on the patient's age as the variable in the calculation. Its simplicity is considered an advantage, making it more accessible and quicker to apply in clinical settings. Notably, the Perlas method has been validated for use in patients with a BMI (body mass index) above 35, demonstrating its applicability to a wide range of individuals, including the morbidly obese [7]. In one study, it accurately predicted gastric residual volume in 53 out of 60 cases, underscoring its reliability. The method sets the threshold for predicting gastric residual volume at 500 mL, higher than the 250 mL threshold of the Bouvet method, and shows a high correlation with the actual residual volume across a broad measurement range.

$$GV = 27 + 14.6 \times RLA\,CSA\left(cm^2\right) - 1.28 \times age(y)$$

Calculation of GRV considering Perlas

The choice between these methods depends on the clinical context, the patient population, and the specific needs of the healthcare provider. While the Bouvet method offers a comprehensive analysis by considering multiple variables, its complexity may limit its utility in fast-paced or resource-constrained environments. Conversely, the Perlas method, with its simplicity and broad applicability, provides a practical alternative for quickly assessing gastric residual volume, particularly in settings where rapid decision-making is crucial.

Incorporating these methods into clinical practice enhances the ability of healthcare professionals to manage enteral nutrition effectively, reducing the risk of complications associated with improper feeding volumes and contributing to better patient care outcomes.

The acknowledgment of gastric juice's lethal dose in pulmonary aspiration, quantified at 1.5 mL/kg body weight, underscores the critical importance of accurately determining gastric residual volume (GRV) in both emergency situations and routine healthcare operations. This measurement not only aids in assessing the risk of significant pulmonary damage due to aspiration but also plays a pivotal role in the management of enteral nutrition.

Despite the current lack of extensive data in adult medicine concerning the regulation of enteral nutrition based on GRV assessments, the rationale for incorporating such evaluations into clinical practice is strong. Visualizing the gastric antrum, along with measuring the diameters and assessing the peristalsis and wall thickness of the small and large intestines, offers a comprehensive approach to understanding the functional status of the gastrointestinal (GI) tract. This methodological approach enables healthcare professionals to gauge the patient's capacity to safely receive enteral nutrition, thereby reducing the risk of aspiration and optimizing nutritional support.

While direct control over nutrition through GRV determination may not be immediately achievable, such evaluations are instrumental in making informed decisions about the initiation or continuation of enteral feeding. By determining a patient's readiness for enteral nutrition and identifying any severe GI tract disorders, clinicians can tailor nutritional interventions to each patient's specific needs and conditions. This not only enhances the safety and effectiveness of enteral nutrition strategies but also contributes to the overall well-being and recovery of patients.

Given the significant implications of GRV for patient care, further research and data collection in this area are essential. Advancing our understanding of GRV's impact on enteral nutrition and aspiration risk will undoubtedly improve clinical practices and patient outcomes in the realm of nutrition management. For the purpose of evaluating gastrointestinal function and readiness for enteral nutrition in critically ill patients, a sonographic assessment adhering to the criteria established by the European Society of Intensive Care Medicine (ESICM) working group on abdominal problems can be conducted [8]. The gastrointestinal ultrasound (GUTS) protocol, which has emerged from this initiative, offers a comprehensive framework for such evaluations. Despite its complexity and the inclusion of 11 distinct parameters, which may pose challenges even for experienced point-of-care sonographers, the GUTS protocol is noted for its high accuracy and predictive capability regarding gastrointestinal function and potential complications.

However, the detailed nature and breadth of the GUTS protocol can limit its feasibility for daily application in an intensive care setting, where time and resources are often constrained. This recognition has led to discussions and efforts to modify the protocol, aiming to retain its diagnostic and predictive strengths while simplifying its application to suit the fast-paced environment of intensive care units.

The modified form of the GUTS protocol could focus on a subset of the original parameters that are most indicative of gastrointestinal dysfunction or readiness for enteral nutrition, thus streamlining the evaluation process. Such an adaptation would allow healthcare providers to quickly and effectively assess the gastrointestinal status of critically ill patients, facilitating timely and appropriate nutritional interventions while minimizing the risk of complications associated with enteral feeding.

Table 12.1 Acute gastric injury score [8]

AGI grade 0	AGI grade I	AGI grade II	AGI grade III
Risk of GI dysfunction Known cause Function is partially impaired No therapeutic interventions needed	Gastrointestinal dysfunction No ability for GI tract to perform digestion Therapeutic interventions or drugs needed	Gastrointestinal failure Loss of GI function despite interventions Diagnosis of intraabdominal problems	Gastrointestinal failure with severe impact on organ function Life-threatening MODS and shock with possibility of GI necrosis or ischemia Laparotomy or other interventions

This approach underscores the importance of flexibility and adaptation in the application of diagnostic protocols, ensuring that they meet the practical demands of clinical settings without compromising the quality of patient care (Table 12.1).

Based on the AGI (abdominal gastrointestinal) score, the GUTS (gastrointestinal ultrasound) protocol assigns specific sonographic measurements [9]. The AGI Score is a grading system designed to assess the gastrointestinal function and potential dysfunction in critically ill patients using ultrasound. While the specific measurements and criteria can vary depending on the version of the protocol and the patient's condition, generally, the AGI Score incorporates a range of sonographic evaluations, including:

1. Gastric antrum size and volume: Assessing the cross-sectional area (CSA) of the gastric antrum to estimate the gastric residual volume. This involves measuring the anteroposterior and longitudinal diameters of the antrum.
2. Small and large intestine diameters: Measuring the diameters of the small and large intestines to evaluate for distension, which may indicate ileus or obstruction.
3. Peristalsis: Observing the peristaltic movements of the intestines to assess their functionality. A lack of peristalsis may indicate a severe gastrointestinal dysfunction.
4. Bowel wall thickness: Measuring the thickness of the bowel walls of the small and large intestines. Increased wall thickness can be a sign of inflammation, infection, or other pathologies.
5. Presence of free fluid: Checking for the presence of free fluid in the abdominal cavity, which can be a sign of inflammation, infection, or injury.
6. Ascites: Evaluating for the presence and amount of ascites, which may indicate liver disease, heart failure, or peritoneal carcinomatosis, among other conditions.
7. Extra-intestinal findings: Identifying any abnormalities outside the intestines that may affect gastrointestinal function, such as enlarged lymph nodes, masses, or organomegaly.

These measurements are used to grade the gastrointestinal function on a scale (e.g., AGI 0 to AGI 3), with higher scores indicating greater dysfunction. The AGI Score helps in the clinical assessment of patients, guiding therapeutic decisions

12 Gastrointestinal Sonography in Nutritional Management: A Clinical Perspective

Table 12.2 GUTS Score equivalent to AGI Score

AGI grade 0	AGI grade I	AGI grade II	AGI grade III
gCSA < 200 mL	gCSA 200–500 or >500 mL	gCSA > 500	gCSA > 500
SBD < 20 mm	SBD >20 < 30 mm	SBD > 30 mm	SBD > 30 mm
LBD < 50 mm	LBD 60 mm	LBD > 60 mm	LBD > 60 mm
MT < 5 mm	MT < 5 mm	MT > 5 mm	MT > 5 mm
Peristalsis absent or noneffective	Peristalsis absent augmented or non-effective	Peristalsis absent	Peristalsis absent
Blood flow resent	Blood flow present	Blood flow altered	Blood flow absent
RI > 0.6 < 1.2	RI >0.6 < 1.2	MBF > 200	No doppler detectable signal
Bladde full	MBF < 200	IAP 15–20 mm Hg	IAP > 20 mm Hg
MBF < 200	IAP 12–15 mm Hg	APP < 60 mm Hg	APP < 60 mm Hg
		RI > 1.2	RI > 1.2
		Bladder with low volume	Bladder empty

such as the readiness for enteral nutrition or the need for further diagnostic evaluations and interventions (Table 12.2).

The AGIUS (abdominal gastrointestinal ultrasound) protocol represents a modification and simplification of the original GUTS protocol but is equipped with a similar predictive power [10, 11]. It focuses specifically on three key sonographic measurements: intestinal diameter, bowel wall thickness, and peristalsis. From these measurements, a score is derived, which can predict enteral feeding intolerance if any of the parameters show abnormalities. Here's a closer look at each component:

12.3.3 Intestinal Diameter

The measurement of the diameter of the intestines (both small and large) is crucial in identifying distension that may be indicative of ileus, obstruction, or other conditions affecting the normal flow and processing of intestinal contents.

12.3.4 Bowel Wall Thickness

This parameter assesses the thickness of the intestinal walls. Increased thickness can be a marker of inflammation, infection, ischemia, or other pathological processes that might contraindicate the initiation or continuation of enteral nutrition due to the risk of intolerance or exacerbation of the underlying condition.

12.3.5 Peristalsis

Observing the peristaltic activity of the intestines provides insight into the functional state of the gastrointestinal tract. Normal peristalsis indicates a likely tolerance to enteral feeding, while reduced or absent peristaltic waves suggest dysfunction or paralysis, which may lead to feeding intolerance.

The AGIUS Score [11] simplifies the evaluation of gastrointestinal function and the risk of enteral feeding intolerance by focusing on these three parameters. A disturbance in any one of these measurements may indicate a potential intolerance to enteral nutrition, thereby guiding clinicians in their decision-making process regarding the initiation or adjustment of nutritional support in critically ill patients. This streamlined approach aims to facilitate quicker and more efficient bedside assessments, allowing for timely interventions tailored to the patient's current gastrointestinal functional status.

A further study by Lai et al. also focused on similar parameters [12]. In this prospective analysis, the gastric residual volume was assessed through the absolute cross-sectional area of the gastric antrum (CSA), alongside stomach peristalsis and the diameter of the colon frame. The findings revealed that the absence of peristalsis, combined with one other parameter, could predict enteral feeding intolerance with a sensitivity of over 88% and a specificity of over 84%. These results are comparably predictive to those obtained using the GUTS protocol, reinforcing the validity and utility of ultrasound-based assessments in predicting enteral feeding intolerance.

The study underscores the importance of evaluating both structural and functional aspects of the gastrointestinal system in critically ill patients. The combined assessment of gastric antrum size (as a proxy for residual volume), peristaltic activity, and colon diameter provides a comprehensive view of the gastrointestinal tract's capacity to handle enteral nutrition. The high sensitivity and specificity demonstrated in this study highlight the potential of ultrasound as a noninvasive, bedside tool for guiding nutritional management decisions in the intensive care setting, offering a practical alternative to more invasive or less readily available methods.

Indeed, the specific score or protocol used is not as crucial as the implementation of a method to assess gastrointestinal tract dysfunction and readiness for enteral nutrition. The key is to have a systematic approach in place that allows healthcare providers to evaluate the gastrointestinal (GI) system's status efficiently and accurately. Whether it's the GUTS protocol, AGIUS algorithm, or the approach described by Lai et al., each provides valuable insights into the GI tract's functional capacity, helping to predict enteral feeding tolerance.

The overarching goal is to ensure that critically ill patients receive the most appropriate nutritional support at the right time. Enteral nutrition, when feasible, is preferred for its benefits in maintaining gut integrity and function. However, it's essential to identify patients who may not tolerate this form of nutrition due to GI dysfunction, to avoid complications like aspiration pneumonia or exacerbation of GI symptoms.

Implementing a protocol for evaluating GI function and readiness for enteral feeding into the routine assessment of critically ill patients can help guide nutritional management decisions, potentially improving outcomes. It allows for a more personalized approach to nutrition, considering the patient's current physiological state and reducing the risks associated with inappropriate feeding.

12.4 Sonographic Assessment of Nasogastric Tubes Positioning

The gold standard for verifying the correct placement of a nasogastric tube is thoracic radiography. However, this method can lead to increased radiation exposure, especially since patients may unintentionally or intentionally remove their nasogastric tubes, necessitating repeated checks. Moreover, while X-ray equipment is often available in intensive care units, its use requires significant personnel resources.

As an alternative, ultrasound can be employed to ensure the correct placement of nasogastric tubes. This can be achieved through a stepwise protocol, allowing for the direct visualization of the tube or the identification of indirect signs, such as the presence of administered air or fluid.

According to Zatelli and Vezzali [13], during the placement of the tube, the ultrasound transducer can be positioned on the left lateral side of the neck to visualize the esophagus posterior to the trachea (Fig. 12.3). In both intubated and nonintubated patients, as the nasogastric tube is advanced, it can be visualized within the esophagus by a sonographic reflection similar to that of the trachea (Fig. 12.3, no. 1, 2). This ultrasound artifact serves as direct evidence of the nasogastric tube's presence, helping to prevent the tube from coiling in the mouth since its

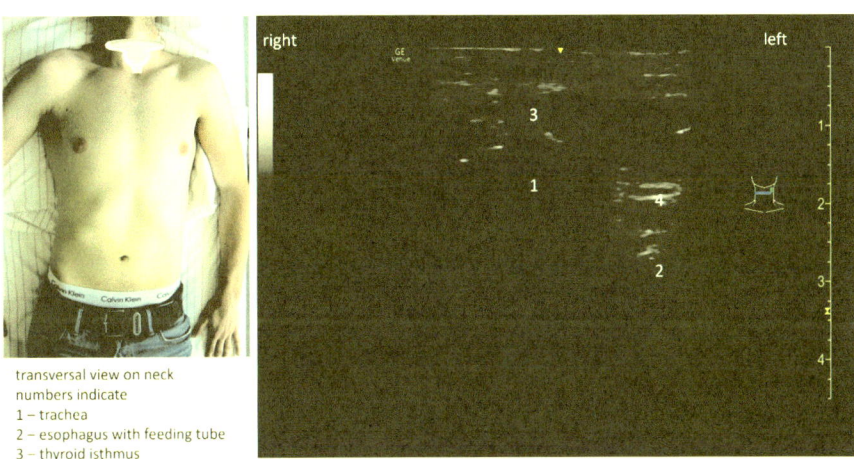

transversal view on neck
numbers indicate
1 – trachea
2 – esophagus with feeding tube
3 – thyroid isthmus
4 – thyroid gland, left lobe

Fig. 12.3 Transversal view of ventral neck, esophagus is visualized with intraluminal fluid and double reflex of gastric tube

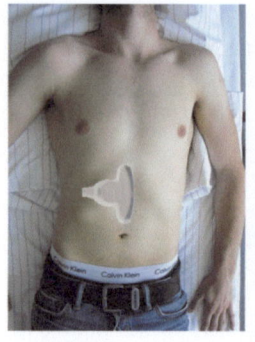
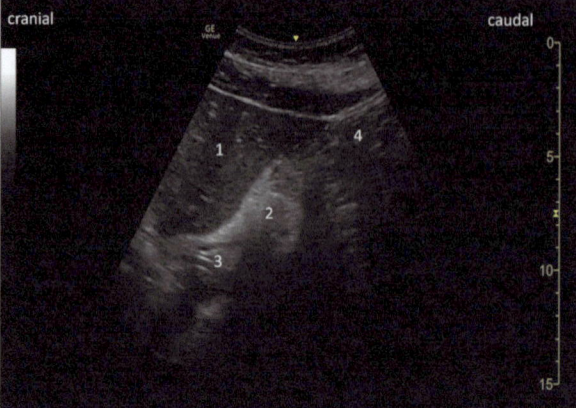

subcostal view – cranio-caudal orientation
numbers idicate
1 – liver, left lobe
2 – pancreas
3 – stomach, filled with air and solid content
4 – kardia, gastric tube inside

Fig. 12.4 Subcostal view at level of left liver lobe and aortic hiatus, aorta is not seen due to visualization of cardia of the stomach where the feeding tube as double lined artefact inside the stomach

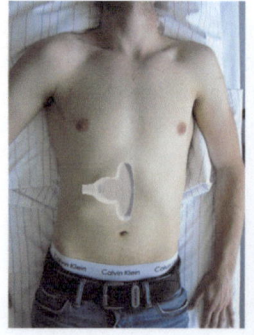
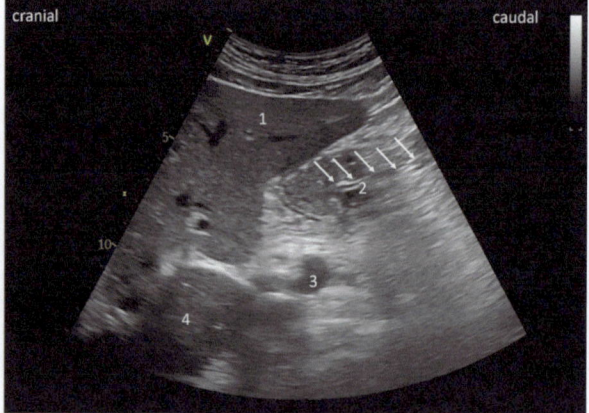

subcostal view – cranio-caudal orientation
numbers idicate
1 – liver, left lobe
2 – stomach with gastric tube
3 – portal vein
4 – lobus caudatus

Fig. 12.5 Subcostal visualization of stomach corpus, arrows indicate gastric tube within solid gastric content

advancement can be visualized. This technique is recommended not only in cases of difficult insertion but as a general practice to enhance safety and accuracy in nasogastric tube placement.

Further along, the distal esophagus and the cardia can be visualized (Fig. 12.4). At this position, it is also possible to display the nasogastric tube as a double contour, distinguishing it from the gastric wall layers (Fig. 12.4, no. 3).

By using a lateral view of the fundus (Fig. 12.5), the nasogastric tube can be visualized in either cross-section or longitudinal section. If this proves challenging, which may occur due to the presence of gastric air, visualization can sometimes be achieved through indirect signs. Applying gentle pressure to the stomach area to allow the air to escape below the transducer is one method.

If the stomach is filled with air and this air can be displaced, the introduction of fluid can help in visualization. The phenomenon of a swarm of echoes caused by the inflowing fluid through the nasogastric tube can also be observed.

If the gastric content is solid or liquid, the introduction of air or fluid can help visualize it. It is advisable to insufflate amounts between 20 and 50 mL to achieve clear visualization.

These sonographic techniques offer a noninvasive, immediate way to confirm the correct placement of nasogastric tubes and assess gastric contents, providing valuable information for managing patient care effectively.

References

1. Goyal RK, Guo Y, Mashimo H. Advances in the physiology of gastric emptying. Neurogastroenterol Motil. 2019;31:e13546.
2. Abell TL, et al. Consensus recommendations for gastric emptying scintigraphy: a joint report of the American Neurogastroenterology and Motility Society and the Society of Nuclear Medicine. J Nucl Med Technol. 2008;36:44–54.
3. Jahreis T, et al. Sonographic evaluation of gastric residual volume during enteral nutrition in critically ill patients using a miniaturized ultrasound device. J Clin Med. 2021;10:4859.
4. Bainbridge D, McConnell B, Royse C. A review of diagnostic accuracy and clinical impact from the focused use of perioperative ultrasound. Can J Anaesth. 2018;65:371–80.
5. Bouvet L, et al. Could a single standardized ultrasonographic measurement of antral area be of interest for assessing gastric contents? A preliminary report. Eur J Anaesthesiol. 2009;26:1015–9.
6. Perlas A, et al. Validation of a mathematical model for ultrasound assessment of gastric volume by gastroscopic examination. Anesth Analg. 2013;116:357–63.
7. Van de Putte P, Perlas A. Gastric sonography in the severely obese surgical patient: a feasibility study. Anesth Analg. 2014;119:1105–10.
8. Reintam Blaser A, et al. Gastrointestinal function in intensive care patients: terminology, definitions and management. Recommendations of the ESICM Working Group on Abdominal Problems. Intensive Care Med. 2012;38:384–94.
9. Perez-Calatayud AA, et al. Point-of-care gastrointestinal and urinary tract sonography in daily evaluation of gastrointestinal dysfunction in critically ill patients (GUTS protocol). Anaesthesiol Intensive Ther. 2018;50:40–8.
10. Pérez-Calatayud ÁA, Carillo-Esper R. Role of gastric ultrasound to guide enteral nutrition in the critically ill. Curr Opin Clin Nutr Metab Care. 2023;26:114–9.
11. Gao T, et al. Predictive value of transabdominal intestinal sonography in critically ill patients: a prospective observational study. Crit Care. 2019;23:378.
12. Lai J, et al. Bedside gastrointestinal ultrasound combined with acute gastrointestinal injury score to guide enteral nutrition therapy in critically patients. BMC Anesthesiol. 2022;22:231.
13. Zatelli M, Vezzali N. 4-Point ultrasonography to confirm the correct position of the nasogastric tube in 114 critically ill patients. J Ultrasound. 2017;20:53–8.

Part III

Organ Dysfunction and Specific Conditions

Nutrition in Patients with Kidney Disease

Wilfred Druml

Acute kidney injury (AKI) is a heterogenous syndrome, a systemic disease process which induces an inflammatory, pro-oxidative, and hypercatabolic state which exerts profound effects on the course of disease and on short- /long-term outcome [1]. AKI is defined by three distinct stages (AKI-1, AKI-2; AKI-3). The metabolic care and nutrition therapy must be adapted meticulously to these distinctly different stages with fundamentally differing metabolic environment and requirements.

It is of fundamental importance that there is no uniform "Nutrition for AKI": In patients with normal kidney function and risk stadium AKI-1, it is all about prevention, in AKI stadium 2 and 3 without renal replacement therapy (RRT) to moderate nutrition to avoid aggravation of renal injury and in AKI 3b and RRT to enable adequate nutrition support by taking into consideration the therapy-associated nutrient losses, but also potential increased intake of energy substrates (lactate, citrate) [2, 3].

Patients with chronic kidney disease (CKD) and patients on regular hemodialysis (HD) therapy, respectively, who acquire an acute intermittent disease process—from a nutritional and metabolic point of view—share many similarities to patients with AKI-3b. In these patients, nutrition support also has to be adapted to the relevant stages of CKD (CKD-3 to CKD-5), but should follow analog principles to those with AKI in comparable kidney dysfunction groups.

High-quality, systematic investigations on nutrition support in patients with AKI or critically ill patients with CKD/HD mostly are lacking. Thus, many statements and recommendations for nutrition in patients with AKI are based on expert opinion [4].

W. Druml (✉)
Klinik für Innere Medizin III, Abteilung für Nephrologie, Vienna, Austria
e-mail: wilfred.druml@meduniwien.ac.at

© The Author(s), under exclusive license to Springer Nature Switzerland AG 2025
A. Rümelin et al. (eds.), *Nutrition in ICU Patients*,
https://doi.org/10.1007/978-3-032-00818-3_13

13.1 Common Metabolic Alterations in Patients with Renal Insufficiency (AKI/CKD)

The metabolic environment and the nutrient requirements in acutely ill patients with renal insufficiency (AKI/CKD) are not only determined by the kidney dysfunction per se and by the type and intensity of renal replacement therapy (RRT) but also by intermittent acute disease process and associated complications and other organ dysfunctions [5].

Nevertheless, it should be noted that AKI/CKD share a specific pattern of alterations of metabolism which become relevant when glomerular filtration falls below 60 ml/min and thus, have to be regarded when designing a nutrition regimen (Table 13.1).

13.2 Metabolic Factors in the Prevention of AKI and Therapy of Risk Stage AKI-1

Considering its profound impact on the evolution of complications and impairment of short- and long-term outcome, the prevention of AKI must present a continued effort. In the absence of effective pharmacological interventions, the general management of the patient, the optimization of hemodynamics, of the volume state, of respiratory function, the avoidance of nephrotoxic drugs, are of outmost importance to preserve or restore kidney function [5]. In this context, the metabolic management and nutrition support play a (often overlooked) major role.

The relevant factors are summarized in Table 13.2. Electrolyte dysbalances and acidosis have been shown to promote kidney injury. Chloride-rich infusion regimens (especially when using (ab)normal saline) may increase the risk of AKI. Avoidance or therapy of hyperglycemia is included into the KDIGO AKI-prevention bundle [6]. An excessive energy or protein intake in the acute phase of disease may increase the risk of kidney breakdown [7]. Preexisting deficiency states, such as of thiamine should be corrected.

A large number of randomized controlled trial have demonstrated that an early high nutrient intake, in an unstable phase of disease, which is characterized by an increased mobilization of endogenous substrates (amino acids, glucose, fatty acids),

Table 13.1 Common metabolic alterations in AKI and CKD

Induction/ augmentation of an inflammatory state
Activation of protein catabolism
Peripheral insulin resistance
Inhibition of lipolysis
Depletion of antioxidative systems
Impairment of immunocompetence
Impairment of potassium disposal
Hormonal derangements: hyperparathyroidism, increased FGF-23, insulin resistance, EPO resistance, GH resistance, etc.

Table 13.2 Metabolic factors in prevention and therapy of AKI

Avoidance of a chloride overload
Maintenance of electrolyte balance (phosphate, potassium, magnesium)
Avoidance/correction of severe acidosis
Preference of enteral nutrition
Avoidance/therapy of hyperglycemia
Avoidance of excessive energy intake
Avoidance of a high protein intake in presence of AKI-1-2
Prevention by a higher amino acid or protein intake (?)
Correction of potential nutrient deficiencies (thiamine, antioxidants)

is associated with a series of complications and especially AKI and potentially worse outcome [8, 9]. Thus, there is a broad agreement that nutrition intake in the acute phase of disease should be restricted [10].

There is an ongoing discussion whether a higher protein intake exerts a nephroprotective effect by increasing renal perfusion and function (activation of "renal reserve capacity"). This certainly should not be done in the early acute phase of disease when a high protein intake is associated with serious side effects but could be effective in a further stable course of disease.

Resent reports have suggested that an isolated high amino acid load (2 g/kg/day for up to 3 days) during surgery may prevent the evolution of AKI [11]. However, this certainly is not a nutritional intervention and may be effective in specific patient groups only.

Taken together we have learned that an early full nutrition, all a high protein, or energy intake any hyperglycemia actually can aggravate renal injury, increase the risk of AKI and the need and duration of RRT and worsen prognosis [8].

Beyond giving attention to these points, the nutrition and metabolic management of the ICU patient should follow the general recommendations for nutrition in the ICU patient [12]. No specific enteral diets or parenteral nutrition preparations should be used in these patients.

13.3 Nutrition Support in AKI Stages 2 and 3 Without the Need of Kidney Replacement Therapy (RRT)

The more severe stages of AKI, AKI-2, and AKI-3 without need of RRT are by definition unstable phases of diseases. The primary goal must be the preservation or better, the restoration of kidney function, and avoidance of further kidney injury and progression to the need of RRT.

The factors listed in Table 13.1 must be meticulously observed also in this stage. Actually, these measures do not fundamentally differ from those followed in the management of other unstable critically ill patients.

Volume management is crucial in this phase, the avoidance of too little or too much of balanced cristalloid solutions and the avoidance of chloride rich solutions. Nevertheless, the risk of overhydration is much higher in these patients, which increases the risk of kidney injury and actually has become a leading cause of initiation of RRT, factors closely associated with a worse outcome.

Any "metabolic overload" should also be avoided in this unstable stage of AKI. Again, energy intake should start or kept below the calculated or measured energy expenditure. However, most interest has received the problem of optimal protein intake. A high protein intake (>1.g kg/BW/day?) during ongoing renal injury aggravates kidney injury and increases the need for RRT and mortality [8, 13]. Individually adapting energy and protein intake and avoiding hyperglycemia must be strictly observed to prevent further kidney damage [8].

One must stress that the long-held dogma to further a full nutrition and accept an increased need for RRT is absolutely wrong. We have learned that RRT is associated with a complex pattern of untoward side effects. Initiation of an otherwise unnecessary RRT can exert profound negative side effects on the further course of disease and prognosis [8].

The novel implication of these recent findings is that nutrition support in this unstable phase of disease must also avoid "overnutrition," should also take into account the kidney function, and should be individually adapted to the grade of renal injury [8]. Any inadequate high nutrition intake in a period where endogenous mobilization of endogenous substrates (glucose, amino acids, fatty acids) will cause a metabolic overload and an aggravation of renal injury (for nutrient requirements, see Table 13.3).

Giving attention to these points should be integrated into the general recommendations for nutrition in the ICU patient. No kidney-specific enteral diets or parenteral nutrition preparations are recommended in these patients.

13.4 Nutrition Support in AKI Stages 3b with the Need Replacement Therapy (RRT) and CKD-5b with the Need of Chronic HD

In these advanced stages of kidney injury, RRT is needed to compensate the systemic consequences of uremia, to maintain volume and electrolyte balances, to support hemodynamics and respiratory functions. In these patients, the specific consequences of kidney dysfunction and of the type and intensity of RRT on metabolism and nutrient requirements have to be taken into consideration.

All modalities of RRT exert a profound impact on metabolism and nutrient balances (Table 13.3) [14]. On one side, this presents unspecific effects of any extracorporeal circulation per se as obligatory consequences of bioincompatibility and the induction of a (low-grade) inflammatory reaction. On the other side, various

Table 13.3 Metabolic effects of renal replacement therapies

Intermittent hemodialysis (iHD)
Loss of water-soluble molecules:
Amino acids, water-soluble vitamins, L-carnitine, etc.
Stimulation of low-grade inflammation/ protein catabolism:
Loss of amino acids, proteins, blood
Secretion of cytokines (TNF-a, etc.)
Inhibition of protein synthesis
Loss of antioxidants
Increased production of reactive oxygen species (ROS)
Continuous renal replacement therapies (CRRT)
Loss of heat (= energy)
Excessive uptake of substrates
Lactate, citrate, glucose
Loss of nutrients
Amino acids, vitamins, selenium, etc.
Loss of albumin
Loss of electrolyte (phosphate, magnesium, potassium)
Elimination of peptides
Hormones, cytokines
Elimination of electrolytes (phosphate, magnesium, calcium)
Elimination of antibiotics
Metabolic consequences of bioincompatibility (Induction of a "low-grade" inflammation, stimulation of protein catabolism, formation of ROS, etc.)

modalities are associated with specific effects, most importantly, the loss of various nutrients, electrolytes but also an increased infusion of energy substrates (lactate, citrate). Especially, continuous RRTs (CRRTs)—because of the prolonged therapy and the associated high fluid turnover—have relevant implications for electrolyte (observe phosphate) and nutrient requirements (Table 13.3).

In these stages, an adequate nutrition is more or less similar to other ICU patients, but design of nutrition solutions must take into consideration the therapy-induced electrolyte and nutrient losses, especially of amino acids/protein and water-soluble vitamins, and the higher energy intake from lactate and citrate.

13.5 Nutritional Requirements

Nutritional requirements in these patient groups are determined by the stage of renal dysfunction and the modality and the dose of RRT but also by the type and severity of underlying acute disease process and further associated complications and organ dysfunctions [15].

It should be stressed that patients with AKI/ CKD—from a metabolic and nutritional point of view—present an extremely heterogenous group of subjects. Nutrient requirements can vary considerably between the patients but also in the same patient during the often dynamic course of disease. Much more than in other patients, nutrition support must be tailored to the individual needs of the patient assessed on a day-to-day basis (Table 13.4).

13.6 Enteral Nutrition (EN)

Even when most studies on nutrition support in patients with AKI have been performed using PN, there can be no doubt that also in this patient group enteral nutrition presents the route of choice, which should be aimed at whenever possible [16]. Besides the many well-described beneficial effects in various patient groups, enteral nutrition is associated with specific effects in patients with renal dysfunction, i.e., an increase in renal perfusion and function.

One limitation to enteral nutrition in patients with AKI/CKD, however, is the fact that renal insufficiency augments the impairment of gastrointestinal motility. In order to improve the tolerance to EN, the use of prokinetics should be considered early (or even prophylactically). Drugs that stimulate both gastric emptying and intestinal motility should be preferred.

In the case that prokinetics are insufficient to stimulate gastrointestinal motility and tolerance, placement of a jejunal tube should be considered. Modern tubes can be placed rapidly and safely also without the need of endoscopy.

Table 13.4 Nutrition requirements for patients with AKI and acutely ill patients with CKD[a]

Energy intake	18–max. 24	kcal/kg/day
Glucose	3–max. 4	g/kg/day
Lipids[b]	0.8–1.0 (max. 1.2)	g/kg/day
Amino acids/protein		
AKI-1-AKI-3a[c]	0.6–0.8	g/kg/day
+ RRT (AKI-3b, CKD-5b)	1.2–1.4	g/kg/day
+ hypercatabolism	(max. 1.5?)	g/kg/day
Vitamins (combination products containing RDA)		
Water soluble	2 × RDA/ day (higher for thiamine??)	
Lipid soluble	1–2 × RDA/day (higher for vitamin D?)	
Trace elements (combination products containing RDA)		
	1 × RDA/day (higher for selenium 200–500 µg/day?)	
Electrolytes (must be adapted individually) (Cave: refeeding hypophosphatemia also in AKI-3b; CKD-5))		

RRT renal replacement therapy, *RDA* recommended dietary allowances
[a]Please note: These are (and can only be) approximate values; requirements can fundamentally vary between the stages of AKI/CKD, between individual patients but also within a patient during the mostly dynamic course of disease! Consider the stage of kidney dysfunction, observe a lower intake during ongoing renal injury!
[b]Consider lipid intake by propofol infusion
[c]Initial of unstable phases of disease

EN should be started at a low rate (about 30% of the final target), and infusion rate should be increased slowly to ensure gastrointestinal tolerance and to avoid the evolution of metabolic complications, but should be avoided in the presence of a dysfunctional gut (risk of nonocclusive bowel ischemia).

Even when provision of a quantitatively sufficient enteral nutrition is not possible (and also during parenteral nutrition), "trophic nutrition" (covering ca. 15% of requirements) should be provided whenever possible to support intestinal functions and barrier.

Enteral diets

Standard high molecular diets as for other ICU patients are recommended also for patients with AKI/CKD. Specific diets adapted to the needs of CKD/HD patients are available but are not indicated in acute phases of disease. These preparations may be used in more chronic phases of diseases and advanced stages of renal dysfunction where these specific diets may facilitate the metabolic management of patients but are not associated with outcome-relevant advantages.

13.7 Parenteral Nutrition

When a (quantitatively sufficient) enteral nutrition is not possible and tolerance cannot be increased by provision of prokinetics and/or placement of a jejunal tube, a supplementary or total parenteral nutrition should be provided.

When enteral nutrition is not desired or possible at all, parenteral nutrition should be started early (within 24 h). It should be kept in mind that many renal patients have preexisting malnutrition. Moreover, in AKI-3b and CKD-5b, several nutrients are eliminated during RRT in relevant amounts. Thus, when buildup of enteral nutrition is retarded, supplementary parenteral nutrition should started at day 3.

When the energy intake due to citrate anticoagulation is increased and the infusion rate of the all-in-one solution must be reduced, an extra infusion may become necessary to compensate the therapy induced losses.

Parenteral nutrition should be started at a low rate (i.e., 30% of the final infusion rate), and infusion rate should be increased individually in order to monitor the utilization of the nutrients provided and to avoid the development of metabolic and organ complications.

Parenteral Nutrition Solutions

For parenteral nutrition, the use of commercially available standard nutrition solutions is recommended [15]. These usually are three-chamber bags containing the macronutrients glucose, amino acids, and a lipid emulsion. Some solutions also contain basic requirements of electrolytes. Water-soluble vitamins, lipid-soluble vitamins, trace elements, and electrolytes (Note: phosphate!) must be added to these basal solutions as required. For patients on RRT, the double dose of water-soluble vitamins should be added and phosphate containing replacement fluids should be used.

13.8 Monitoring and Complications of Nutrition Support

Because of the reduced tolerance to volume and electrolyte infusions and the impairment of the utilization of several substrates, metabolic disturbances, such as electrolyte imbalances, hyperglycemia, hypertriglyceridemia, or excessive rises in BUN, can develop in patients with impaired renal function much more often and faster than in other patient groups.

It has become clear that an inadequate nutrition during unstable phases of AKI can aggravate renal injury and increase the requirement of RRT. Thus, nutrition support of patients with AKI/CKD requires a much closer clinical and metabolic monitoring than other patient groups and individual adaptation of nutrition accordingly [8].

Moreover, because of the interference of renal dysfunction with gastrointestinal motility, also enteral nutrition may be associated with a higher complication rate in these patients with AKI/CKD.

Most side effects and complications can be prevented when infusion of the nutrition solution is started at a low rate and gradually increased according to the "renal tolerance." This practice facilitates the monitoring of nutrition support and the adaptation to needs of the individual patient and avoid aggravation of renal injury.

References

1. Druml W. Systemic consequences of acute kidney injury. Curr Opin Crit Care. 2014;20:613–9.
2. Druml W, Joannidis M, John S, Jorres A, Schmitz M, Kielstein J, Kindgen-Milles D, Oppert M, Schwenger V, Willam C, Zarbock A. Metabolic management and nutrition in critically ill patients with renal dysfunction: recommendations from the renal section of the DGIIN, OGIAIN, and DIVI. Med Klin Intensivmed Notfmed. 2018;113:393–400.
3. Druml W, Kalantar-Zadeh K. The metabolic management and nutrition of acute kidney injury. In: Koyner J, Topf J, Lerma E, editors. Handbook of crital care nephrology. Philadelphia: Wolters Kluwer; 2021. p. 169–79.
4. Sabatino A, Fiaccadori E, Barazzoni R, Carrero JJ, Cupisti A, De Waele E, Jonckheer J, Cuerda C, Bischoff SC. ESPEN practical guideline on clinical nutrition in hospitalized patients with acute or chronic kidney disease. Clin Nutr. 2024;43:2238–54.
5. Druml W. Metabolic alterations in acute renal failure. Contrib Nephrol. 1992;98:59–66.
6. Gunst J, Debaveye Y, Guiza F, Dubois J, De Bruyn A, Dauwe D, De Troy E, Casaer MP, De Vlieger G, Haghedooren R, Jacobs B, Meyfroidt G, Ingels C, Muller J, Vlasselaers D, Desmet L, Mebis L, Wouters PJ, Stessel B, Geebelen L, Vandenbrande J, Brands M, Gruyters I, Geerts E, De Pauw I, Vermassen J, Peperstraete H, Hoste E, De Waele JJ, Herck I, Depuydt P, Wilmer A, Hermans G, Benoit DD, Van den Berghe G, Collaborators TG-F. Tight blood-glucose control without early parenteral nutrition in the ICU. N Engl J Med. 2023;389:1180–90.
7. Al-Dorzi HM, Albarrak A, Ferwana M, Murad MH, Arabi YM. Lower versus higher dose of enteral caloric intake in adult critically ill patients: a systematic review and meta-analysis. Crit Care. 2016;20:358.
8. Druml W, Staudinger T, Joannidis M. The kidney: the critical organ system for guiding nutrition therapy in the ICU-patient? Crit Care. 2024;28:266.
9. Yue HY, Peng W, Zeng J, Zhang Y, Wang Y, Jiang H. Efficacy of permissive underfeeding for critically ill patients: an updated systematic review and trial sequential meta-analysis. J Intensive Care. 2024;12:4.

10. de Man AME, Gunst J, Reintam Blaser A. Nutrition in the intensive care unit: from the acute phase to beyond. Intensive Care Med. 2024;50:1035–48.
11. Landoni G, Monaco F, Ti LK, Baiardo Redaelli M, Bradic N, Comis M, Kotani Y, Brambillasca C, Garofalo E, Scandroglio AM, Viscido C, Paternoster G, Franco A, Porta S, Ferrod F, Calabro MG, Pisano A, Vendramin I, Barucco G, Federici F, Severi L, Belletti A, Cortegiani A, Bruni A, Galbiati C, Covino A, Baryshnikova E, Giardina G, Venditto M, Kroeller D, Nakhnoukh C, Mantovani L, Silvetti S, Licheri M, Guarracino F, Lobreglio R, Di Prima AL, Fresilli S, Labanca R, Mucchetti M, Lembo R, Losiggio R, Bove T, Ranucci M, Fominskiy E, Longhini F, Zangrillo A, Bellomo R, Group PS. A randomized trial of intravenous amino acids for kidney protection. N Engl J Med. 2024;391:687–98.
12. Singer P, Blaser AR, Berger MM, Alhazzani W, Calder PC, Casaer MP, Hiesmayr M, Mayer K, Montejo JC, Pichard C, Preiser JC, van Zanten ARH, Oczkowski S, Szczeklik W, Bischoff SC. ESPEN guideline on clinical nutrition in the intensive care unit. Clin Nutr. 2019;38:48–79.
13. Stoppe C, Patel JJ, Zarbock A, Lee ZY, Rice TW, Mafrici B, Wehner R, Chan MHM, Lai PCK, MacEachern K, Myrianthefs P, Tsigou E, Ortiz-Reyes L, Jiang X, Day AG, Hasan MS, Meybohm P, Ke L, Heyland DK. The impact of higher protein dosing on outcomes in critically ill patients with acute kidney injury: a post hoc analysis of the EFFORT protein trial. Crit Care. 2023;27:399.
14. Fishman G, Singer P. Metabolic and nutritional aspects in continuous renal replacement therapy. J Intensive Med. 2023;3:228–38.
15. Fiaccadori E, Sabatino A, Barazzoni R, Carrero JJ, Cupisti A, De Waele E, Jonckheer J, Singer P, Cuerda C. ESPEN guideline on clinical nutrition in hospitalized patients with acute or chronic kidney disease. Clin Nutr. 2021;40:1644–68.
16. Fiaccadori E, Maggiore U, Giacosa R, Rotelli C, Picetti E, Sagripanti S, Melfa L, Meschi T, Borghi L, Cabassi A. Enteral nutrition in patients with acute renal failure. Kidney Int. 2004;65:999–1008.

Nutrition in Liver Disease

Jule K. Adams and Alexander Koch

14.1 Nutrition in ICU–Nutrition in Liver Disease

1. *What It's About—the Liver's Central Role in Nutrition and Metabolism*

The liver plays a vital role in metabolism and detoxification (Fig. 14.1). Besides synthesizing and storing macronutrients, it also serves as a depot for several micronutrients. One of its crucial functions is maintaining glucose homeostasis by providing glycogen. Over 90% of plasma proteins are synthesized in the liver. The production and excretion of bile salts ensures the absorption of dietary fat and fat-soluble vitamins. Another essential task is the detoxification of substances that are ingested as side effects of a normal diet. The liver exerts a significant role in inflammatory response, as it synthesizes numerous cytokines and chemokines [1].

2. *What to Face: Liver Disease in Critically Ill Patients*

In the intensive care setting, it is crucial to distinguish the different types of hepatopathy including acute decompensation (AD) in advanced or end-staged liver disease, acute-on-chronic liver failure (ACLF), or acute liver failure (ALF). An early and correct diagnosis allows an adjusted therapy to patients' needs and hereby improves the overall outcome. In the field of nutritional therapy, liver injury or impaired liver function are accompanied by similar metabolic challenges.

J. K. Adams · A. Koch
Department of Gastroenterology, Metabolic Disorders and Intensive Care Medicine,
University Hospital RWTH Aachen, Aachen, Germany
e-mail: akoch@ukaachen.de

© The Author(s), under exclusive license to Springer Nature
Switzerland AG 2025
A. Rümelin et al. (eds.), *Nutrition in ICU Patients*,
https://doi.org/10.1007/978-3-032-00818-3_14

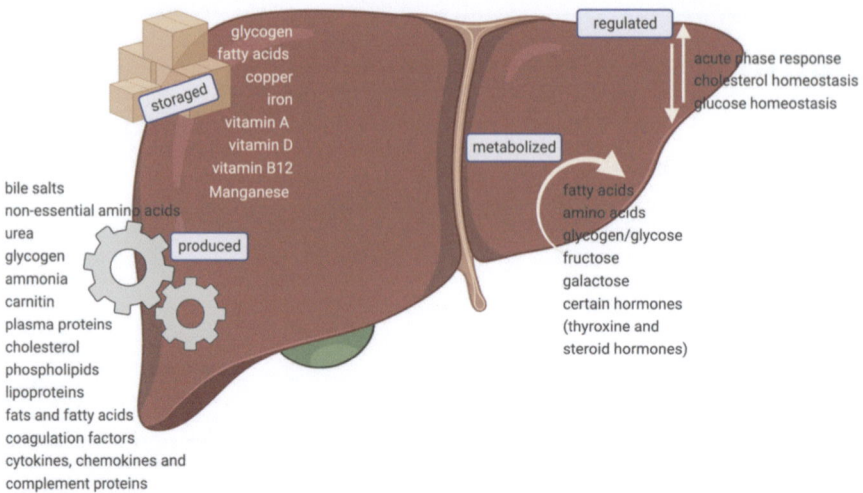

Fig. 14.1 Overview of production, storage, metabolism, and regulation of essential nutrients in the liver [1]. (Created using biorender.com)

14.2 Acute Decompensation of Cirrhosis and Acute-on-Chronic Liver Failure

The acute decompensation in advanced or end-staged liver disease is defined as the acute development of overt clinical symptoms. At this stage, patients typically present with ascites, bleedings, encephalopathy, and jaundice as consequence of complex pathophysiological processes [2]. Intravasal hypovolemia due to hypoalbuminemia, portal hypertension, and peripheral arterial vasodilation activate mechanisms of fluid and sodium retention and contribute to extravasal fluid overload (e.g., anasarca and ascites) as well as hepatorenal syndrome (HRS), a specific type of prerenal acute kidney failure.

Besides hemodynamic dysfunction, decompensated cirrhosis is understood as a proinflammatory syndrome and immune dysfunction. Accompanied by changes in the microbiome and increased intestinal permeability, it is characterized by a high susceptibility for infections such as spontaneous bacterial peritonitis (SBP) and sepsis, commonly due to pneumonia and urogenital infections [3].

Intestinal bleedings, mainly esophageal variceal bleeding, and hepatic encephalopathy due to ammonium accumulation are further important clinical signs of decompensation. Once cirrhosis is classified as decompensated, a notable prognostic deterioration can be observed. For example, ascites in patients with cirrhosis has been associated with a median survival of 1.1 years [4].

In case of ACLF, the acute hepatic decompensation is resulting in multi-organ failure [2]. There are a variety of potential triggers (hepatic and extrahepatic) for AD and ACLF. Bacterial infections, active alcohol intake, or use of new medication are the major precipitating events in Western countries, while the exacerbation of

Table 14.1 The CLIF-C-(Chronic Liver Failure-Consortium)-organ failure score system for the calculation of the CLIF-C- ACLF-Score [6].

Organ system	Biomarker	Score = 1	Score = 2	Score = 3
Liver	Bilirubin (mg/dL)	<6	6 to ≤12	≥12
Kidney	Creatinine (mg/dL)	<2	2 to ≤3.5	≥3.5 or RRT
Brain	Encephalopathy grade (West-Haven)	0	1–2	3–4
Coagulation	INR	<2	2 to ≤2.5	≥2.5
Circulation	MAP (mmHg)	≥70	<70	Vasopressors
Respiratory	PaO_2/FiO_2 or SpO_2/FiO_2	>300	≤300 and >200	≤200

FiO₂ fraction of inspired oxygen, *PaO₂* partial pressure of arterial oxygen, *SpO₂* pulse oximetric saturation, *RRT* renal replacement therapy

hepatitis B also plays an important role in Eastern countries. Other possible trigger factors are viral or fungal infections, hemorrhage, or surgery [2].

In general, ACLF is causing a mortality rate up to 50% [5]. The CLIF-C-ACLF score (modified from the well-established Sequential Organ Failure Assessment score, SOFA) is used to classify different severity levels of ACLF and to predict the probability of death within 28 days. For the calculation of the CLIF-C-ACLF score, the CLIF-organ failure score system (Table 14.1) as well as white blood cell count and patients' age are used [6].

14.3 Acute Liver Failure

Acute (primary) liver failure is defined as a severe hepatopathy with an acute onset of jaundice, coagulopathy (INR >1,5) and hepatic encephalopathy (HE). The definition requires the exclusion of preexisting chronic liver disease, as well as secondary causes such as sepsis or cardiogenic shock. The interval from jaundice to HE appearance helps to differentiate between hyperacute (7 days), acute (8–28 days), and subacute (5–12 weeks) ALF [7]. Due to a lack of epidemiological data, incidence is estimated with 200–500 cases per year in Germany [8]. Major causes are acetaminophen toxicity, other drugs (e.g., antibiotics), or acute viral infections with a variance in distribution depending on the geographic area (Table 14.2). ALF is associated with a high in-hospital mortality of 23–59% [8]. As prognostic tools for estimating the need of a high-urgency liver transplantation, the Kings' college criteria and the Clichy criteria (for viral hepatitis) are clinically used.

In acute manifestation of autoimmune hepatitis, Morbus Wilson, or Budd-Chiari syndrome, although they are related to chronic preexisting disease, high-urgency liver transplantation is also therapeutic option. Secondary acute liver failure can occur due to conditions like lymphoma infiltration, sepsis, or hypoxic hepatitis (e.g., in cardiogenic shock), where high-urgency transplantation is not feasible [9].

Table 14.2 Primary and secondary causes of ALF [9]

	Primary ALF	Secondary ALF
Acute liver failure	Drug toxicity Acute viral hepatitis A, B, E Mushroom poisoning Budd-Chiari syndrome Pregnancy-associated liver disease	Hypoxic hepatitis Hemophagocytic syndrome Sepsis Lymphoma infiltration
Preexisting liver disease presenting as acute liver failure	Morbus Wilson Autoimmune hepatitis Budd-Chiari syndrome Hepatitis-B reactivation *High-urgency transplantation possible*	Liver metastasis Status post liver resection Alcoholic hepatitis Acute-on-chronic liver failure *High-urgency transplantation not possible*

Table 14.3 Laboratory parameters and the formula used for the MELD score [13]

Laboratory parameters	MELD formula
Bilirubin	$9.57 \times \log_e (\text{creatinine}) + 3.78 \times \log_e (\text{total bilirubin}) + 11.2 \times \log_e (\text{INR}) + 6.43$
Creatinine	
INR	

14.4 Liver Transplantation

Liver transplantation is considered as the definitive treatment option for end-stage liver disease. Whether a patient is eligible for it depends on several criteria that need to be carefully assessed beforehand. The Model of End-Stage Liver Disease (MELD) score is used to prioritize the patients depending on their clinical condition and to simplify the organ allocation (Table 14.3). The MELD score is updated regularly to ensure any dynamic in course of the disease is reflected [10, 11]. In Germany, 780 liver transplants were performed in 2021 [12].

14.5 Metabolic Consequences of Liver Disease

Impaired liver function leads to a variety of changes in metabolism. Particularly, patients with chronic liver disease have a high risk of malnutrition and sarcopenia (Fig. 14.2). A recent meta-analysis points out that 37.5% of patients with liver cirrhosis suffer from sarcopenia, with higher prevalence in males, patients with alcohol-related liver disease, and higher severity of cirrhosis, as expressed by MELD [14].

Reduced dietary intake results, among other factors, from early satiety, anorexia of chronic disease, and nausea. Impaired production and secretion of bile salts lead to malabsorption of fat and fat-soluble vitamins [15]. The early transition from

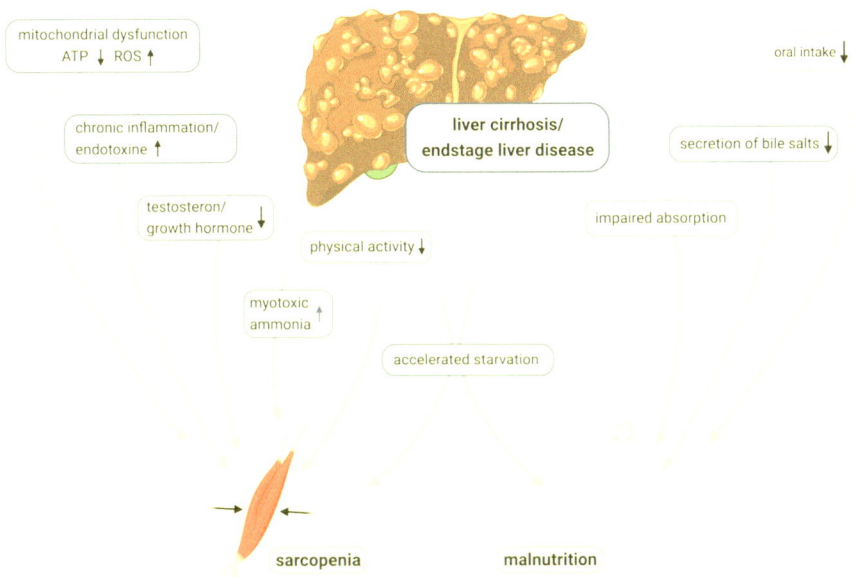

Fig. 14.2 Pathophysiological processes leading to malnutrition and sarcopenia in end-stage liver disease [15]. (Created using biorender.com)

glycogenolysis to gluconeogenesis from amino acids and fatty acid oxidation in the postprandial state goes along with heightened rates of whole-body protein breakdown and is termed "accelerated starvation" [15]. Changes in protein metabolism and decreased levels of branched-chain amino acids cause a reduction in ammonia detoxification and elevated systemic levels of myotoxic ammonia. Moreover, chronic systemic inflammation is not only associated with chronic liver disease but is likely to negatively impact muscle protein synthesis. Lowered testosterone and growth hormone levels also potentially promote the development of sarcopenia [15, 16]. In the intensive care setting, significantly reduced physical activity and possible difficulties occurring in terms of enteral nutrition, for example, in case of HE episodes or gastrointestinal bleeding, should also be taken into consideration. Besides a reduced intake, impaired absorption can also cause micronutrient deficiencies and affect patients' outcome. An overview of micronutrients with likely lowered levels in liver disease is given in Fig. 14.1.

3. *What to Address—Impact of Malnutrition and Sarcopenia in Liver Disease*

The pathophysiological mechanisms and clinical consequences of liver disease cause several challenges in the treatment of liver patients in general and particularly in critical ill patients. While acute liver injury can result in multi-organ failure reducing resilience within a short period of time, chronic liver disease is highly associated with permanently limited physical reserves. The severity of liver dysfunction directly correlates with the level of nutrition risk. Patients with cirrhosis simultaneously suffering from sarcopenia are more likely to develop AD and ACLF and have a significantly increased risk of death, approximately doubling their mortality rate [14].

Still malnutrition and sarcopenia are often overlooked or not sufficiently addressed in the clinical routine. Patients with ALF do not have prior liver injury, so that the chronic condition of malnutrition and sarcopenia can be missing. But like in patients with a predamaged liver, metabolic derangements causing acidosis or alkalosis and affecting glucose levels and electrolyte balance are common complications [17]. In the intensive care treatment of acute or chronic liver disease, it is imperative to assess the nutritional condition of every patient and address the individual nutritional need to optimize the overall outcome.

4. *How to Assess—Nutritional Assessment in Liver Patients*

To assess sarcopenia beyond physical examination, quantifying skeletal muscle mass can be useful. The psoas muscle and potentially the paraspinal and abdominal wall muscles are classified as core skeletal muscles that are relatively independent by activity and water retention, but consistently affected by the metabolic and molecular dysfunctions caused by cirrhosis.

Computed tomography (CT) is an often-used imaging tool in the intensive care setting, and whenever a CT scan has been performed, its data can also be used for nutritional assessment. CT-assessed skeletal muscle mass has a predictive value in terms of mortality risk for patients with liver cirrhosis, although cutoff values still require further validation [15].

Other tools for body mass assessment suggested by the EASL guideline on nutrition in chronic liver disease are mid-arm circumference (MAMC, defined as mid-arm circumference minus [triceps skinfold (TSF) $\times$ 0.314]), mid-arm muscle area [MAMA = (MAMC)^2/4 $\times$ 0.314] and triceps skinfold. Anthropometric measurements are low-cost, rapid, and are not affected by fluid retention. Current studies suggest that mortality prediction by these tools is more accurately in men than in women. Another simple way to quantify sarcopenia, but less relevant in the ICU setting, is measuring the handgrip strength [15].

An increasing number of obese patients with metabolic dysfunction-associated steatotic liver disease (MASLD), formerly known as nonalcoholic fatty liver disease (NAFLD) [18], related cirrhosis are treated on ICU. It is important to consider potential presence of sarcopenic obesity as it is a common phenomenon in patients with advanced liver disease. The term sarcopenic obesity describes the increase of adipose tissue combined with a loss of skeletal muscle. It is important to note that a BMI equal or higher than 30 kg/m^2 does not rule out malnutrition or sarcopenia [15].

Besides that, fluid retention can affect BMI so that the estimated patient's dry weight instead of the measured bodyweight should be used. For this purpose, the post-paracentesis weight, the weight before decompensation or subtracting a percentage of weight depending on the degree of ascites (mild 5%, moderate 10%, severe 15%) can be referred to. If bilateral pedal edema is present, it is recommended to subtract an additional 5%. Although this method is not yet validated, it is part of the EASL practice guidelines on nutrition in liver disease [15].

Monitoring of macro- and micronutrient levels as well as vitamin levels should be part of a comprehensive nutritional assessment. Decreased levels of serum albumin imply an impaired liver synthesis in patients with advanced or end-stage liver disease. With an elimination half-life of 14–20 days, albumin has limited value for reflecting rapid changes in nutritional status. As an acute phase protein, albumin levels can be furthermore influenced by sepsis or trauma.

Since patients with advanced liver disease often present with a deficiency of fat-soluble vitamins, vitamin A, D, E, and K levels should be monitored and substituted if needed. In patients with chronic alcohol abuse, lowered thiamine (vitamin B1) levels are common. An early substitution of thiamine is crucial to prevent severe complications like Wernicke's encephalopathy or Korsakoff syndrome. Thiamine should be administered intravenously at a daily dosage of 300 mg. In case of lowered micronutrient levels such as zinc, selenium, vitamin B12, and folic acid, a substitution can improve the patients' outcome [19].

Both patients with chronical alcohol abuse and patients with critical illness are at elevated risk for refeeding syndrome. After nutrition (enteral or parenteral) is reintroduced in malnourished patients, refeeding syndrome can cause life-threatening conditions such as cardiac arrythmia and decompensation, severe mental deterioration, seizures, electrolyte disturbances, and volume overload, up to a fatal outcome. Refeeding syndrome is defined as the decrease of magnesium, phosphorus, or potassium levels and/or organ dysfunction resulting from a decrease in any of the three micronutrients and/or due to thiamin deficiency. First clinical symptoms or changes in micronutrient levels usually occur within the first 5 days after reinitiating or significantly increasing energy intake. To reduce the risk of refeeding syndrome, the energy intake should be increased slowly or on the other hand reduced if necessary. Micronutrients like magnesium, phosphorus, and potassium should be adequately substituted [20].

5. *How to Treat—Practice of Clinical Nutrition*

In general, critically ill patients with acute, chronic, or acute-on-chronic liver disease pose a challenge in clinical management. In the field of nutritional medicine, concrete evidence-based recommendations for this specific patient group are often missing. In the following, recommendations from current guidelines are summarized and provide an overview of the key pillars of nutritional medicine in intensive care patients with liver disease.

In the clinical course of critically ill patients, different stages of disease with specific nutritional needs have been defined. The early acute phase of a critical disease (1–3 days) comprises a catabolic state including metabolic instability, followed by a late acute phase (2–4 days) with protein catabolism. The postacute phase includes a convalescence (>7 days) and a rehabilitation phase (several months) or results in a prolonged inflammatory and catabolic syndrome (PICS) as a possible long-term complication of critical illness [21]. Depending on the respective guideline, recommendations for medical nutrition therapy may vary. In the absence of indirect calorimetry, the Germany Society of Nutrition Medicine (DGEM) proposes a daily caloric need of 24 kcal/kg/d. In consideration of the individual metabolic tolerance, it is advised to start with 75% of the calculated daily caloric need (to prevent hyperalimentation) and reach the full caloric intake at the end of the acute phase (100% on days 4–7). After overcoming the acute stage of disease, the daily calory intake can be increased up to 36 kcal/kg/d [21]. The American Society for Parenteral and Enteral Nutrition (ASPEN) guideline proposes feeding with a caloric target of 12–25 kcal/kg/d in the first 7–10 days of ICU treatment without considering different clinical phases [22]. The recommendations for critically ill patients also apply to patients with acute and chronic liver failure under the condition of using dry weight for calculations [23].

To quantify the metabolic dynamic in critically ill patients, the resting energy expenditure (REE) can be assessed by indirect calorimetry (IC). Its primary usage for objectifying the individual caloric needs is recommended by several nutrition guidelines [15, 21, 23, 24].

Until recently, its standardization was limited by lacking commercially available IC devices that were accurate and convenient enough in the clinical setting. Recent innovations are promising and could help to prevent under- or overfeeding [25]. Limitations regarding the use in patients with continuous renal replacement therapy (CRRT) or on extracorporeal membrane oxygenation (ECMO) have to be considered [21, 25]. Up-to-date investigations on the validity of indirect calorimetry in critically ill patients with liver disease are lacking and urgently needed in future.

Different guidelines show consensus on providing high-dose protein (1.2–2.0 g/kg) in critically ill patients with liver disease based on the patient's dry weight [23, 26].

Protein restriction as a strategy to reduce hepatic encephalopathy showed no benefit or even harm [13, 23]. A recent double-blind RCT on nutrition in nonhospitalized patients with liver cirrhosis confirms previous study results [27–29]. Patients with history of overt HE, receiving a diet including 1–1.5 g/kg protein per day for 6 months, showed a significant reversal of mild hepatic encephalopathy and were less likely to develop overt HE in comparison to patients without nutritional therapy [30]. Only for patients with severe overt HE (ammonia levels >150 μmol/l), a short-time (24–48 h) reduction of protein feeding may be beneficial to lower the risk of cerebral edema [31].

In a recently published, multicentered RCT (NUTRIREA-3), early calorie and protein restriction had no impact on mortality, but was associated with faster recovery and fewer complications, such as bowl ischemia and liver dysfunction, in critical ill patients receiving invasive mechanical ventilation and vasopressor therapy for shock [32]. In conclusion, in the early acute phase of critical disease, overfeeding has to be avoided, but in patients with predominant hepatic disorders, protein targets should be adjusted to high-protein delivery after initial stabilization and overcoming the (early) acute phase.

The data and recommendations on the oral and intravenous use of branched-chain amino acids (BCAA) remain controversial. A Cochrane systemic review analyzing 16 RCTs and comparing oral and intravenous BCAA supplementation in noncritically ill patients with HE with a control intervention showed no significant impact on mortality or nutritional status, while having positive effects on the mental status [33]. The EASL guideline on nutrition in patients with chronic liver disease recommends BCAA-enriched nutrition in treatment of HE and sarcopenia [15]. Since more data on BCAA-supplementation in critically ill patients is needed, most guidelines recommend against its standardized use in the ICU setting [15, 23, 24].

Regarding the question of the most appropriate way for nutrition delivery, the main principles in liver patients do not differ from other critically ill patients. Even if evidence is low, there is an expert consensus on using "enteral over parenteral nutrition" in critically ill patients [23, 24]. As soon as potentially fatal disruptions in metabolic function and other possible contraindications are clinically controlled, low-dose EN should be implemented also in liver patients and standard enteral formulations can be used [26]. For patients with oral food intake without need for enteral nutrition, it is essential to ensure they receive a "late evening snack" to reduce the duration of nocturnal fasting which contributes to muscular wasting and sarcopenia [15].

The regular assessment and adjustment of fluid management is crucial. Patients with liver disease often experience ascites and edema, while their intravascular volume is depleted due to hypalbuminemia and portal hypertension.

While an improved overall survival in nonhospitalized patients with cirrhosis and long-term albumin administration [34] has been shown, there is conflicting data on albumin replacement in critically ill patients or patients with septic shock. Nevertheless, albumin substitution can be considered in critically ill patients with liver failure based on its antioxidant, immunological, and osmotic effects [26].

Due to accelerated starvation, patients with advanced hepatic disorders are highly susceptible for hypoglycemia. Owing to that, their blood glucose levels should be monitored regularly [15]. The Critical Care Medical Guidelines for the Management of Adult Acute and Acute-on-Chronic Liver Failure in the ICU suggests targeting serum blood glucose levels between 110–180 mg/dL [26]. A meta-analysis of blood glucose management in critically ill patients did not show a mortality benefit of tight glycemic control in critically ill patients, but fivefold increase rate of hypoglycemia [35]. Accordingly, ESPEN guideline recommends starting insulin therapy as soon as glucose levels exceed 180 mg/dl [24].

14.6 Special Situations

14.6.1 Esophageal Bleeding

Gastrointestinal bleeding and specifically variceal bleeding are common complications of liver cirrhosis and a potential trigger event for ACLF. In hemodynamically stable patients, it is generally recommended to wait for a minimum of 48–72 h after an episode of acute variceal bleeding before reintroducing enteral nutrition. The presence of nonbleeding esophageal varices does not contraindicate feeding via a gastric tube [15].

14.6.2 Parenteral Nutrition-Associated Liver Disease (PNALD)

Especially long-term parenteral nutrition (PN) can cause liver disease, occurring more often in newborns and children than in adults. PNALD is difficult to diagnose due to varying clinical presentation and unspecific elevations of liver enzymes. In general, liver injury through PN is reversible but can also result in cirrhosis or long-term liver injury. The early implementation of enteral feeding plays a crucial role in the prevention of PNALD [36].

14.6.3 Liver Transplantation

In the pre- and postoperative setting in the ICU, parenteral and enteral nutrition should be implemented to reduce complication rates, time on mechanical ventilation, and ICU stay. Both, enteral and parenteral nutrition, are combined in most of the centers [37]. Chronic dilutional hyponatremia is a frequent phenomenon in patients with liver cirrhosis, so that tight monitoring of natrium levels in the perioperative setting should ensure the prevention of a rapid alterations and cerebral pontine myelinolysis. Regular measurements of serum magnesium levels enable an early detection of immunosuppression-induced hypomagnesemia [15].

6. *What's important?—conclusion*

The main principles of nutritional therapy in critically ill patients with liver disease do not differ from the general ICU population. Currently, there is no evidence for different caloric or protein needs. Nevertheless, liver disease or impaired liver function are often accompanied by metabolic derangements, nutritional deficiencies, and a heightened risk of malnutrition and sarcopenia. Typical signs of acute decompensation such as hepatic encephalopathy, hydropic decompensation, and infections as consequence of immune dysfunction potentially complicate the nutritional management. A detailed assessment is crucial to address individual nutritional needs and prevent patients from further complications (Fig. 14.3). More data on critically ill patients with liver disease is urgently needed to adapt nutritional therapy and improve the overall outcome for this specific patient population in the ICU.

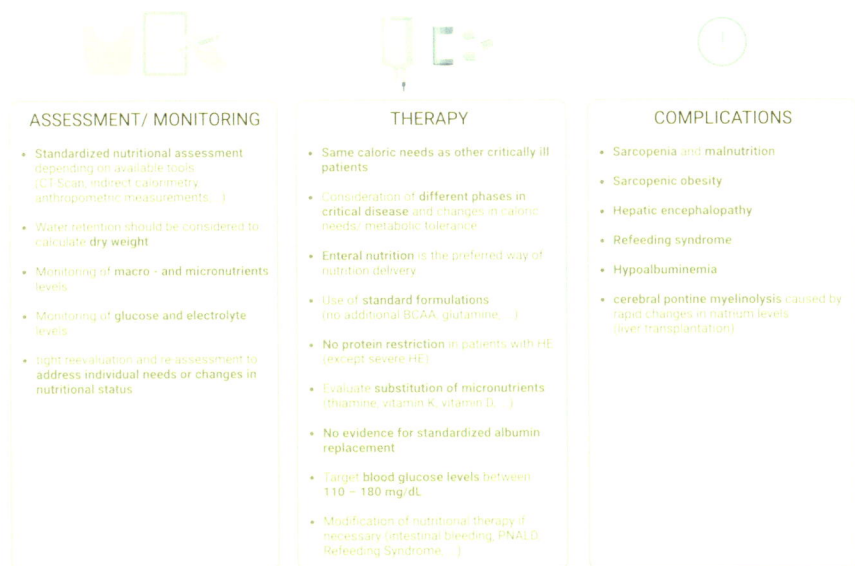

Fig. 14.3 Principles of nutritional assessment and nutritional therapy in critically ill patients with liver disease. BCAA branched-chain amino acids, HE hepatic encephalopathy. (Created using biorender.com)

References

1. Palmer LB, Kuftinec G, Pearlman M, Green CH. Nutrition in cirrhosis. Curr Gastroenterol Rep. 2019;21(8):38.
2. European Association for the Study of the Liver. Electronic address eee. European Association for the Study of the L. EASL clinical practice guidelines for the management of patients with decompensated cirrhosis. J Hepatol. 2018;69(2):406–60.
3. Bernardi M, Moreau R, Angeli P, Schnabl B, Arroyo V. Mechanisms of decompensation and organ failure in cirrhosis: from peripheral arterial vasodilation to systemic inflammation hypothesis. J Hepatol. 2015;63(5):1272–84.
4. Tapper EB, Parikh ND. Diagnosis and management of cirrhosis and its complications: a review. JAMA. 2023;329(18):1589–602.
5. Piano S, Tonon M, Vettore E, Stanco M, Pilutti C, Romano A, et al. Incidence, predictors and outcomes of acute-on-chronic liver failure in outpatients with cirrhosis. J Hepatol. 2017;67(6):1177–84.
6. Jalan R, Saliba F, Pavesi M, Amoros A, Moreau R, Gines P, et al. Development and validation of a prognostic score to predict mortality in patients with acute-on-chronic liver failure. J Hepatol. 2014;61(5):1038–47.
7. European Association for the Study of the Liver, Wendon J, Panel M, Cordoba J, Dhawan A, et al. EASL clinical practical guidelines on the management of acute (fulminant) liver failure. J Hepatol. 2017;66(5):1047–81.
8. Canbay A, Tacke F, Hadem J, Trautwein C, Gerken G, Manns MP. Acute liver failure: a life-threatening disease. Dtsch Arztebl Int. 2011;108(42):714–20.

9. Koch A, Trautwein C, Tacke F. Acute liver failure. Med Klin Intensivmed Notfmed. 2017;112(4):371–81.
10. European Association for the Study of the Liver. EASL clinical practice guidelines: liver transplantation. J Hepatol. 2016;64(2):433–85.
11. Eurotransplant; M de Rosner vR. Chapter 5 – ET liver allocation system (ELAS); 2022.
12. Organtransplantation DS. Jahresbericht – Organspende und Transplantation in Deutschland; 2022.
13. Kamath PS, Kim WR, Advanced Liver Disease Study G. The model for end-stage liver disease (MELD). Hepatology. 2007;45(3):797–805.
14. Tantai X, Liu Y, Yeo YH, Praktiknjo M, Mauro E, Hamaguchi Y, et al. Effect of sarcopenia on survival in patients with cirrhosis: a meta-analysis. J Hepatol. 2022;76(3):588–99.
15. European Association for the Study of the Liver. European Association for the Study of the L. EASL clinical practice guidelines on nutrition in chronic liver disease. J Hepatol. 2019;70(1):172–93.
16. Lai JC, Tandon P, Bernal W, Tapper EB, Ekong U, Dasarathy S, et al. Malnutrition, frailty, and sarcopenia in patients with cirrhosis: 2021 practice guidance by the American Association for the study of liver diseases. Hepatology. 2021;74(3):1611–44.
17. Kappus MR. Acute hepatic failure and nutrition. Nutr Clin Pract. 2020;35(1):30–5.
18. Rinella ME, Lazarus JV, Ratziu V, Francque SM, Sanyal AJ, Kanwal F, et al. A multisociety Delphi consensus statement on new fatty liver disease nomenclature. Ann Hepatol. 2023;101133:E93.
19. Weimann MPA. Ernährungsmedizin: Nach dem Curriculum Ernährungsmedizin der Bundesärztekammer Thieme; 2017 13.12.2017.
20. De Silva A, Nightingale JMD. Refeeding syndrome: physiological background and practical management. Frontline Gastroenterol. 2020;11(5):404–9.
21. Elke G, Hartl WH, Kreymann KG, Adolph M, Felbinger TW, Graf T, et al. Clinical nutrition in critical care medicine – guideline of the German Society for Nutritional Medicine (DGEM). Clin Nutr ESPEN. 2019;33:220–75.
22. Compher C, Bingham AL, McCall M, Patel J, Rice TW, Braunschweig C, et al. Guidelines for the provision of nutrition support therapy in the adult critically ill patient: The American Society for Parenteral and Enteral Nutrition. JPEN J Parenter Enteral Nutr. 2022;46(1):12–41.
23. McClave SA, Taylor BE, Martindale RG, Warren MM, Johnson DR, Braunschweig C, et al. Guidelines for the provision and assessment of nutrition support therapy in the adult critically ill patient: Society of Critical Care Medicine (SCCM) and American Society for Parenteral and Enteral Nutrition (A.S.P.E.N.). JPEN J Parenter Enteral Nutr. 2016;40(2):159–211.
24. Singer P, Blaser AR, Berger MM, Alhazzani W, Calder PC, Casaer MP, et al. ESPEN guideline on clinical nutrition in the intensive care unit. Clin Nutr. 2019;38(1):48–79.
25. Wischmeyer PE, Molinger J, Haines K. Point-counterpoint: indirect calorimetry is essential for optimal nutrition therapy in the intensive care unit. Nutr Clin Pract. 2021;36(2):275–81.
26. Nanchal R, Subramanian R, Karvellas CJ, Hollenberg SM, Peppard WJ, Singbartl K, et al. Guidelines for the management of adult acute and acute-on-chronic liver failure in the icu: cardiovascular, endocrine, hematologic, pulmonary, and renal considerations. Crit Care Med. 2020;48(3):e173–e91.
27. Cordoba J, Lopez-Hellin J, Planas M, Sabin P, Sanpedro F, Castro F, et al. Normal protein diet for episodic hepatic encephalopathy: results of a randomized study. J Hepatol. 2004;41(1):38–43.
28. Gheorghe L, Iacob R, Vadan R, Iacob S, Gheorghe C. Improvement of hepatic encephalopathy using a modified high-calorie high-protein diet. Rom J Gastroenterol. 2005;14(3):231–8.
29. Maharshi S, Sharma BC, Sachdeva S, Srivastava S, Sharma P. Efficacy of nutritional therapy for patients with cirrhosis and minimal hepatic encephalopathy in a randomized trial. Clin Gastroenterol Hepatol. 2016;14(3):454–60. e3; quiz e33.
30. Sharma BC, Maharshi S, Sachdeva S, Mahajan B, Sharma A, Bara S, et al. Nutritional therapy for persistent cognitive impairment after resolution of overt hepatic encephalopathy in

patients with cirrhosis: a double-blind randomized controlled trial. J Gastroenterol Hepatol. 2023;38:1917.
31. Bischoff SC, Bernal W, Dasarathy S, Merli M, Plank LD, Schutz T, et al. ESPEN practical guideline: clinical nutrition in liver disease. Clin Nutr. 2020;39(12):3533–62.
32. Reignier J, Plantefeve G, Mira JP, Argaud L, Asfar P, Aissaoui N, et al. Low versus standard calorie and protein feeding in ventilated adults with shock: a randomised, controlled, multicentre, open-label, parallel-group trial (NUTRIREA-3). Lancet Respir Med. 2023;11(7):602–12.
33. Gluud LL, Dam G, Les I, Marchesini G, Borre M, Aagaard NK, et al. Branched-chain amino acids for people with hepatic encephalopathy. Cochrane Database Syst Rev. 2017;5(5):CD001939.
34. Caraceni P, Riggio O, Angeli P, Alessandria C, Neri S, Foschi FG, et al. Long-term albumin administration in decompensated cirrhosis (ANSWER): an open-label randomised trial. Lancet. 2018;391(10138):2417–29.
35. Yamada T, Shojima N, Noma H, Yamauchi T, Kadowaki T. Glycemic control, mortality, and hypoglycemia in critically ill patients: a systematic review and network meta-analysis of randomized controlled trials. Intensive Care Med. 2017;43(1):1–15.
36. Madnawat H, Welu AL, Gilbert EJ, Taylor DB, Jain S, Manithody C, et al. Mechanisms of parenteral nutrition-associated liver and gut injury. Nutr Clin Pract. 2020;35(1):63–71.
37. Weimann A, Braga M, Carli F, Higashiguchi T, Hubner M, Klek S, et al. ESPEN guideline: clinical nutrition in surgery. Clin Nutr. 2017;36(3):623–50.

Nutrition in Lung Disease

Matthias Hecker

Acute or chronic respiratory insufficiency is a major cause of morbidity and mortality in patients on intensive care units (ICU) worldwide. Especially against the background of the recent COVID-19 pandemic situation, the importance to respiratory critical care medicine gained attention to a larger audience. Besides respiratory and hemodynamic support, the early establishment of an adequate nutritional regime is an integral component of supportive care for these patients. The acute respiratory distress syndrome (ARDS) and exacerbations of chronic obstructive pulmonary disease (COPD) are two major respiratory disorders with relevance for intensivists, which should be addressed in the following concerning disease-specific nutritional support.

15.1 Acute Respiratory Distress Syndrome (ARDS)

ARDS is characterized by the uncontrolled formation of a noncardiogenic pulmonary edema leading to severe hypoxemia due to an impaired integrity of the alveolo-capillary integrity [1]. Another pathophysiological hallmark of ARDS is a progressive ventilation-perfusion mismatch with the development of intrapulmonary shunting as a consequence [2]. Main causes for the development of ARDS are severe pneumonia, aspiration, or sepsis. Lung-protective ventilation, prone positioning, and in individual cases the establishment of an extracorporeal membrane oxygenation (ECMO) are essential life-saving therapeutic options for ARDS patients [2, 3]. The nutritional and metabolic aspects of ARDS pathophysiology are an hyperinflammatory state associated with hypercatabolism and increases energy

M. Hecker (✉)
Medizinische Klinik und Poliklinik II, Universitätsklinikum Gießen und Marburg GmbH, Gießen, Germany
e-mail: Matthias.Hecker@innere.med.uni-giessen.de

expenditure. As a consequence, ARDS patients are at major risk of malnutrition and sarcopenia. Thus, ARDS patients should be considered for malnutrition upon admission on ICU and assessed by a nutritional evaluation. As in other intensive care patients, the determination of the energy requirements for ARDS patients is challenging. To define the energy expenditure of intensive care patients, most guidelines recommend the use of indirect calorimetry [4, 5]. If indirect calorimetry is not available, calculation of resting energy expenditure (REE) from VCO_2 (carbon dioxide production) obtained from ventilators, VO_2 (oxygen consumption) assessed by pulmonary arterial catheter, or the simple weight-based equations (such as 20–25 kcal/kg/day) are recommended [4, 5]. Although malnutrition is a constant threat to ARDS patient, rather hypocaloric nutrition (up to 70% estimated needs) should be administered in the early phase of acute illness due to the decreased metabolism in the initial phase of stress response [4, 6]. Entering the catabolic phase, caloric delivery should likely match expended energy (LL) to avoid malnutrition and muscle wasting. Concerning the route of administration, the same principles applied to a general intensive care patient are valid in case of ARDS: If possible, early enteral nutrition (EN), starting within 48 h after ICU admission, should be preferred over delayed EN due to a reduction of infectious complications [4]. In case of contraindications for EN the implementation of nutritional regime based on parenteral nutrition (PN) should be performed within the first 3–7 days after ICU admission. Early and progressive PN is reserved for severely malnourished patients with contraindication for EN [4]. For all routes of administration, the following principle is essential: Avoid full EN or PN in the first 3 days after admission to prevent overfeeding but try to achieve the individual energy goal thereafter!

Concerning the composition of macronutrients, the upper limit for carbohydrates should be 5 g/kg body weight/day. For intravenous lipids, the upper recommendation is 1 g/kg body weight/day with a tolerance up to 1.5 g/kg/day [7, 8]. Parenteral lipid emulsions enriched omega-3 fatty acids (fish oil dose 0.1–0.2 g/kg/day) can be provided in patients receiving PN [4, 8]. When applying PN, micronutrients (i.e., trace elements and vitamins) should be provided daily with PN. Nevertheless, the use of antioxidant micronutrients (e.g., vitamins C + E, selenium, zinc), high-dose omega-3-enriched formulars, or glutamine supplementation in terms of an immunonutrition is generally not recommended in ARDS patients [4].

15.2 Exacerbated COPD

Chronic obstructive pulmonary disease (COPD) is one of the leading causes of morbidity and mortality affecting an increasing number of patients worldwide. Besides other environmental factors, the major risk factor for the development of COPD is former or current tobacco smoking, leading to a chronic inflammation of the small airways [9]. In the progression to the disease, airway remodeling with narrowing of the peripheral airways can lead to airflow limitations and emphysema formation, thus causing severe dyspnea and finally an impaired gas exchange [9, 10]. Shortness of breath is often associated with a progressive loss of physical activity in the cause of the disease leading in combination with increased resting metabolic rate due to respiratory insufficiency, tissue hypoxia and a chronic inflammatory state to malnutrition, unintentional weight loss, and pronounced cachexia [9, 11]. Several studies revealed that between 25% and 40% of patients with advanced COPD are malnourished [12, 13]. In addition, underweight and low fat-free mass are independently associated with a poor prognosis in patients with COPD, especially when suffering from an exacerbation [11, 12].

An acute exacerbation of COPD is regarded as an acute worsening of symptoms characterized clinically by increased dyspnea, cough, sputum production, and sputum purulence [14]. Pharmacologic management includes bronchodilators, corticosteroids, and in some cases antibiotics. Supplemental oxygen, physical therapy, and mucolytics may be useful in selected patients [14]. In severe cases, treatment on intensive care units for invasive or noninvasive ventilatory support might be necessary. In general, nutritional guidelines for ICU patients are also valid for critically ill COPD patients [4]. Nevertheless, as mentioned above, COPD patients are especially at-risk for suffering from malnutrition and muscle wasting having a significant prognostic impact. For this reason, exacerbated COPD patients should be assessed by a nutritional evaluation upon ICU admission in order to adequately treat malnutrition and sarcopenia especially in an intensive care setting.

References

1. Hecker M, Weigand MA, Mayer K. Acute respiratory distress syndrome. Internist (Berl). 2012;53(5):557–66.
2. Ware LB, Bastarache JA, Calfee CS. ARDS: new mechanistic insights, new therapeutic directions. Clin Chest Med. 2014;35(4):xv–xvi.
3. Hecker M, et al. Clinical aspects of acute lung insufficiency (ALI/TRALI). Transfus Med Hemother. 2008;35(2):80–8.
4. Singer P, et al. ESPEN practical and partially revised guideline: clinical nutrition in the intensive care unit. Clin Nutr. 2023;42(9):1671–89.
5. McClave SA, et al. Guidelines for the provision and assessment of nutrition support therapy in the adult critically ill patient: Society of Critical Care Medicine (SCCM) and American Society for Parenteral and Enteral Nutrition (A.S.P.E.N.). JPEN J Parenter Enteral Nutr. 2016;40(2):159–211.
6. Biolo G, et al. Metabolic response to injury and sepsis: changes in protein metabolism. Nutrition. 1997;13(9 Suppl):52S–7S.
7. Hecker M, Felbinger TW, Mayer K. Nutrition and acute respiratory failure. Med Klin Intensivmed Notfmed. 2013;108(5):379–83.
8. Hecker M, Mayer K. Intravenous lipids in adult intensive care unit patients. World Rev Nutr Diet. 2015;112:120–6.
9. Leap J, et al. Pathophysiology of COPD. Crit Care Nurs Q. 2021;44(1):2–8.
10. Anzueto A, Miravitlles M. Pathophysiology of dyspnea in COPD. Postgrad Med. 2017;129(3):366–74.
11. Collins PF, et al. Nutritional support in chronic obstructive pulmonary disease (COPD): an evidence update. J Thorac Dis. 2019;11(Suppl 17):S2230–7.

12. Anker SD, et al. ESPEN guidelines on enteral nutrition: cardiology and pulmonology. Clin Nutr. 2006;25(2):311–8.
13. Vermeeren MA, et al. Prevalence of nutritional depletion in a large out-patient population of patients with COPD. Respir Med. 2006;100(8):1349–55.
14. Viniol C, Vogelmeier CF. Exacerbations of COPD. Eur Respir Rev. 2018;27(147):170103.

Pancreatic Disease in ICU

Johann Ockenga

Diseases of the pancreas are among the most common diseases in everyday clinical practice. Essentially, a distinction is made between acute and chronic pancreatitis.

Nutritional care requirements of patients with acute or chronic pancreatitis differ significantly. While the patient with acute pancreatitis suffers from a highly acute clinical picture up to severe SIRS or sepsis, which is treated in hospital or in an intensive care unit, chronic pancreatitis is a disease that drags on for years or decades, which predominantly takes place in an outpatient setting. An acute flare-up of a chronic pancreatitis may be handled like an acute pancreatitis, which is the topic of this chapter.

The incidence of acute pancreatitis varies between 5 and 80 per 100,000 inhabitants per year. In parallel with increasing alcohol consumption and changing life circumstances, there is a trend toward an increasing incidence of acute pancreatitis over the last 40 years. A certain lack of clarity in the available data is due, among other things, to the fact that there is usually no histological diagnosis, but the diagnosis is made on the basis of clinical, laboratory, and radiological criteria, which have limits in their sensitivity and specificity.

In the sex distribution, males slightly dominate over females with 1.4:1. This difference increases when alcoholic pancreatitis is present. The peak in age distribution is between 35 and 45 years [9, 27].

In the western world, gallstone disease (including microlithiasis) with 35%–40% and alcohol abuse with 30–40% are the main causes of acute pancreatitis. In addition, there are a variety of other rare causes of acute pancreatitis responsible for another 10%–20% [27].

J. Ockenga (✉)
Medizinische Klinik II m.S. Gastroenterologie, Endokrinologie und Ernährungsmedizin, Klinikum Bremen Mitte, Bremen, Germany
e-mail: johann.ockenga@klinikum-bremen-mitte.de

© The Author(s), under exclusive license to Springer Nature Switzerland AG 2025
A. Rümelin et al. (eds.), *Nutrition in ICU Patients*,
https://doi.org/10.1007/978-3-032-00818-3_16

In approximately 20% of patients with acute pancreatitis, a severe course develops. While interstitial, edematous pancreatitis usually progresses rapidly and without complications, hemorrhagic, necrotizing pancreatitis is linked to substantial morbidity and mortality. The Ranson score and APACHE II score have been established for assessing the severity of acute pancreatitis. Imaging by computed tomography and ultrasound has an important role in detecting pancreatic necrosis, which is of prognostic importance [19]. Especially, necrotizing pancreatitis requires special nutritional attention due to its relevant morbidity and mortality.

16.1 Nutrition Strategy

For a long time, nutritional therapy in patients with acute pancreatitis was determined by the dogma that oral or enteral nutrition worsened the course of the disease. This recommendation was based on the assumption that enteral nutrition is an excretory stimulus for pancreatic acinar cells. This would result in increased release of intracellular pancreatic enzymes, thereby exacerbating pancreatitis. Additionally, there was a fear of inducing increased pain in patients by early enteral feeding. Based on these seemingly plausible considerations, the recommendation was made to exclusively feed patients with acute pancreatitis parenterally. However, until the early 1990s, there were no appropriately designed randomized trials to substantiate this dogma with clinical data. On the contrary, as early as 1987, Sax et al. published a study in the American Journal of Surgery that showed no benefit for early total parenteral nutrition in patients with acute pancreatitis [22]. In this nonrandomized retrospective study, a delayed oral diet and longer hospital stay were found in patients receiving early parenteral nutrition compared with a control group receiving only fluid and electrolyte replacement initially.

Approximately 80%–90% of patients hospitalized for acute pancreatitis present with edematous pancreatitis, which usually resolves without major complications after 5–7 days. These patients usually do not require an admission to an intensive care unit and no specific nutritional therapy [2]. The possibilities of resuming oral nutrition will be discussed again later in the text.

In the remaining 10%–20%, a severe course develops often accompanied with necrosis of the pancreatic tissue or in the retroperitoneum, resulting in a much worse course of the disease with prolonged hospitalization and intensive care unit stay [7]. A feared complication of these patients is secondary infection of the necrosis areas with bacteria from the gastrointestinal tract [19]. The larger the necrosis area, the greater the risk of this feared complication is [23]. In this group of critical ill patients, nutrition is part of the multimodal intensive care therapy [2].

It is well known from studies of critically ill patients that early enteral nutrition has a favorable effect on the course of the disease (see Chap. 7). Therefore, it seemed conclusive to test this concept also in patients with acute pancreatitis; also considering the hypothesis that early enteral nutrition is favorable for the gastrointestinal barrier and may prevent secondary infection of necrotic parts. Since the early 1990s, several studies have been published comparing enteral versus parenteral nutrition in acute pancreatitis [1].

The main findings of these studies are that enteral nutrition is associated with (i) a reduction in risk of infectious complications, (ii) a reduction in hospital length of stay, (iii) a reduction in the risk of organ failure compared to parenteral nutrition. An effect on mortality could not be shown in the individual studies, but is evident in the meta-analysis of eight studies (see Table 16.1) [1]. In the initial studies, results indicated that the beneficial effect occurred particularly with early enteral feeding commencing within 48 h of disease progression [18]. In contrast, a prospective Dutch multicenter study showed that in moderate to severe acute pancreatitis, it is also possible to wait up to 72 h before starting enteral nutrition [4]. Among other things, this study showed that in a relevant proportion of patients, oral nutrition was already possible again on day 3, although this population did not show such a severe course. As shown in a recent meta-analysis, especially severe acute pancreatitis may benefit from early enteral nutrition [20].

Overall, therefore, the dogma that enteral nutrition is not feasible in patients with acute pancreatitis has changed to the clear recommendation that when nutritional therapy is indicated, enteral nutrition is primarily indicated in patients with severe acute pancreatitis.

In the European guideline on nutrition in pancreatic disease published by ESPEN (European Society for Enteral, Parenteral Nutrition and Metabolism) [2], as well as in the accompanying German Guideline published by DGEM (Deutsche Gesellschaft für Ernährungsmedizin) [15], it is recommended that parenteral nutrition should only be given if enteral nutrition to meet requirements is not possible within 5–7 days in ICU. However, if the patient present already at onset of the acute pancreatitis with severe malnutrition and/or adequate enteral nutrition is not feasible, early parenteral nutrition or a combination of enteral and parenteral nutrition may be indicated to reach the nutritional goals [2, 12].

There is no specific guideline for nutritional support in acute pancreatitis from ASPEN (American Society for Parenteral and Enteral Nutrition), but this approach is also supported by the general American Guideline on Nutrition in Intensive Care [12].

Table 16.1 Results of a Cochrane analysis (8 studies, 348 patients) regarding the effect of enteral nutrition compared to parenteral nutrition in acute pancreatitis [1]

	Odds ratio	95% CI
Infection	0.50	0.23–0.65
Surgery	0.44	0.29–0.67
Mortality	0.50	0.28–0.91
Morbidity (Severe pancreatitis)	0.18	0.06–0.58

16.2 Nutritional Requirements

In the most recent ESPEN guideline [2], an energy supply of 25–35 kcal/kg/day and protein supply range over 1.2–1.5 g/kg/day is recommended. A mixed source of energy from carbohydrates, fat, and protein should be provided. In severe AP, administration of carbohydrates/day should be 3–6 g/kg and of lipids/day up to 2 g/kg. Acute pancreatitis is characterized by an overwhelming inflammation. It produces increased protein catabolism, characterized by a decremented production of gluconeogenesis by exogenous glucose. In addition, an increased energy expenditure and insulin resistance, and an augmented dependence of fatty acid oxidation for energy substrates can be observed. Therefore, energy requirements during the clinical course of AP are changing according to the severity and stage of AP, comorbidities, as well as complications. Thus, the nutritional goals must be defined on a daily basis.

Micronutrients should be given at least due to the recommend daily doses to avoid a shortage. Especially in patients with chronic alcohol consumption or patients with malnutrition, severe micronutrient deficiency is frequent and includes vitamins B1, B2, B3, B12, C, A, folic acid, and zinc. In this case, a higher substitution is necessary.

16.3 Implementation of Enteral Nutrition

Almost all initial studies on enteral nutrition in acute pancreatitis were performed with jejunal application of a predominantly elementary (low-molecular-weight) tube diet. The clinical observation that some of the patients received the intended jejunal nutrition accidental into the stomach without significant disadvantages led to the approach of primary gastric nutrition. For example, in the work of Kumar et al., 31 patients with moderate to severe acute pancreatitis (mean APACHE II about 10) were randomized into a group receiving nasogastric tube feeding (15 patients) and another intervention group receiving nasojejunal tube feeding (16 patients) [11]. Both groups received an elementary diet. Start of feeding was within 72 h after the onset of clinical symptoms of pancreatitis. The goal of 1800 kilocalories of enteral nutrition was achieved within 7 days in all patients. No significant difference in clinical course (incidence of diarrhea, incidence of pain, infected necrosis, positive blood cultures, need for surgical necrosectomy, or mortality) was found between the two groups.

Overall, the authors conclude that enteral feeding in acute pancreatitis is possible both nasojejunal and nasogastric. Therefore, it makes sense to start with gastric feeding and switch to a jejunal tube only in cases of high reflux or severe motility disorders. This conclusion is also supported by a meta-analysis of a total of four studies and one recent study [17, 24]. This approach has the decisive advantage for clinical practice that the placement of a nasogastric tube is significantly easier than achieving a safe nasojejunal tube position.

In recent years, minimal endoscopic necrosectomy has become a preferred procedure for the treatment of infected pancreatic necrosis. No systematic studies are available on the appropriate nutritional approach in these cases. From our own experience, we can report that these patients usually tolerate oral or enteral nutrition and that this should be preferred.

Although the vast majority of studies have used low-molecular-weight tube feeds, new data suggest that a high-molecular-weight tube feed can be used and that a switch to a low-molecular-weight tube feed should be made only in cases of intolerance [5]. There is no indication for the use of immunonutrition based on the data.

In conclusion, enteral nutrition should be the preferred route of nutritional therapy in patients with acute pancreatitis. Certainly, there will always be patients who cannot be completely fed enterally due to gastrointestinal contraindications (severe ileus, high reflux, intestinal ischemia, etc.). Then, a combination of enteral and parenteral nutrition or complete parenteral nutrition while maintaining metabolic homeostasis should be pursued. Such a combined approach in patients who cannot be adequately fed enteral nutrition certainly has the potential to improve the clinical course of the patients. The optimal timing of initiation of parenteral nutrition and caloric intake, analogous to critically ill patients, is not yet well defined (see Table 16.2).

If parenteral nutrition is indicated, it should be provided as total parenteral nutrition with the substrates carbohydrates, lipids, and amino acids and is based on the known rules for nutrition of critically ill patients (see Chaps. 3, 4, 5). Protein intake should be estimated at 1.2 g/kg body weight. In case of long-term absence of enteral nutrition, the supply of parenteral glutamine in a dose of 0.3–0.5 g/kg body weight alanine–glutamine is recommended. Figure 16.1 provides a summary of this algorithm.

Table 16.2 Nutritional recommendations for severe acute pancreatitis

Question	Recommendation
Enteral vs. parenteral nutrition	Enteral preferred
Timing of feeding	Enteral feeding within 24–72 h[a]
Gastric vs. jejunal route	Start gastral feeding, if intolerance change to jejunal
Oral food	Start soft diet with liquid or solid
Enteral formula	No general benefit of semi-elemental vs. polymeric formula
Enteral infusion	Continuous feeding
Probiotics/immunonutrition	Not recommend with exception of glutamine in long term exclusive parenteral feeding

[a]Start early in malnourished patients and in patients who will not be able to be fed oral or enteral in the next 5 days

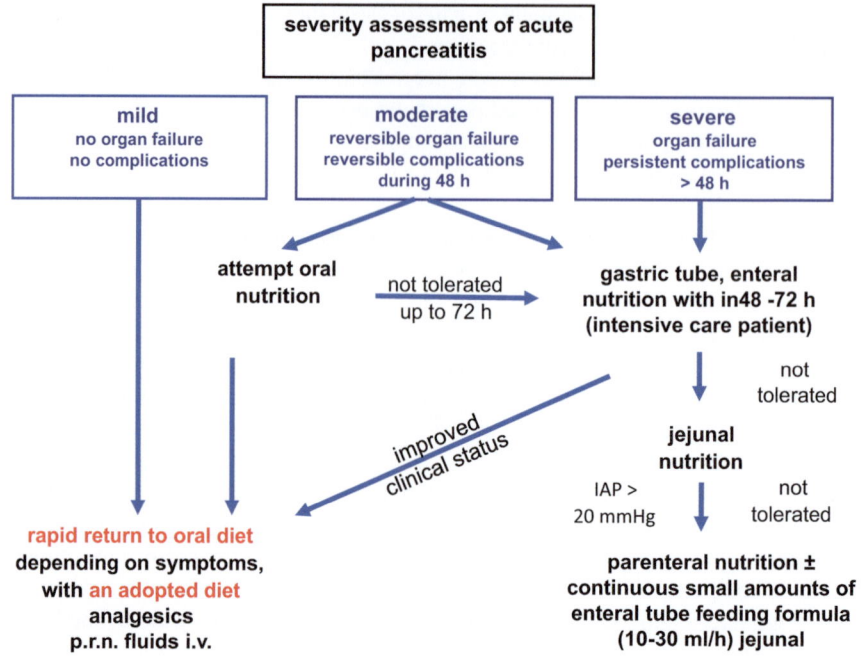

Fig. 16.1 Nutritional algorithm in acute pancreatitis

16.4 Role of Special Substrates

Various specific supplements such as high doses of antioxidants, probiotics, glutamine, and omega-3 fatty acids have been studied. The majority of data shows inconclusive results.

In a Cochrane analysis, no clear benefit for pharmacological intervention with vitamins or antioxidants in acute pancreatitis could be demonstrated [13].

In acute pancreatitis, microbiome alterations and increased intestinal permeability have been described and may be one reason for infectious complications such as superinfection of necrosis [8]. Recovering the intestinal microbiome leads to the idea of using probiotics.

The hypothesis that administration of probiotics might reduce the rate of infectious complications has been investigated in smaller pilot studies with tendentially positive results [16]. However, a Dutch multicenter study showed that the use of a probiotic cocktail together with the administration of prebiotics resulted in a significantly worse outcome in patients with severe necrotizing pancreatitis [6]. The extent to which this represents only a specific effect of the study design or a general effect of probiotics in severely ill patients is currently the subject of further discussion and investigation. However, probiotics should currently only be used in controlled studies in acute pancreatitis.

Dietary polyunsaturated fatty acids, especially lipoxins, resolvins, and protectins, might have immunomodulatory effects. There are some randomized studies with enteral formula or parenteral solutions enriched with ω-3 fatty acids in the treatment of AP, which showed some positive effects on total time of jejunal feeding and hospital length. A meta-analysis of RCTs showed that omega-3 fatty acids supplementation was beneficial in reduction the risk of new-organ failure in patients with AP [26]. However, before a clear recommendation can be given, further more large and well-designed RCTs are required to elucidate the efficacy of omega-3 FA supplementation.

Glutamine has been discussed as a semi essential amino acid, especially in parenteral fed patients. A meta-analysis of 12 RCTs has been shown that glutamine can be associated with a decrease in infectious complications (RR = 0.58; 95% CI: 0.39–0.87) and mortality (RR = 0.30, 95% CI: 0.15–0.60) among patients who received total PN but not EN [3]. The above findings were confirmed in another study that determined the advantages of intravenous glutamine [28]. Therefore, intravenous glutamine appears to be beneficial in patients with total PN; however, the beneficial effects of enteral glutamine should be investigated in the future. Glutamine is recommended as a supplement in the following doses: 0.3–0.5 g/kg/day.

16.5 Increased Abdominal Pressure

In patients with severe AP and intra-abdominal pressure (IAP) >15 mmHg, EN should be initiated via nasojejunal route starting at 20 mL/h, increasing the rate according to the tolerance. Temporary reduction or discontinuation of EN should be considered when IAP values further increase under EN.

When IAP >20 mmHg or in the presence of abdominal compartment syndrome, EN should be (temporarily) stopped and PN should be initiated according to the metabolic competence of the patient. In patients with severe AP and open abdomen, EN should be administered, at least in a small amount. If required for achievement of nutritional requirements, supplementary or total PN should be added [2].

16.6 Diet After Recovery or in Mild Acute Pancreatitis

As outlined earlier, most patients present with mild or moderate acute pancreatitis that heals within 5–7 days with restitutio ad integrum. Again, a rather cautious approach to resumption of oral food intake was previously recommended with the idea of avoiding stimulation of pancreatic secretion, and food buildup was often started only after normalization of serum lipase. Complicated diet buildup schemes with gradual expansion of diet composition were designed and propagated for a long time. However, prospective data supporting this approach are not available.

Studies have investigated a simplified and patient-centered approach to diet buildup after pancreatitis [10, 14]. In a German open randomized multicenter trial, we showed that in mild acute pancreatitis, the patient's desire to resume oral nutrition may play a more important role than previously and that this can be done independently of normalization of serum lipase [25]. This has been confirmed by a recent multicenter trial [21].

This leads to the recommendation that in mild acute pancreatitis and after recovery of a severe acute pancreatitis, in addition to parenteral hydration and electrolyte replacement, a light whole food diet can be started early according to individual preference and tolerance. Specific dietary regimens are not necessary. However, this approach may result in some patients to a recurrence of pain exacerbation (approximately one in six patients), which then delays recovery [7].

References

1. Al-Omran M, Albalawi ZH, Tashkandi MF, Al-Ansary LA. Enteral versus parenteral nutrition for acute pancreatitis. Cochrane Database Syst Rev. 2010;2010(1):CD002837.
2. Arvanitakis M, Ockenga J, Bezmarevic M, Gianotti L, Krznaric Z, Lobo DN, Loser C, Madl C, Meier R, Phillips M, Rasmussen HH, Van Hooft JE, Bischoff SC. ESPEN guideline on clinical nutrition in acute and chronic pancreatitis. Clin Nutr. 2020;39(3):612–31.
3. Asrani V, Chang WK, Dong Z, Hardy G, Windsor JA, Petrov MS. Glutamine supplementation in acute pancreatitis: a meta-analysis of randomized controlled trials. Pancreatology. 2013;13(5):468–74.
4. Bakker OJ, van Brunschot S, van Santvoort HC, Besselink MG, Bollen TL, Boermeester MA, Dejong CH, van Goor H, Bosscha K, Ali UA, Bouwense S, van Grevenstein WM, Heisterkamp J, Houdijk AP, Jansen JM, Karsten TM, Manusama ER, Nieuwenhuijs VB, Schaapherder AF, van der Schelling GP, Schwartz MP, Spanier BW, Tan A, Vecht J, Weusten BL, Witteman BJ, Akkermans LM, Bruno MJ, Dijkgraaf MG, van Ramshorst B, Gooszen HG, G. Dutch Pancreatitis Study. Early versus on-demand nasoenteric tube feeding in acute pancreatitis. N Engl J Med. 2014;371(21):1983–93.
5. Baron TH, DiMaio CJ, Wang AY, Morgan KA. American Gastroenterological Association clinical practice update: management of pancreatic necrosis. Gastroenterology. 2020;158(1):67–75 e61.
6. Besselink MG, van Santvoort HC, Buskens E, Boermeester MA, van Goor H, Timmerman HM, Nieuwenhuijs VB, Bollen TL, van Ramshorst B, Witteman BJ, Rosman C, Ploeg RJ, Brink MA, Schaapherder AF, Dejong CH, Wahab PJ, van Laarhoven CJ, van der Harst E, van Eijck CH, Cuesta MA, Akkermans LM, Gooszen HG, G. Dutch Acute Pancreatitis Study. Probiotic prophylaxis in predicted severe acute pancreatitis: a randomised, double-blind, placebo-controlled trial. Lancet. 2008;371(9613):651–9.
7. Bevan MG, Asrani VM, Bharmal S, Wu LM, Windsor JA, Petrov MS. Incidence and predictors of oral feeding intolerance in acute pancreatitis: a systematic review, meta-analysis, and meta-regression. Clin Nutr. 2017;36(3):722–9.
8. Brubaker L, Luu S, Hoffman K, Wood A, Navarro Cagigas M, Yao Q, Petrosino J, Fisher W, Van Buren G. Microbiome changes associated with acute and chronic pancreatitis: a systematic review. Pancreatology. 2021;21(1):1–14.
9. Gullo L, Migliori M, Pezzilli R, Olah A, Farkas G, Levy P, Arvanitakis C, Lankisch P, Beger H. An update on recurrent acute pancreatitis: data from five European countries. Am J Gastroenterol. 2002;97(8):1959–62.
10. Jacobson BC, Vander Vliet MB, Hughes MD, Maurer R, McManus K, Banks PA. A prospective, randomized trial of clear liquids versus low-fat solid diet as the initial meal in mild acute pancreatitis. Clin Gastroenterol Hepatol. 2007;5(8):946–51; quiz 886.

11. Kumar A, Singh N, Prakash S, Saraya A, Joshi YK. Early enteral nutrition in severe acute pancreatitis: a prospective randomized controlled trial comparing nasojejunal and nasogastric routes. J Clin Gastroenterol. 2006;40(5):431–4.
12. McClave SA, Taylor BE, Martindale RG, Warren MM, Johnson DR, Braunschweig C, McCarthy MS, Davanos E, Rice TW, Cresci GA, Gervasio JM, Sacks GS, Roberts PR, Compher C, M. Society of Critical Care, P. American Society for and N. Enteral. Guidelines for the provision and assessment of nutrition support therapy in the adult critically ill patient: Society of Critical Care Medicine (SCCM) and American Society for Parenteral and Enteral Nutrition (A.S.P.E.N.). JPEN J Parenter Enteral Nutr. 2016;40(2):159–211.
13. Moggia E, Koti R, Belgaumkar AP, Fazio F, Pereira SP, Davidson BR, Gurusamy KS. Pharmacological interventions for acute pancreatitis. Cochrane Database Syst Rev. 2017;4(4):CD011384.
14. Moraes JM, Felga GE, Chebli LA, Franco MB, Gomes CA, Gaburri PD, Zanini A, Chebli JM. A full solid diet as the initial meal in mild acute pancreatitis is safe and result in a shorter length of hospitalization: results from a prospective, randomized, controlled, double-blind clinical trial. J Clin Gastroenterol. 2010;44(7):517–22.
15. Ockenga J, Fromhold-Treu S, Löser C, Madl C, Martignoni M, Meier R, Rubin D, Schütte K, Stang K, Török HP, Wehle L, Weimann A. S3-Leitlinie Klinische Ernährung bei Pankreaserkrankungen. Aktuel Ernährungsmed. 2024; https://doi.org/10.1055/a-2328-6190.
16. Olah A, Belagyi T, Poto L, Romics L Jr, Bengmark S. Synbiotic control of inflammation and infection in severe acute pancreatitis: a prospective, randomized, double blind study. Hepato-Gastroenterology. 2007;54(74):590–4.
17. Petrov MS, Correia MI, Windsor JA. Nasogastric tube feeding in predicted severe acute pancreatitis. A systematic review of the literature to determine safety and tolerance. JOP. 2008;9(4):440–8.
18. Petrov MS, Pylypchuk RD, Uchugina AF. A systematic review on the timing of artificial nutrition in acute pancreatitis. Br J Nutr. 2009;101(6):787–93.
19. Petrov MS, Shanbhag S, Chakraborty M, Phillips AR, Windsor JA. Organ failure and infection of pancreatic necrosis as determinants of mortality in patients with acute pancreatitis. Gastroenterology. 2010;139(3):813–20.
20. Qi D, Yu B, Huang J, Peng M. Meta-analysis of early enteral nutrition provided within 24 hours of admission on clinical outcomes in acute pancreatitis. JPEN J Parenter Enteral Nutr. 2018;42(7):1139–47.
21. Ramirez-Maldonado E, Lopez Gordo S, Pueyo EM, Sanchez-Garcia A, Mayol S, Gonzalez S, Elvira J, Memba R, Fondevila C, Jorba R. Immediate oral refeeding in patients with mild and moderate acute pancreatitis: a multicenter, randomized controlled trial (PADI trial). Ann Surg. 2021;274(2):255–63.
22. Sax HC, Warner BW, Talamini MA, Hamilton FN, Bell RH Jr, Fischer JE, Bower RH. Early total parenteral nutrition in acute pancreatitis: lack of beneficial effects. Am J Surg. 1987;153(1):117–24.
23. Schmid SW, Uhl W, Friess H, Malfertheiner P, Buchler MW. The role of infection in acute pancreatitis. Gut. 1999;45(2):311–6.
24. Singh N, Sharma B, Sharma M, Sachdev V, Bhardwaj P, Mani K, Joshi YK, Saraya A. Evaluation of early enteral feeding through nasogastric and nasojejunal tube in severe acute pancreatitis: a noninferiority randomized controlled trial. Pancreas. 2012;41(1):153–9.
25. Teich N, Aghdassi A, Fischer J, Walz B, Caca K, Wallochny T, von Aretin A, von Boyen G, Gopel S, Ockenga J, Leodolter A, Ruddel J, Weber E, Mayerle J, Lerch MM, Mossner J, Schiefke I. Optimal timing of oral refeeding in mild acute pancreatitis: results of an open randomized multicenter trial. Pancreas. 2010;39(7):1088–92.
26. Wolbrink DRJ, Grundsell JR, Witteman B, Poll MV, Santvoort HCV, Issa E, Dennison A, Goor HV, Besselink MG, Bouwense SAW, G. Dutch Pancreatitis Study. Are omega-3 fatty acids safe and effective in acute pancreatitis or sepsis? A systematic review and meta-analysis. Clin Nutr. 2020;39(9):2686–94.

27. Xiao AY, Tan ML, Wu LM, Asrani VM, Windsor JA, Yadav D, Petrov MS. Global incidence and mortality of pancreatic diseases: a systematic review, meta-analysis, and meta-regression of population-based cohort studies. Lancet Gastroenterol Hepatol. 2016;1(1):45–55.
28. Yong L, Lu QP, Liu SH, Fan H. Efficacy of glutamine-enriched nutrition support for patients with severe acute pancreatitis: a meta-analysis. JPEN J Parenter Enteral Nutr. 2016;40(1):83–94.

17. Nutritional Management in Patients with Severe Traumatic Brain Injury

Maximilian Fichtl and Thomas W. Felbinger

17.1 Introduction

Severe traumatic brain injury (TBI) occurs about 5.5 million times a year worldwide. Even if survived, it often requires long-term intensive care and long-term rehabilitation. Nutritional management as an integral part of the treatment strategy for critically ill patients and in particular for those with TBI and consecutive long-term stay in the ICU has been neglected for many years. However, many excellent performed and statistically well-powered studies in the last two decades lead to publication of very detailed international guidelines as well as an increased understanding of the importance of nutrition therapy.

Whereas most studies were performed in a general critically ill population, there are some studies or post hoc analysis dealing with neurotrauma patients. Therefore, specific recommendations can be made for these patients after TBI. The following chapter will summarize our current knowledge in nutritional management in patients with TBI.

17.2 Metabolic Response to TBI and Energy Requirements

The primary local result of TBI to the brain is direct brain tissue damage, impaired cerebral blood flow and metabolism, vasospasm, edema, oxidative stress, and release of cytokines.

On a systemic level, activation of the sympathetic nerve system after adrenaline release from the adrenal medulla, effector hormone production like corticosteroids after activation of the hypothalamic–pituitary gland system, and proinflammatory

---

M. Fichtl · T. W. Felbinger (✉)
Department of Anesthesiology, Perioperative and Pain Medicine, Harlaching and Neuperlach Medical Center, The Munich Hospitals Ltd, Munich, Germany
e-mail: thomas.felbinger@muenchen-klinik.de

© The Author(s), under exclusive license to Springer Nature Switzerland AG 2025
A. Rümelin et al. (eds.), *Nutrition in ICU Patients*,
https://doi.org/10.1007/978-3-032-00818-3_17

cytokine production are consequences of TBI. This leads to a high metabolic rate (75%–200% of REE) with uncontrolled catabolism and resistance to anabolic signals like insulin, all of which result in increased energy expenditure, changed substrate use and in the long term in a changed body composition due to excessive loss of energy and protein. Hypermetabolism and therefore a catabolic state after TBI may persist for several weeks or months and generally plateaus at 2 months.

Protein and energy wasting is worsened with the severity of TBI and in the presence of high gastric residuals and unsuccessful enteral nutrition. The actual energy expenditure during the acute phase may be difficult to predict since it is influenced by multiple concomitant factors (i.e., body temperature, severity of the injury, possible accompanying injuries, sedation, and ventilation).

Thus, many patients with long-term stay in the ICU due to TBI develop severe energy and protein deficit. Most patients with severe traumatic brain injury regain their nutritional independence within the first 6 months after injury, but also most develop signs of malnutrition. As Krakau et al. have shown, up to 68% of TBI patients exhibited signs of malnourishment with weight loss of up to 10–29% [1].

Sunderland et al. reported in an older study that estimating energy expenditure in TBI with predictive formulas often are very inaccurate [2], therefore, especially during the acute phase indirect calorimetry where available should be used routinely as recommended by APSEN-SCCM and ESPEN. Nutrient requirement and metabolic rate can vary in particular during the initial phase of TBI due to the above-mentioned factors. As a result, repetitive measurements using indirect calorimetry may be necessary.

17.3 Indication for Artificial Nutrition Support After TBI

It is well known that malnutrition (in particular when body mass index <18,5 in postoperative patients) worsens outcome [3]. Patients with TBI demonstrate a significant loss of muscle mass which correlates with length of hospitalization and 3-month function level [4]. Improved nutrient intake may therefore improve outcome [5].

In a study including nearly 800 patients with TBI, those who were not fed within 5 and 7 days after TBI had a two- and fourfold increased mortality. The amount of nutrition in the first 5 days correlated with outcome. Every 10-kcal/kg decrease in caloric intake was associated with a 30–40% increase in mortality rates. This holds up even after controlling for factors known to affect mortality, including arterial hypotension, age, pupillary status, initial GCS score, and CT scan findings [6].

Early enhanced enteral nutrition (EN) with reaching nutritional goal at day 1 or when started within 48 h compared to a later start of EN also resulted in lower mortality and improved neurologic outcome in other studies [7, 8].

As a result of these studies, SCCM and ASPEN recommended in their current guidelines that, like other critically ill patients, early enteral feeding be initiated in TBI in the immediate post-trauma period (within 24–48 h of injury) once the patient is hemodynamically stable [9].

17.4 Route of Nutritional Support After TBI

A Cochrane review and a meta-analysis by Wang et al. demonstrated no significant difference in outcome between routes of feeding (EN vs PN) in patients with TBI [10]. In a prospective clinical trial comparing EN, PN, and EN + PN, the combined approach EN + PN was able to decrease length of stay, mechanical ventilation, and mortality [11].

SCCM and ASPEN suggest that EN is the preferred route of feeding in TBI, alluding to the beneficial effects of EN on immunologic responses and preservation of gut integrity as seen in other critical ill patient populations [9]. A combined EN + PN approach is indicated whenever EN alone is insufficient to meet caloric and protein goals.

Delayed gastric emptying and gastric hypo−/akinesia are a common dysfunction in patients with TBI [1]. To avoid overfeeding, regurgitation, and aspiration, initial EN rate should be chosen accordingly and can be increased every 6–8 h until the target amount is achieved. In certain scenarios, prokinetic agents may be used to avoid regurgitation. Nevertheless, it must be noted that the use of prokinetic agents does not automatically result in an improvement of nutrient uptake. Hence, EN rate should be started slowly and may be increased within the process.

Postpyloric feeding when compared to gastric feeding may be associated with a decrease of pneumonia and a higher caloric supply [9, 12]. Therefore, a postpyloric access may be preferred in patients after the acute phase with prolonged gastric intolerance or those with preexisting malnutrition to avoid a further energy deficit.

However, it must be noted that the placement of a transpyloric tube may be more difficult compared to a gastric tube. Additionally, it should be taken into consideration that gastric tubes typically have a larger lumen, which reduces the risk of clogging and dysfunction.

Even after transferal to the general ward, resumption of oral diet can be impaired due to the use of opioids, facial trauma, or prolonged cervical immobilization, which can be taken into consideration.

17.5 Macronutrients and Glycemic Control

A meta-analysis of 24 studies revealed that energy expenditure in TBI can result from 75%–200% of baseline-predicted resting energy expenditure (REE), depending on severity of TBI, level of sedation, delirium, or hyperthermia [13]. Therefore, 20–25 kcal/kgBW/d energy is recommended in the acute phase and 25–30 kcal/kgBW/d in the stable or chronic phase. Like the recommendations in general critically ill patients, those after TBI require higher protein supply (1–1.5 g/kg BW) [14]. Some authors recommend even higher protein dose due to the excessive losses [15].

One must be aware that despite these recommendations, actual delivery in patients with TBI often is much lower. Taylor et al. reported the actual delivery of only 58% of protein and 53% of energy requirements, respectively. Gastric intolerance due to the trauma, the use of opioids, sedatives, or vasopressors, the stop of EN for diagnostic or therapeutic procedures in intubated patients and swallowing disorders or agitation in extubated patients are common reasons. A stop of enteral nutrition in TBI patients was found in 63% of days in the ICU [16].

Hyperglycemia and higher glucose variability have long been known to deteriorate outcome after TBI [17]. To avoid this, glucose intakes should be applied continuously and be controlled. Intravenous insulin often is necessary to avoid plasma glucose levels >180 mg/dL and to therefore exert beneficial effects on neuroprotection, inflammation, ROS and NO metabolism, polyneuropathy, and coagulation [18].

Intensive insulin treatment is no longer recommended due to a higher incidence of hypoglycemic events. Moreover, plasma glucose levels do not correlate directly with brain tissue glucose levels as obtained by microdialysis technique. During hypoglycemia in the brain, lactate, ketone bodies, and BCAA are being metabolized to avoid further energetic damage to the brain. However, severe hypoglycemic events are as deleterious as severe hyperglycemia.

Accordingly, and especially during the initial phase of artificial nourishment, blood glucose levels should be measured repetitively during the day. Furthermore, blood lipids (triglycerides, high-density lipoprotein, low-density lipoprotein, and cholesterol) combined with ammonia should be measured on daily basis to identify insufficient metabolism as well as overfeeding.

17.6 Immunomodulating Formula

Only one trial in 36 adult patients compared the use of immune-modulating formulations (containing arginine, glutamine, prebiotic fiber, and omega-3 fatty acids) with standard tube feed in TBI patients. As a result, the use of immune-modulating formulations led to reduced cytokines and increased antioxidant indices [31]. Another enteral immunonutrition formula reduced in a small study the number of infections and length of stay [34].

Despite only few data, based on expert consensus, SCCM and ASPEN recommend the use of either arginine-containing immune-modulating formulations or EPA/DHA supplement with standard enteral formula in patients with TBI [9]. This stands in contrast to general recommendations by ESPEN and DGEM not to use immune-modulating formulas in critically ill patients.

17.7 Omega-3-Fatty Acids (Polyunsaturated Fatty Acids (PUFAs))

Docosahexaenic acid (DHA) but not eicosapentaenic acid (EPA) when applied after mild TBI decreased cell death under experimental conditions [27] and improved recovery [28]. DHA may protect neurons by decreasing ROS directly and indirectly by increased glutathione-mediated antioxidants activity [29]. Clinical studies with patients after TBI are missing, but PUFA-enriched diet was able to reduce the recurrence of ischemic stroke [32, 33]. Whether this was due to changed eicosanoid synthesis or just due to the antithrombotic effects of PUFA is not clear. Dose response trials or other clinical studies using this strategy are still missing [30].

17.8 Vitamins

The supply of some vitamins has been proposed to improve outcome after TBI. Vitamins are essential for the general metabolism and often have antioxidative effects.

Vitamin D deficiency is associated with worse outcome [19]. Administration of vitamin D, alone or together with progesterone, has reduced proinflammatory cytokines under experimental conditions [20]. Further effects of vitamin D supplementation may be the reduction of oxidative stress and modulation of apoptosis. However, these effects are often deducted from data of patients with vitamin D deficiency. It remains unclear whether patients without concomitant vitamin D deficiency benefit from vitamin D supplementation likewise [23].

Similarly, vitamin E supplementation reduced reactive oxygen species (ROS) and improved neurological outcome in an animal model [21]. Similar results have been shown after vitamin B3 administration [22, 23].

Since large confirming clinical trials are still missing, vitamins can best be seen today only as adjuvants of nutritional therapy. Further research is necessary to confirm the neuroprotective properties of specific vitamin supplementation.

17.9 Minerals

Plasma levels of magnesium often are decreased after TBI, maybe by interacting with transient receptor potential melastatin (TRPM) resulting in neuronal cell death [24]. Magnesium supplementation in patients with TBI improved somatic scores [5].

Zink is involved in many neurobiological functions. Low zinc levels after TBI may be a consequence of low albumin levels after a shift of protein synthesis from transport proteins like albumin toward acute phase proteins or excessive urinary losses. Zinc, with its antioxidant properties, has been a promising supplement after TBI by decreasing oxidative stress, inflammatory parameters, markers of apoptosis and autophagy, and eventually improved neurologic outcome [14, 35]. Low zinc levels have been correlated with more depression after TBI, which could be reversed in an animal model by zinc supplements [25, 26]. In contrast, some data suggest that an increase in zinc levels may contribute to excitotoxic cell death and should therefore be avoided and treated.

However, due to the limited clinical data available, no strong recommendation for mineral supplementation can be made so far.

17.10 Summary

Patients after TBI often are prone to undernutrition. Therefore, early nutritional support is strongly recommended since insufficient nutrition is associated with poor outcomes for patients with TBI.

If indicated, artificial nutrition should be started within 48 h and adjusted individually based on the metabolic rate if necessary. During initial phase, the target amount may be determined using indirect calorimetry. Enteral nutrition is preferred due to its physiological properties to the gut. Supplemental parenteral nutrition will often be necessary due to prolonged gastric intolerance.

Generally, 20–25 kcal/kgBW during the acute phase and 25–30 kcal/kgBW during the chronic phase should be provided, while considering that many factors such as severity of TBI, the level of sedation and catecholamines, the actual requirement can be increased or decreased. Blood glucose levels above 180 mg/dl should be avoided by using continuous administration of insulin. Recommended target values for protein intake are at 1–1.5 g/kgBW.

Low levels of minerals or vitamins shall be corrected and may improve neurologic function. However high-dose supplementation of these micronutrients or other immune-modulating substrates like glutamine or omega-3-fatty acids cannot be recommended at this time due to limited clinical data in patients with TBI.

References

1. Krakau K, Hansson A, Karlsson T, de Boussard CN, Tengvar C, Borg J. Nutritional treatment of patients with severe traumatic brain injury during the first six months after injury. Nutrition. 2007 Apr;23(4):308–17.
2. Sunderland PM, Heilbrun MP. Estimating energy expenditure in traumatic brain injury: comparison of indirect calorimetry with predictive formulas. Neurosurgery. 1992 Aug;31(2):246–52.
3. Finkielman JD, Gajic O, Afessa B. Underweight is independently associated with mortality in post-operative and non-operative patients admitted to the intensive care unit: a retrospective study. BMC Emerg Med. 2004;4:3.
4. Chapple LS, Deane AM, Williams LT, Strickland R, Schultz C, Lange K, Heyland DK, Chapman MJ. Longitudinal changes in anthropometrics and impact on self-reported physical function after traumatic brain injury. Crit Care Resusc. 2017;19(1):29–36.
5. Wahls T, Rubenstein L, Hall M, Snetselaar L. Assessment of dietary adequacy for important brain micronutrients in patients presenting to a traumatic brain injury clinic for evaluation. Nutr Neurosci. 2014 Nov;17(6):252–9.
6. Härtl R, Gerber LM, Ni Q, Ghajar J. Effect of early nutrition on deaths due to severe traumatic brain injury. J Neurosurg. 2008 Jul;109(1):50–6.
7. Taylor SJ, Fettes SB, Jewkes C, Nelson RJ. Prospective, randomized, controlled trial to determine the effect of early enhanced enteral nutrition on clinical outcome in mechanically ventilated patients suffering head injury. Crit Care Med. 1999 Nov;27(11):2525–31.
8. Chiang YH, Chao DP, Chu SF, Lin HW, Huang SY, Yeh YS, Lui TN, Binns CW, Chiu WT. Early enteral nutrition and clinical outcomes of severe traumatic brain injury patients in acute stage: a multi-center cohort study. J Neurotrauma. 2012;29(1):75–80.
9. McClave SA, Taylor BE, Martindale RG, Warren MM, Johnson DR, Braunschweig C, McCarthy MS, Davanos E, Rice TW, Cresci GA, Gervasio JM, Sacks GS, Roberts PR, Compher C. Society of Critical Care Medicine; American Society for Parenteral and Enteral

Nutrition. Guidelines for the Provision and Assessment of Nutrition Support Therapy in the Adult Critically Ill Patient: Society of Critical Care Medicine (SCCM) and American Society for Parenteral and Enteral Nutrition (A.S.P.E.N.). JPEN J Parenter Enteral Nutr. 2016;40(2):159–211.
10. Wang X, Dong Y, Han X, Qi XQ, Huang CG, Hou LJ. Nutritional support for patients sustaining traumatic brain injury: a systematic review and meta-analysis of prospective studies. PLoS One. 2013;8(3):e58838.
11. Fan M, Wang Q, Fang W, Jiang Y, Li L, Sun P, Wang Z. Early Enteral Combined with Parenteral Nutrition Treatment for Severe Traumatic Brain Injury: Effects on Immune Function, Nutritional Status and Outcomes. Chin Med Sci J. 2016;31(4):213–20.
12. Acosta-Escribano J, Fernández-Vivas M, Grau Carmona T, Caturla-Such J, Garcia-Martinez M, Menendez-Mainer A, Solera-Suarez M, Sanchez-Payá J. Gastric versus transpyloric feeding in severe traumatic brain injury: a prospective, randomized trial. Intensive Care Med. 2010 Sep;36(9):1532–9.
13. Foley N, Marshall S, Pikul J, Salter K, Teasell R. Hypermetabolism following moderate to severe traumatic acute brain injury: a systematic review. J Neurotrauma. 2008 Dec;25(12):1415–31.
14. Scrimgeour AG, Condlin ML. Nutritional treatment for traumatic brain injury. J Neurotrauma. 2014;31(11):989–99.
15. Dickerson RN, Pitts SL, Maish GO, Schroeppel TJ, Magnotti LJ, Croce MA, Minard G, Brown RO. A reappraisal of nitrogen requirements for patients with critical illness and trauma. J Trauma Acute Care Surg. 2012 Sep;73(3):549–57.
16. Chapple LAS, Chapman MJ, Lange K, Deane AM, Heyland DK. Nutrition support practices in critically ill head-injured patients: a global perspective. Crit Care. 2016 Jan;7(20):6.
17. Matsushima M, Peng M, Velasco C, Schaefer E, Diaz-Arrastia R, Frankel H. Glucose variability negatively impacts long-term functional outcome in patients with traumatic brain injury. J Crit Care. 2012 Apr;27(2):125–31.
18. Garg R, Chaudhuri A, Munschauer F, Dandona P. Hyperglycemia, insulin, and acute ischemic stroke: a mechanistic justification for a trial of insulin infusion therapy. Stroke. 2006 Jan;37(1):267–73.
19. Cekic M, Cutler SM, VanLandingham JW, Stein DG. Vitamin D deficiency reduces the benefits of progesterone treatment after brain injury in aged rats. Neurobiol Aging. 2011;32(5):864–74.
20. Tang H, Hua F, Wang J, Yousuf S, Atif F, Sayeed I, Stein DG. Progesterone and vitamin D combination therapy modulates inflammatory response after traumatic brain injury. Brain Inj. 2015 Sep;29(10):1165–74.
21. Aiguo W, Ying Z, Gomez-Pinilla F. Vitamin E protects against oxidative damage and learning disability after mild traumatic brain injury in rats. Neurorehabil Neural Repair. 2010;24(3):290–8.
22. Peterson TC, Hoane MR, McConomy KS, Farin FM, Bammler TK, MacDonald JW, Kantor ED, Anderson GD. A combination therapy of nicotinamide and progesterone improves functional recovery following traumatic brain injury. J Neurotrauma. 2015;32(11):765–79.
23. Vonder Haar C, Anderson GD, Hoane MR. Continuous nicotinamide administration improves behavioral recovery and reduces lesion size following bilateral frontal controlled cortical impact injury. Behav Brain Res. 2011;224(2):311–7.
24. Cook NL, Van Den Heuvel C, Vink R. Are the transient receptor potential melastatin (TRPM) channels important in magnesium homeostasis following traumatic brain injury? Magnes Res. 2009 Dec;22(4):225–34.
25. Cope EC, Morris DR, Scrimgeour AG, VanLandingham JW, Levenson CW. Zinc supplementation provides behavioral resiliency in a rat model of traumatic brain injury. Physiol Behav. 2011;104(5):942–7.
26. Maes M, D'Haese PC, Scharpé S, D'Hondt P, Cosyns P, De Broe ME. Hypozincemia in depression. J Affect Disord. 1994 Jun;31(2):135–40.
27. Ménard C, Patenaude C, Gagné AM, Massicotte G. AMPA receptor-mediated cell death is reduced by docosahexaenoic acid but not by eicosapentaenoic acid in area CA1 of hippocampal slice cultures. J Neurosci Res. 2009 Mar;87(4):876–86.

28. Desai A, Kevala K, Kim HY. Depletion of brain docosahexaenoic acid impairs recovery from traumatic brain injury. PLoS One. 2014;9(1):e86472.
29. Wang X, Zhao X, Mao ZY, Wang XM, Liu ZL. Neuroprotective effect of docosahexaenoic acid on glutamate-induced cytotoxicity in rat hippocampal cultures. Neuroreport. 2003;14(18):2457–61.
30. Hasadsri L, Wang BH, Lee JV, Erdman JW, Llano DA, Barbey AK, Wszalek T, Sharrock MF, Wang HJ. Omega-3 fatty acids as a putative treatment for traumatic brain injury. J Neurotrauma. 2013;30(11):897–906.
31. Rai VRH, Phang LF, Sia SF, Amir A, Veerakumaran JS, Kassim MKA, Othman R, Tah PC, Loh PS, Jailani MIO, Ong G. Effects of immunonutrition on biomarkers in traumatic brain injury patients in Malaysia: a prospective randomized controlled trial. BMC Anesthesiol. 2017;17(1):81.
32. Dyall SC, Michael-Titus AT. Neurological benefits of omega-3 fatty acids. NeuroMolecular Med. 2008;10(4):219–35.
33. Tanaka K, Ishikawa Y, Yokoyama M, Origasa H, Matsuzaki M, Saito Y, Matsuzawa Y, Sasaki J, Oikawa S, Hishida H, Itakura H, Kita T, Kitabatake A, Nakaya N, Sakata T, Shimada K, Shirato K, JELIS Investigators, Japan. Reduction in the recurrence of stroke by eicosapentaenoic acid for hypercholesterolemic patients: subanalysis of the JELIS trial. Stroke. 2008;39(7):2052–8.
34. Falcão de Arruda IS, de Aguilar-Nascimento JE. Benefits of early enteral nutrition with glutamine and probiotics in brain injury patients. Clin Sci (Lond). 2004;106(3):287–92.
35. Young B, Ott L, Kasarskis E, Rapp R, Moles K, Dempsey RJ, Tibbs PA, Kryscio R, McClain C. Zinc supplementation is associated with improved neurologic recovery rate and visceral protein levels of patients with severe closed head injury. J Neurotrauma. 1996 Jan;13(1):25–34.

Sepsis 18

Benjamin Tan and Markus A. Weigand

In cases of sepsis, metabolic maladaptation occurs, resulting in stress hyperglycemia, acute muscle breakdown, and increased recycling of endogenous amino acids. These events lead to accelerated hepatic glucose production accompanied by insulin resistance [1–3].

A known consequence of these changes is the dysfunction of the mitochondria. This dysfunction manifests as a reduction in oxygen utilization capacity and an inability to utilize exogenously supplied nutrients. This initial stage of sepsis is marked by insulin resistance and a significant mobilization of caloric reserves that can supply up to 50–75% of glucose requirements and up to 500–1400 kcal/d [1–4].

Supplying external nutrition cannot inhibit these catabolic processes and may even heighten oxidative stress, exacerbating mitochondrial dysfunction and cell death [5] Furthermore, early nutrition has been demonstrated to inhibit autophagy [3]. Autophagy is a cellular mechanism that digests and recycles cellular particles and proteins. Additionally, it can also dispose of viral and bacterial components, indicating a potential role in resolving infections and sepsis [3].

Autophagy is a highly regulated process that can be manipulated by nutritional therapy. It is suppressed by feeding and enhanced by starvation.

While these theoretical considerations may support a no-feeding approach in sepsis, the increased metabolic needs related to stress observed in sepsis outweigh the massive endogenous mobilization of caloric reserves. As a result, sepsis promotes malnutrition, and withholding exogenous nutrition could exacerbate postseptic malnutrition, which could potentially lead to an increase in mortality [6].

B. Tan
Department of Pediatric Cardiology, University Hospital Heidelberg, Heidelberg, Germany

M. A. Weigand (✉)
Department of Anaesthesiology, University Hospital Heidelberg, Heidelberg, Germany
e-mail: markus.weigand@med.uni-heidelberg.de

The cytokine release in sepsis directly impedes the function of intestinal myocytes, inhibits enteric neuromuscular transmission, resulting in a dysregulation of gastrointestinal hormones, and disrupts the balance between gut epithelium and microbiome, promoting intestinal edema and multiple organ dysfunctions [1, 7–10].

The absorption of enteral nutrition in sepsis thus becomes unpredictable. In fact, enteral nutrition may be a risk factor for worsening sepsis-induced intestinal dysfunction.

From a pathophysiological standpoint, several questions must be addressed when prescribing artificial nutrition to septic patients.

1. The first question pertains to the most suitable route of administration. Which is better, enteral or parenteral feeding?
2. How much should be given, and what should the caloric and protein goals be? When is the appropriate time to initiate feeding?
3. Are there any specific macronutrient or micronutrient supplements that should be utilized in the case of sepsis?

18.1 Route of Administration: Enteral or Parenteral?

The debate regarding enteral versus parenteral nutrition for critically ill patients is thoroughly examined in Part II Clinical Application. However, when addressing this question in sepsis, special attention must be given to specific details. As stated in the introduction, the cytokine release in sepsis may lead to gastrointestinal dysfunction, even if the primary source of infection is not found in the gastrointestinal tract.

While no randomized controlled trial (RCT) has specifically investigated septic patients, the NUTRIREA-2 trial is the most comparable and therefore warrants further attention [11]. The NUTRIREA-2 trial investigated the impact of early parenteral versus early enteral nutrition on mortality in adult patients who required mechanical ventilation for at least 48 h and also required vasoactive support via a central line. The trial was an open-label, parallel-group, multicenter RCT conducted in 44 intensive care units (ICUs) throughout France. Patients who had undergone previous gastrointestinal surgery and/or had gastrointestinal pathologies such as small bowel syndrome were excluded. Nutritional therapy began within 24 h after intubation, with a target of 20–25 kcal/kg/d for the initial 7 days and 25–30 kcal/kg/d thereafter. The parenteral group received pure parenteral nutrition for the first 7 days, while the enteral group received only pure enteral nutrition. After 7 days, both groups were given enteral nutrition, and parenteral nutrition was supplemented in the enteral group only if energy targets were not met by pure enteral nutrition. The primary outcome was 28-day mortality. A total of 1202 individuals were enrolled in the enteral group and 1208 in the parenteral group. The mean age was 66 years, with an average SOFA-score of 11. Among the participants, 61% in the enteral group and 64% in the parenteral group had sepsis as their cause of vasoactive therapy. The primary outcome and most secondary outcomes, such as ICU length of stay, time on vasoactive support, and ventilation days, demonstrated no significant difference. Nevertheless, notable discrepancies appeared in gastrointestinal complications. A significantly higher number of patients in the enteral group experienced vomiting (34% vs. 24%, $p < 0.0001$), diarrhea (36% vs. 33%, $p = 0.009$), as well as more concerning complications such as bowel ischemia (2% vs. 1%, $p = 0.007$) and acute colonic pseudo-obstruction (1% vs. <1%, $p = 0.004$). While the numbers are relatively small in this large patient cohort (bowel ischemia in 19 patients and acute colonic pseudo-obstruction in 11 patients), the observed differences are significant and worrisome due to the severity of both complications and their high mortality rates [12, 13]. Furthermore, these observations are intriguing because patients at risk for gastrointestinal complications were excluded, and the primary sources of infections were ICU-acquired infections, primarily ventilator-associated pneumonia.

These findings may represent clinical evidence of the previously described sepsis-induced gastrointestinal dysfunction and suggest a potential advantage of parenteral nutrition in sepsis.

Based on the available evidence, both enteral and parenteral routes can be used to provide nutritional support in sepsis. In addition, the current ESPEN guidelines recommend an early and gradual enteral approach as long as there are no contraindications for enteral nutrition [14]. Regardless of which route is selected, the crucial aspect is to introduce nutrition slowly and in a stepwise manner (see the following section).

18.2 How Much Should Be Given, and What Should the Caloric and Protein Goals Be? When Is the Appropriate Time to Initiate Feeding?

Directly related to the choice of nutritional route, consideration should be given to the amount of nutrition to be provided. According to a meta-analysis conducted by Elke et al., the observed benefits and differences between enteral and parenteral nutrition, such as reduced instances of infectious complications, are more likely linked to the caloric energy supplied rather than the chosen route of administration. The meta-analysis revealed notable variations in infectious complications among the subgroups of RCTs considered. In instances where the parenteral group received a significantly higher amount of calories than the enteral group, infections were more prevalent. However, when the caloric intake was similar in both groups, no difference in infectious complications was observed [15]. Based on the introductory theoretical considerations and the observed data, it is evident that there exists a correlation between caloric intake and complications with a potential impact on the outcome. In the context of sepsis, the administration of nutrition necessitates a careful evaluation of the potential risks associated with overfeeding, which can result from the endogenous energy release during the early phase of sepsis, and the risks of malnutrition during the later stage of the condition. Beginning enteral feeding during sepsis is crucial, however, following general nutritional targets and normative values established for other critically ill patients is not ideal. It is important to note that these values should be utilized with discretion and reassessed regularly to ensure optimal patient care. Elke et al. conducted a secondary analysis using a large international database consisting of 2,270 patients to investigate calorie and protein intake by enteral nutrition in patients with sepsis. The mean prescribed energy and protein amounts were 23.9 kcal/kg/d and 1.2 g/kg/d, respectively. However, the received calories and protein amounts on average were only 14.5 kcal/kg/d and 0.7 g/kg/d, respectively, which is approximately 60% of the prescribed goals. Additionally, the majority of patients did not achieve this amount within the first 3 days of ICU admission, and throughout the 12-day observation period, no more than 80% of the prescribed goals were met [16]. These findings indicate that providing nutrition in sepsis improves outcomes, but it should likely be delivered gradually during the first week with lower calorie and protein targets than typically recommended. One technique that may be effective in achieving these goals is permissive underfeeding, which was studied in the PermiT RCT of 894 mechanically ventilated patients, 30% of whom were diagnosed with severe sepsis on admission. The group undergoing intervention received 40–60% of their required calories for a span of 14 days. This was found to be noninferior in the primary outcome of 90-day mortality when compared to those receiving standard feeding (70–100% of caloric needs). In fact, the underfed group even exhibited a potential nephroprotective effect as the need for renal replacement therapy was significantly lower [17]. Unlike Elke et al.'s analysis, the underfed group in this study received complete protein support of 1.2–1.5 g/kg/d from the first day.

Similar findings were shown in the EpaNIC trial, which compared early and late parenteral nutrition in 4,460 patients, 22% of whom had sepsis. A delayed parenteral nutrition strategy, which commenced only after 8 days of ICU stay, if enteral nutrition failed to meet the designated goals, exhibited no mortality difference in comparison to an early parenteral nutrition strategy, which initially provided for 100% of the nutritional needs from day 3 on. However, the former led to a lesser incidence of organ dysfunctions (such as the need for renal replacement therapy and ventilation days), shorter stays in the ICU and hospital, and fewer occurrences of new infections [18].

These findings have been replicated in numerous other observational and randomized controlled trials within the general ICU population, particularly in those with acute lung injury. It has been demonstrated that initial underfeeding is safe, while early full feeding may even result in harm [19–26]. As previously stated, the inhibition of autophagy, particularly in cases of sepsis, may contribute to the adverse effects of early full dose nutrition. This phenomenon was demonstrated in a subanalysis of the EPaNIC trial that was prospectively planned [18, 21]. Hermans et al. demonstrated that early implementation of full parenteral nutrition inhibits autophagy, resulting in increased muscle weakness and prolonged muscle recovery time compared to the late parenteral nutritional protocol. This effect is particularly crucial in septic patients, as 60% of the patients who underwent muscle biopsy for immunohistochemical investigation for autophagy had sepsis. Moreover, the markers for autophagy were twice as high in the late parenteral group compared to the muscle biopsies from a healthy control group, indicating that underfeeding could potentially stimulate autophagy.

The significance of protein intake in critical illness and sepsis has become increasingly evident alongside caloric intake. Early studies suggested that higher protein intake had a positive impact on critical illness [27–32]; however, recent retrospective observational studies suggest that this effect might be time-dependent and may even yield harm from increased protein intake (>0.8 g/kg/day) during the first 3 days of critical illness [33, 34].

New evidence regarding caloric and protein targets in the early stages of sepsis has been published in the NUTRIREA-3 trial [35]. This multicenter, open-label, parallel-group randomized controlled trial was carried out in 61 French intensive care units. The study examined 3,036 patients who were intubated within the last 24 h and required ventilator support for at least 48 h and vasopressor support. 58% of patients had sepsis as the cause of circulatory shock. The study compared two feeding strategies during the first 7 days of ICU hospitalization. In the permissive underfeeding group, patients were administered 6 kcal/kg/d and 0.2–0.4 g/kg/d protein while the standard group received 25 kcal/kg/d and 1.0–1.3 g/kg/d protein. On day 7 or after extubation, whichever came first, both groups were prescribed 30 kcal/kg/d and 1.2–2.0 g/kg/d. The mean time from intubation to the initiation of nutrition was 17 h for both groups. Enteral nutrition was received by 60% of patients, while 23% received parenteral nutrition exclusively. Both groups adhered closely to their prescribed caloric and protein goals. The primary outcome, 90-day mortality, did not differ significantly, but several secondary outcomes reached statistical significance. The permissive group experienced significantly fewer days of mechanical ventilation, as well as fewer gastrointestinal complications, notably less bowel ischemia, and less liver dysfunction. The standard group showed a notable increase in the occurrence of hypophosphatemia, suggesting a potential refeeding syndrome and the incapacity of critically ill organisms to metabolize heightened amounts of energy and protein.

Based on the available evidence, it is suggested that an initial permissive underfeeding for the first 5–7 days and a stepwise increase in caloric and protein supply over several days is the safest way to prescribe nutrition in septic patients.

A possible feeding plan is illustrated in Fig. 18.1.

18.2.1 Guideline Statements

The 2021 Surviving Sepsis Campaign (SSC) guidelines weakly recommend early enteral feeding within 72 h for sepsis or septic shock patients who are able to receive enteral feeding, backed by low-quality evidence [36]. The guidelines do not address specific details regarding calorie and protein goals or the timing of parenteral nutrition.

The latest guidelines from the European Society for Clinical Nutrition and Metabolism (ESPEN) recommend using early gradual enteral nutrition in septic patients after hemodynamic stabilization and replacing or supplementing enteral

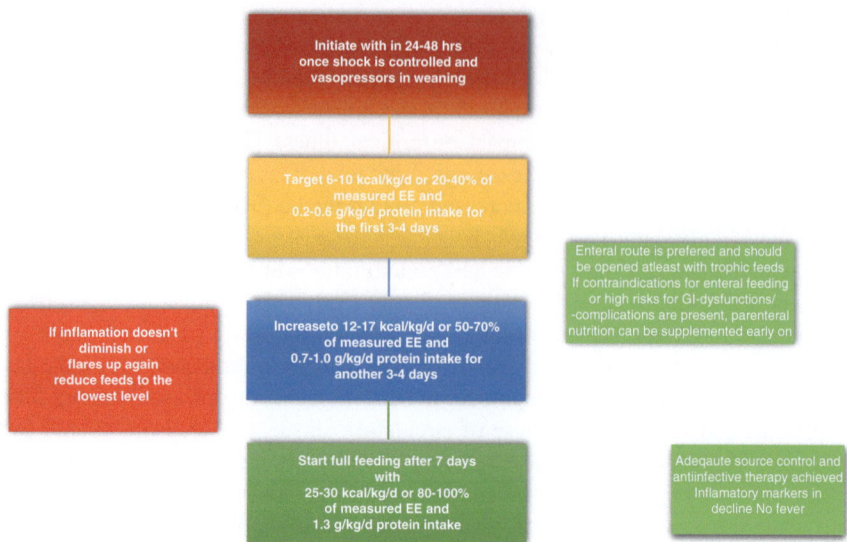

Fig. 18.1 Gradual feeding chart for patients with sepsis/septic shock. (EE: energy expenditure)

nutrition with parenteral nutrition if enteral nutrition is contraindicated. Enteral nutrition should not exceed 20–50% of the nutritional requirements, and parenteral nutrition should be prescribed only after 3 days and should not exceed 50% of the nutritional needs [14].

The previous guidelines of the American Society for Parenteral and Enteral Nutrition (ASPEN) indicate that enteral nutrition should be administered to sepsis/septic shock patients within 24–48 h as soon as resuscitation is completed, and the patient becomes hemodynamically stable. In the early stages of sepsis or septic shock, regardless of nutritional risk, parenteral nutrition, either exclusively or as a supplement to enteral nutrition, should not be utilized. According to expert consensus, it is suggested to implement trophic feeding during the initial phase of sepsis, which is defined as 10–20 kcal/h or up to 500 kcal/d. After 24–48 h, the feeding can be advanced as tolerated to reach over 80% of the target energy goal within the first week. Additionally, it is recommended to intake 1.2–2 g of protein per kilogram of body weight per day [37].

Although the American Society issued an update recently for the general critical ill, accepting lower calorie targets of 12–25 kcal/kg/d for 7–10 days and announcing that early parenteral nutrition was now considered equal to early enteral nutrition, they made no changes to the protein targets and did not publish any updated recommendations for patients with sepsis and septic shock [38].

Based on the abundance of recent studies and findings that are discussed in this context, it is necessary to update the American guidelines to ensure they align with the latest base of knowledge. In this regard, the most accurate reflection of current evidence is provided by the updated ESPN recommendations.

18.3 Are There Any Specific Macronutrient or Micronutrient Supplements That Should Be Utilized in the Case of Sepsis?

For further information, please refer to the chapters on macronutrition, micronutrition, and immunonutrition.

Metabolic resuscitation using micronutrients in the treatment of sepsis appears to be a rational option [39, 40], especially the use of vitamin C, which was widely heralded as a cure for sepsis in the second half of the 2010s [41–44]. However, subsequent years of extensive clinical research have not demonstrated a clear benefit of vitamin C supplementation on relevant variables, and in some cases have even shown the possibility of harm [45–50]. Therefore, the current SSC guidelines weakly recommend against the use of vitamin C in sepsis and septic shock due to low-quality evidence [36].

On the contrary, the 2022 ESPEN guidelines on micronutrients suggest a high daily dose of vitamin C, ranging between 2 and 3 g, for critically ill patients during the acute phase of inflammation [51].

Out of the macronutrient components, fatty acids have been found to have immunomodulatory effects. Generally, omega-6 fatty acids are considered to be pro-inflammatory while omega-3 fatty acids are known to be anti-inflammatory [52–54].

Although high-dose omega-3 supplementation is not recommended, current guidelines suggest enriching enteral and parenteral formulas with omega-3 fatty acids [14]. Moreover, mounting evidence favors the utilization of parenteral fat emulsions based on fish oil rather than the traditional soybean oil solutions, which have been linked to pro-inflammatory effects and liver malfunction. On the other hand, omega-3 fatty acid-based solutions derived from fish oil have been connected with reduced mortality rates among sepsis patients [55–60].

In conclusion, patients with sepsis should receive enteral and parenteral formulas enriched with omega-3 acids.

For parenteral solutions, it is advisable to use fish oil-based fat emulsions rather than soybean oil-based emulsions.

References

1. Kott M, Hartl WH, Elke G. Enteral vs. parenteral nutrition in septic shock: are they equivalent? Curr Opin Crit Care. 2019;25(4):340–8.
2. Moonen H, Van Zanten ARH. Mitochondrial dysfunction in critical illness during acute metabolic stress and convalescence: consequences for nutrition therapy. Curr Opin Crit Care. 2020;26(4):346–54.
3. McClave SA, Weijs PJ. Preservation of autophagy should not direct nutritional therapy. Curr Opin Clin Nutr Metab Care. 2015;18(2):155–61.
4. Iapichino G, Radrizzani D, Armani S, Noto A, Spanu P, Mistraletti G. Metabolic treatment of critically ill patients: energy balance and substrate disposal. Minerva Anestesiol. 2006;72(6):533–41.

5. McKeever L, Peterson SJ, Cienfuegos S, Rizzie J, Lateef O, Freels S, et al. Real-time energy exposure is associated with increased oxidative stress among feeding-tolerant critically ill patients: results from the FEDOX trial. JPEN J Parenter Enteral Nutr. 2020;44(8):1484–91.
6. Singer P, Blaser AR, Berger MM, Alhazzani W, Calder PC, Casaer MP, et al. ESPEN guideline on clinical nutrition in the intensive care unit. Clin Nutr. 2019;38(1):48–79.
7. Lyons JD, Coopersmith CM. Pathophysiology of the gut and the microbiome in the host response. Pediatr Crit Care Med. 2017;18(3_suppl Suppl 1):S46–S9.
8. Meng M, Klingensmith NJ, Coopersmith CM. New insights into the gut as the driver of critical illness and organ failure. Curr Opin Crit Care. 2017;23(2):143–8.
9. Wan YD, Zhu RX, Wu ZQ, Lyu SY, Zhao LX, Du ZJ, et al. Gut microbiota disruption in septic shock patients: a pilot study. Med Sci Monit. 2018;24:8639–46.
10. Deane AM, Chapman MJ, Reintam Blaser A, McClave SA, Emmanuel A. Pathophysiology and treatment of gastrointestinal motility disorders in the acutely ill. Nutr Clin Pract. 2019;34(1):23–36.
11. Reignier J, Boisrame-Helms J, Brisard L, Lascarrou JB, Ait Hssain A, Anguel N, et al. Enteral versus parenteral early nutrition in ventilated adults with shock: a randomised, controlled, multicentre, open-label, parallel-group study (NUTRIREA-2). Lancet. 2018;391(10116):133–43.
12. Trompeter M, Brazda T, Remy CT, Vestring T, Reimer P. Non-occlusive mesenteric ischemia: etiology, diagnosis, and interventional therapy. Eur Radiol. 2002;12(5):1179–87.
13. Saunders MD, Kimmey MB. Systematic review: acute colonic pseudo-obstruction. Aliment Pharmacol Ther. 2005;22(10):917–25.
14. Singer P, Blaser AR, Berger MM, Calder PC, Casaer M, Hiesmayr M, et al. ESPEN practical and partially revised guideline: clinical nutrition in the intensive care unit. Clin Nutr. 2023;42(9):1671–89.
15. Elke G, van Zanten AR, Lemieux M, McCall M, Jeejeebhoy KN, Kott M, et al. Enteral versus parenteral nutrition in critically ill patients: an updated systematic review and meta-analysis of randomized controlled trials. Crit Care. 2016;20(1):117.
16. Elke G, Wang M, Weiler N, Day AG, Heyland DK. Close to recommended caloric and protein intake by enteral nutrition is associated with better clinical outcome of critically ill septic patients: secondary analysis of a large international nutrition database. Crit Care. 2014;18(1):R29.
17. Arabi YM, Aldawood AS, Haddad SH, Al-Dorzi HM, Tamim HM, Jones G, et al. Permissive underfeeding or standard enteral feeding in critically ill adults. N Engl J Med. 2015;372(25):2398–408.
18. Casaer MP, Mesotten D, Hermans G, Wouters PJ, Schetz M, Meyfroidt G, et al. Early versus late parenteral nutrition in critically ill adults. N Engl J Med. 2011;365(6):506–17.
19. Arabi YM, Haddad SH, Tamim HM, Rishu AH, Sakkijha MH, Kahoul SH, et al. Near-target caloric intake in critically ill medical-surgical patients is associated with adverse outcomes. JPEN J Parenter Enteral Nutr. 2010;34(3):280–8.
20. National Heart L, Blood Institute Acute Respiratory Distress Syndrome Clinical Trials N, Rice TW, Wheeler AP, Thompson BT, Steingrub J, et al. Initial trophic vs full enteral feeding in patients with acute lung injury: the EDEN randomized trial. JAMA. 2012;307(8):795–803.
21. Hermans G, Casaer MP, Clerckx B, Guiza F, Vanhullebusch T, Derde S, et al. Effect of tolerating macronutrient deficit on the development of intensive-care unit acquired weakness: a subanalysis of the EPaNIC trial. Lancet Respir Med. 2013;1(8):621–9.
22. Tian F, Wang X, Gao X, Wan X, Wu C, Zhang L, et al. Effect of initial calorie intake via enteral nutrition in critical illness: a meta-analysis of randomised controlled trials. Crit Care. 2015;19:180.
23. Braunschweig CA, Sheean PM, Peterson SJ, Gomez Perez S, Freels S, Lateef O, et al. Intensive nutrition in acute lung injury: a clinical trial (INTACT). JPEN J Parenter Enteral Nutr. 2015;39(1):13–20.
24. Rugeles S, Villarraga-Angulo LG, Ariza-Gutierrez A, Chaverra-Kornerup S, Lasalvia P, Rosselli D. High-protein hypocaloric vs normocaloric enteral nutrition in critically ill patients: a randomized clinical trial. J Crit Care. 2016;35:110–4.

25. Allingstrup MJ, Kondrup J, Wiis J, Claudius C, Pedersen UG, Hein-Rasmussen R, et al. Early goal-directed nutrition versus standard of care in adult intensive care patients: the single-Centre, randomised, outcome assessor-blinded EAT-ICU trial. Intensive Care Med. 2017;43(11):1637–47.
26. Braunschweig CL, Freels S, Sheean PM, Peterson SJ, Perez SG, McKeever L, et al. Role of timing and dose of energy received in patients with acute lung injury on mortality in the intensive nutrition in acute lung injury trial (INTACT): a post hoc analysis. Am J Clin Nutr. 2017;105(2):411–6.
27. Weijs PJ, Stapel SN, de Groot SD, Driessen RH, de Jong E, Girbes AR, et al. Optimal protein and energy nutrition decreases mortality in mechanically ventilated, critically ill patients: a prospective observational cohort study. JPEN J Parenter Enteral Nutr. 2012;36(1):60–8.
28. Allingstrup MJ, Esmailzadeh N, Wilkens Knudsen A, Espersen K, Hartvig Jensen T, Wiis J, et al. Provision of protein and energy in relation to measured requirements in intensive care patients. Clin Nutr. 2012;31(4):462–8.
29. Weijs PJ, Looijaard WG, Beishuizen A, Girbes AR, Oudemans-van Straaten HM. Early high protein intake is associated with low mortality and energy overfeeding with high mortality in non-septic mechanically ventilated critically ill patients. Crit Care. 2014;18(6):701.
30. Nicolo M, Heyland DK, Chittams J, Sammarco T, Compher C. Clinical outcomes related to protein delivery in a critically ill population: a multicenter, multinational observation study. JPEN J Parenter Enteral Nutr. 2016;40(1):45–51.
31. Compher C, Chittams J, Sammarco T, Nicolo M, Heyland DK. Greater protein and energy intake may be associated with improved mortality in higher risk critically ill patients: a multicenter, multinational observational study. Crit Care Med. 2017;45(2):156–63.
32. Bendavid I, Zusman O, Kagan I, Theilla M, Cohen J, Singer P. Early Administration of Protein in critically ill patients: a retrospective cohort study. Nutrients. 2019;11(1):106.
33. de Koning MLY, Koekkoek W, Kars J, van Zanten ARH. Association of PROtein and CAloric intake and clinical outcomes in adult SEPTic and non-septic ICU patients on prolonged mechanical ventilation: the PROCASEPT retrospective study. JPEN J Parenter Enteral Nutr. 2020;44(3):434–43.
34. Koekkoek W, van Setten CHC, Olthof LE, Kars J, van Zanten ARH. Timing of PROTein INtake and clinical outcomes of adult critically ill patients on prolonged mechanical VENTilation: the PROTINVENT retrospective study. Clin Nutr. 2019;38(2):883–90.
35. Reignier J, Plantefeve G, Mira JP, Argaud L, Asfar P, Aissaoui N, et al. Low versus standard calorie and protein feeding in ventilated adults with shock: a randomised, controlled, multicentre, open-label, parallel-group trial (NUTRIREA-3). Lancet Respir Med. 2023;11(7):602–12.
36. Evans L, Rhodes A, Alhazzani W, Antonelli M, Coopersmith CM, French C, et al. Surviving sepsis campaign: international guidelines for management of sepsis and septic shock 2021. Intensive Care Med. 2021;47(11):1181–247.
37. McClave SA, Taylor BE, Martindale RG, Warren MM, Johnson DR, Braunschweig C, et al. Guidelines for the provision and assessment of nutrition support therapy in the adult critically ill patient: Society of Critical Care Medicine (SCCM) and American Society for Parenteral and Enteral Nutrition (A.S.P.E.N.). JPEN J Parenter Enteral Nutr. 2016;40(2):159–211.
38. Compher C, Bingham AL, McCall M, Patel J, Rice TW, Braunschweig C, et al. Guidelines for the provision of nutrition support therapy in the adult critically ill patient: the American Society for Parenteral and Enteral Nutrition. JPEN J Parenter Enteral Nutr. 2022;46(1):12–41.
39. Khoshnam-Rad N, Khalili H. Safety of vitamin C in sepsis: a neglected topic. Curr Opin Crit Care. 2019;25(4):329–33.
40. Moskowitz A, Andersen LW, Huang DT, Berg KM, Grossestreuer AV, Marik PE, et al. Ascorbic acid, corticosteroids, and thiamine in sepsis: a review of the biologic rationale and the present state of clinical evaluation. Crit Care. 2018;22(1):283.
41. Rubin R. Wide interest in a Vitamin C drug cocktail for Sepsis despite lagging evidence. JAMA. 2019;322(4):291–3.
42. Marik PE. "Vitamin S" (steroids) and Vitamin C for the treatment of severe Sepsis and septic shock! Crit Care Med. 2016;44(6):1228–9.

43. Marik PE, Farkas JD. The changing paradigm of Sepsis: early diagnosis, early antibiotics, early Pressors, and early adjuvant treatment. Crit Care Med. 2018;46(10):1690–2.
44. Marik PE, Khangoora V, Rivera R, Hooper MH, Catravas J. Hydrocortisone, Vitamin C, and thiamine for the treatment of severe Sepsis and septic shock: a retrospective before-after study. Chest. 2017;151(6):1229–38.
45. Agarwal A, Basmaji J, Fernando SM, Ge FZ, Xiao Y, Faisal H, et al. Administration of Parenteral Vitamin C in patients with severe infection: protocol for a systematic review and meta-analysis. JMIR Res Protoc. 2022;11(1):e33989.
46. Fujii T, Luethi N, Young PJ, Frei DR, Eastwood GM, French CJ, et al. Effect of Vitamin C, hydrocortisone, and thiamine vs hydrocortisone alone on time alive and free of vasopressor support among patients with septic shock: the VITAMINS randomized clinical trial. JAMA. 2020;323(5):423–31.
47. Fowler AA 3rd, Truwit JD, Hite RD, Morris PE, DeWilde C, Priday A, et al. Effect of Vitamin C infusion on organ failure and biomarkers of inflammation and vascular injury in patients with Sepsis and severe acute respiratory failure: the CITRIS-ALI randomized clinical trial. JAMA. 2019;322(13):1261–70.
48. Putzu A, Daems AM, Lopez-Delgado JC, Giordano VF, Landoni G. The effect of Vitamin C on clinical outcome in critically ill patients: a systematic review with Meta-analysis of randomized controlled trials. Crit Care Med. 2019;47(6):774–83.
49. Moskowitz A, Huang DT, Hou PC, Gong J, Doshi PB, Grossestreuer AV, et al. Effect of ascorbic acid, corticosteroids, and thiamine on organ injury in septic shock: the ACTS randomized clinical trial. JAMA. 2020;324(7):642–50.
50. Lamontagne F, Masse MH, Menard J, Sprague S, Pinto R, Heyland DK, et al. Intravenous Vitamin C in adults with Sepsis in the intensive care unit. N Engl J Med. 2022;386(25):2387–98.
51. Berger MM, Shenkin A, Schweinlin A, Amrein K, Augsburger M, Biesalski HK, et al. ESPEN micronutrient guideline. Clin Nutr. 2022;41(6):1357–424.
52. Calder PC. n-3 fatty acids, inflammation, and immunity--relevance to postsurgical and critically ill patients. Lipids. 2004;39(12):1147–61.
53. Djuricic I, Calder PC. Beneficial outcomes of Omega-6 and Omega-3 polyunsaturated fatty acids on human health: an update for 2021. Nutrients. 2021;13(7):2421.
54. Rosa Neto JC, Calder PC, Curi R, Newsholme P, Sethi JK, Silveira LS. The Immunometabolic roles of various fatty acids in macrophages and lymphocytes. Int J Mol Sci. 2021;22(16):8460.
55. Calder PC, Waitzberg DL, Klek S, Martindale RG. Lipids in parenteral nutrition: biological aspects. JPEN J Parenter Enteral Nutr. 2020;44(Suppl 1):S21–S7.
56. Pradelli L, Mayer K, Klek S, Omar Alsaleh AJ, Clark RAC, Rosenthal MD, et al. Omega-3 fatty-acid enriched parenteral nutrition in hospitalized patients: systematic review with meta-analysis and trial sequential analysis. JPEN J Parenter Enteral Nutr. 2020;44(1):44–57.
57. Wang C, Han D, Feng X, Wu J. Omega-3 fatty acid supplementation is associated with favorable outcomes in patients with sepsis: an updated meta-analysis. J Int Med Res. 2020;48(12):300060520953684.
58. Wang H, Su S, Wang C, Hu J, Dan W, Peng X. Effects of fish oil-containing nutrition supplementation in adult sepsis patients: a systematic review and meta-analysis. Burns. Trauma. 2022;10:tkac012.
59. Pradelli L, Klek S, Mayer K, Omar Alsaleh AJ, Rosenthal MD, Heller AR, et al. Omega-3 fatty acid-containing parenteral nutrition in ICU patients: systematic review with meta-analysis and cost-effectiveness analysis. Crit Care. 2020;24(1):634.
60. Haines KL, Ohnuma T, Trujillo C, Osamudiamen O, Krishnamoorthy V, Raghunathan K, et al. Hospital change to mixed lipid emulsion from soybean oil-based lipid emulsion for parenteral nutrition in hospitalized and critically ill adults improves outcomes: a pre-post-comparative study. Crit Care. 2022;26(1):317.

Nutrition Therapy in Major Burns

Mette M. Berger

19.1 Introduction

Among acute diseases, major burns are a devastating traumatic condition that is completely dependent on nutrition therapy for survival and recovery. On admission, the severity of the injury and outcome depends on three factors: the total body surface area (TBSA) burned, the presence of inhalation injury, and the age of the patient [31]. According to the surface affected by the injury, the burn injury will be classified as minor (<20% TBSA), major to severe (20–60% TBSA), or massive (>60% TBSA).

Critically ill patients with major burns have some specificities distinguish them from other trauma patients:

- The destruction of the skin barrier causes significant exudative losses of fluids, proteins, vitamins, and trace elements. It further exposes the patients to thermal losses and microorganism contamination.
- The skin destruction causes a massive oxidative stress, with a major increase of lipid peroxidation which contributes to organ dysfunction. The associated inflammatory response persists for several weeks after injury.
- The immune depression (humoral and cellular) starts within hours after injury and will persist for weeks or months. The destruction of the skin barrier further increases the infectious risk.
- The amount and surface of tissue to repair is enormous: it generally requires multiple hydrotherapy sessions and several surgical procedures (with associated fasting periods).

M. M. Berger
Centre Hospitalier Universitaire Vaudois (CHUV), University of Lausanne, Lausanne, Switzerland
e-mail: Mette.Berger@unil.ch

- Vascular access is difficult due to the limited remaining healthy skin surface: stitching through burns may be required.
- The endocrine and metabolic alterations are the most extreme and long-lasting observed in critically ill patients.
- The patients generally require ICU treatment for prolonged periods of time (0.7–1.3 days per % TBSA burned).

Specialized burn centre treatment has been shown to both increase survival and quality of life, but also to be cost effective. Nutritional therapy is a corner stone of their management: recommendations have been summarized in the ESPEN guidelines [29].

19.2 Nutritional Requirements

Some patients with minor burns <20% BSA suffer inhalation injury and are therefore briefly treated in the ICU until respiratory recovery: they can be managed as any critically ill surgical patient, i.e., fed orally or enterally with standard energy targets (25–30 kcal/kg/day). The situation is very different with major burns.

19.2.1 Energy

The burn injury releases nearly immediately a host of mediators, starting with histamine, which causes the early massive capillary leak. The massive and prolonged release of cytokines that follows triggers a hypermetabolic and hypercatabolic response that will persist until skin closure. The most extreme changes will be observed during the first 2–3 weeks after injury, with a subsequent progressive fading: nevertheless the metabolic alterations persist until several months after injury [16].

In the 1970s, the observation of a hypermetabolic response in major burns, associated with a rapid loss of body weight, lean body mass and obvious massive malnutrition, led to the development of the hyper-alimentation concept which prevailed until the late 1980s. The Curreri formula is a typical example of these excesses which caused numerous complications (hyperglycemia, fatty liver, septic complications, respiratory weaning difficulties, etc.). These equations belong to the past and should be banned from clinical practice due to the automatic overfeeding they cause.

Modern management (see Tables 19.1 and 19.2) has attenuated the magnitude of the hypermetabolic response measured by indirect calorimetry in the 1970s: in those years, the increases in resting energy expenditure (EE) could reach 200–240% of the predicted resting values.

19 Nutrition Therapy in Major Burns

Table 19.1 ESPEN Recommendations for the nutrition of adult major burns

Topic		Grade
Indication	Nutritional therapy should be initiated early within 12 h of injury, preferentially by the enteral route.	B
Route	We recommend giving priority to the enteral route, parenteral nutrition being rarely required and indicated.	C
Energy needs and predictive equations	We recommend considering indirect calorimetry as a gold standard to assess energy requirements. If not available or not suitable, we recommend using the Toronto equation for burn adults.	D
Proteins	Protein requirements are higher than in other categories of patients and should be set around 1.5–2.0 g/kg in adults and 1.5–3 g/kg/day in children. We strongly suggest considering glutamine supplementation (or ornithine alpha-keto-glutarate) but not arginine.	D C
Glucose and glycemia control	We strongly suggest limiting carbohydrate delivery (prescribed for nutritional and drug dilution purpose to 60% of total energy intake and not to exceed 5 mg/kg/min in both adults and children. We strongly suggest keeping glucose levels under 8 mmol/l (and over 4.5 mmol/l), using continuous intravenous infusion of insulin.	D D
Lipids	We suggest monitoring total fat delivery and to keep energy from fat <35% of total energy intake	C
Micronutrients	We strongly suggest associating, in both adults and children, a substitution of zinc, copper, and selenium, as well as of vitamin B1, C, D, and E.	C
Metabolic modulation	We strongly recommend using non nutritional strategies to attenuate hypermetabolism and hypercatabolism in both adults and children (warm ambient temperature, early excision surgery, non-selective beta-blockers, and oxandrolone).	B

Table 19.2 Interventions that attenuate the hypermetabolic response in major burns [4, 37]

Intervention	Timing
Early enteral nutrition	Within 12 h after injury (as early as possible, but progressive)
Early I.V. trace element repletion	Within 12 h after injury (for doses, see Table 19.3) and for 8-21 days according to burned TBSA
Nursing in warm surrounding (25–30 °C)	From admission
Early tangential excision of full thickness burns	Starting within 2–4 days after injury
Beta-blockade (propranolol)	End of first week and continue through to the rehabilitation phase
Insulin therapy: target 6–8(10[a]) mmol/l	From admission

[a] in diabetics

Predicting the EE and the degree of hypermetabolism during the stay is difficult though because many factors in addition to the classical age, weight and sex modify it, such as fever, amount of energy ingested the previous day, and time since injury. Repeated indirect calorimetry is therefore the gold standard in management of the patients with major burns. But this device is not widely available. In its absence, the Toronto equation should be used [1]. This equation was developed in a Canadian burn centre by multiple regression analysis of indirect calorimetry studies in burned patients. Allard et al. calculated that the measured energy expenditure (MEE) was best approximated by the equation:

$$\begin{aligned}\text{Energy requirement}(\text{kcal}) = & -4343 + (10.5 \times \%\text{TBSA}) + (0.23 \times \text{CI}) \\ & + (0.84 \times \text{EBEE}) + (114 \times \text{Temp}(°C)) \\ & - (4.5 \times \text{Postburn days})\end{aligned}$$

where CI is energy intake of the previous day, and EBEE = estimated basal metabolic rate from the Harris Benedict equation. Figure 19.1 shows the results of the Toronto prediction compared to the indirect calorimetry (40 min measurements) in two patients with massive burns: the values (black triangles) do not fit exactly with calorimetry but is a reasonable compromise. The measured values below the Toronto prediction were the result of the patients being beta-blocked with propranolol.

All other formulas invariably cause overfeeding. The Toronto equation also shows the important impact of the time elapsed since injury in reducing the early elevated requirements, largely due to the decrease in lean body mass and decline of the inflammatory response with progressive healing. In a series of 250 surviving burned patients, energy delivery beyond 1.1 x resting EE resulted in increased fat mass without improving in lean body mass [14]: this is a clear disadvantage. Note that recommendation is to measure EE in fed state [32], thereby including diet-induced thermogenesis.

Energy delivery should be closely monitored as a recent study including 493 patients on mechanical ventilation has confirmed that a feeding dose of 20–30 kcal/day may improve survival compared to lower or higher doses [33].

19.2.2 Substrates

19.2.2.1 Carbohydrates
Glucose is the principal energy source for rapidly replicating cells such as the leucocytes and wounds. Glucose should represent about 55–60% of total energy intake. The body's glucose oxidation capacity is the limit to increasing the glucose amounts: this upper limit is around 4–5 mg/kg/min. In an adult 70 kg man, this represents 403 g carbohydrates per day. As dextrose 5% is frequently delivered to treat hypernatremia, this limit is easily reached. It is particularly important to monitor the total doses of glucose delivered both with the enteral feeds and intravenous fluids to

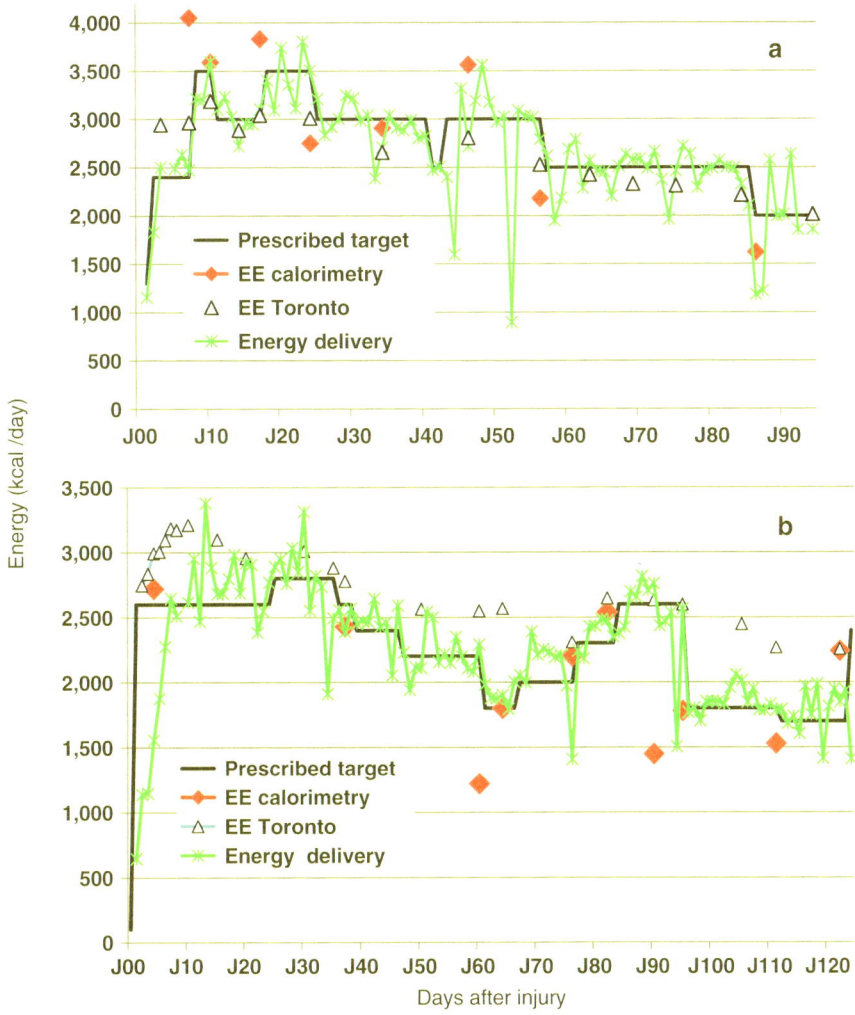

Fig. 19.1 Nutritional follow up in two patients with massive burns: it shows the evolution of indirect calorimetry results, of the Toronto predicted requirements, and of the actual feeding (prescribed energy target and real delivery). (**a**): man 28 years, admission weight 75 kg, burns 72% TBSA, (**b**): man 59 years, admission weight 88 kg, burns 90% TBSA. (*EE* energy expenditure)

avoid causing hepatic de novo lipogenesis and the subsequent fatty liver (hepatic steatosis).

Blood glucose control with insulin belongs to daily practice in burn centres: the targets should be reasonable though and aim at keeping blood glucose between 6 and 8 (10 in diabetics) mmol/l: these limits have been proven to be safe [34]. Doses of insulin required for this control vary between 2 and 6 UI/h., sometimes for a few hours up to 10 UI/h. in diabetics. Increasing doses should trigger a control of the energy intakes and target. A reasonable glucose control is associated with a lower infectious complication rate and a better graft take.

19.2.2.2 Proteins

Catabolism is massively enhanced after major burns, and a daily loss of 250–400 g of muscles per day is a common finding. The clinically available biomarkers of protein catabolism are not many: urinary methyl histidine is precise but is not widely available. Another easily available marker seems promising, the urea to creatinine ratio, according to preliminary data major burns [30]. In trauma patients, this ratio is an indicator of protein catabolism and to be correlated with the L4 psoas and L3 muscle cross-sectional areas—the high ratios accompany skeletal muscle wasting [13]. The urea-to-creatinine ratio has recently been shown to be a good indicator of catabolism, but data in major burns are still missing (Paulus et al. Critical Care (2025) 29:175 https://doi.org/10.1186/s13054-025-05396-6).

Protein requirements and attenuation of catabolism should be addressed in multimodal way combining (1) high protein diets, (2) the delivery of glutamine, (3) a relatively high proportion of carbohydrates (55–60% of total energy supply while respecting the maxima mentioned previously), (4) attenuation of the catecholamine-mediated hypermetabolism using the non-selective beta-blocker propranolol, and finally (5) by promoting early mobilisation and physical exercise.

Since the 1980s, several isotopic studies have shown that protein requirements are significantly increased, ranging between 1.5 and 2.5 g/kg/day [11, 24, 25]. This is higher than in any other disease and represents 20–25% of the total energy intake per day. These elevated requirements imply that standard industrial enteral feeding solutions do not provide sufficient proteins for this condition, and that solutions characterized as "high nitrogen energy" must still be supplemented with protein concentrates or glutamine, the best nitrogen source.

Glutamine (Gln), a conditionally essential amino acid, is of particular importance in burns whether provided as its precursor (ornithine alpha keto glutarate = OKG) [8], or as glutamine [20, 38]. As the precursor of puric and pyrimidic bases and of glutamate (further incorporated into glutathione), glutamine has a key role in immune defence, protein anabolism, and antioxidant defences. Within 48 h of injury, a rapid depletion of the skeletal muscle content is observed. The higher needs are in part caused by the cutaneous losses which are proportional to burn size [5]. Several clinical studies have shown that early Gln supplements reduce infectious complications and improve wound healing [17, 39]. In burns, both enteral and intravenous route have proven efficient. There is a minimal dose and duration of supplementation to respect: 0.3 g/kg/day for at least 10 days, as short-lived (48 h) administration has no effect. In case of acute renal failure, whatever the cause (crush injury or shock) without renal replacement therapy or with blood urea increasing above 20 mmol/l, or in acute liver failure, the administration should be discontinued.

The negative trial RE-ENERGIZE [15] has cast doubt about the benefits of glutamine. The many shortcomings of the study should encourage further research and clinical application:

1. The 10-year duration of the trial recruitment is problematic (May 2011 to June 2021), as clinical practice changes over such a long time. Moreover, burn treatment varies substantially between countries and was not standardized.
2. The cohort was very heterogeneous with a slightly larger burn BSA% in the Gln group it includes numerous low severity patients (BSA 10%, SAPS = 3, APACHEII = 1): the low severity patients have no indication to enteral nutrition nor to glutamine [29] which is not depleted in minor burns.
3. No nutrition protocol was provided/published because it was not unified—resulting in a major heterogeneity: no recommendation was made, not even the use of the Toronto equation for energy target. Not showing the data reflects this major problem, as overfeeding with fixed equation targets may have compromised the outcome by overfeeding.
4. No biological laboratory outwork is available, especially no Gln levels.
5. Once it became clear that the original sample size could not be reached, the protocol was amended to switch the primary and secondary outcomes.
6. Attrition of participants to the 6-month survivor questionnaires.

Practically, the Gln story is not over considering the well identified biological effects, such as in the recent study showing that Gln alleviates tissue injury, promotes redox balance, and restores ATP generation in the liver of burn septic mice [40]. Nevertheless, routine administration of additional Gln in burns affecting <20% BSA is not warranted, as Gln is present in nutritional quantities in all enteral feeding solutions, generally representing 8% of the amino acids in the solution.

19.2.2.3 Lipids
Lipid requirements have been little investigated, being considered a practical energy source. The available data are in favour of a lower proportion of lipids than in healthy subjects, ideally below 20% of total energy. Garrel et al. showed that delivering as low as 15% of total energy as lipids was associated with a decrease in infectious complications, particularly pneumonia [9]. In a paediatric burn cohort including 944 children, retrospective high-quality data confirm the advantages of low-fat diets, with shorter ICU stay per % TBSA burn and lower incidence of sepsis [22]. A randomized study in 92 adult patients with mean burns 38% BSA, a low-fat (18% of energy) omega-3 fatty acid-containing solution was associated with a significant reduction of infectious complication and a better digestive tolerance.

The concomitant delivery of lipids with the sedative propofol should be included in all energy and substrate calculations. Despite not being optimal, during the period of intense hypermetabolism, delivering up to 30–35% of total energy as fat may be the only way to avoid glucose overloading.

19.2.2.4 Micronutrients

Since the 1940s, higher needs for micronutrients have been described in major burns, especially of ascorbic acid and zinc. Their importance is particularly elevated in burns where their functions in antioxidation, immunity, and wound healing are prominent. Also important is to understand that they work as a web.

This was well shown in a Canadian cohort study including 172 patients, aged 49 ± 17 years and burned 33 ± 13% TBSA, compared and multi-micronutrient antioxidant intervention in 81 patients with 91 controls [26]. In the antioxidant group, the authors observed a significantly reduction of inflammatory markers at both early and late time points, ($P < 0.05$). This treatment was also associated with a reduction of measured EE ($P < 0.05$). Morbidity and mortality did not differ significantly between groups. When adjusted for patient demographics and injury characteristics, length of hospital stay was significantly shorter in the antioxidant group (risk ratio (RR), 0.78; 95% confidence interval 0.66–0.92) [26].

19.2.2.4.1 Trace Elements

Early acute trace element deficiencies caused by large exudative losses have been recurrently demonstrated since the 1970s. Three trace elements are particularly involved for obvious biological reasons: as shown by balance studies, the losses persist until wound closer. Copper, which is essential for neurotransmitter synthesis, neutrophil function, and collagen synthesis (via the cuproenzyme lysyloxidase), is lost in particularly high amounts: in a 30% TBSA burn, 20–40% of body content may be lost within 7 days. Selenium is also lost at roughly 10% of body content: selenium is essential for the activity of the glutathione peroxidase enzymes, the primary antioxidants both in the extracellular and intracellular compartments. Zinc, which is involved in nearly any metabolic pathway, the immune system, and wound healing, is lost in the same quantity, with 10% of the body content being lost within the first weeks until wound closure.

In randomised trials providing multi-vitamins to both groups of patients, the early administration of high doses of Cu, Se, and Zn calculated to replete and compensate the exudative losses in the intervention group (Table 19.3) attenuates lipid peroxidation by restoring endogenous antioxidant defences and metabolic function.

Table 19.3 Proposed daily trace element doses in patients with burns >20% TBSA (to be delivered in addition to the basal micronutrient requirements)

Micronutrient	Dose/day—route	Timing
Copper	4 mg—I.V.	From admission for: 8 days (20–40% TBSA)
Selenium	400–500 mcg—I.V.	15 days (41–60% TBSA), or
Zinc	30 mg—I.V.	30 days (>60% TBSA)
Vitamin C	1–2 g—I.V or enteral	From admission and until discharge for the ICU with a multi-micronutrient preparation
Vitamin B1	100 mg—I.V or enteral	From admission and until discharge for the ICU with a multi-micronutrient preparation
Vitamin E	100 mg—enteral	From admission and until discharge for the ICU with a multi-micronutrient preparation

NB: the trace element administration (in 250 ml saline) requires a central venous line for delivery.

The clinical complications which are caused by the biological alterations associated with these acute depletions can be prevented by the early repletion from admission for 8–30 days, depending on burn size [7]. A meta-analysis has confirmed the benefits on infections, reducing the incidence of nosocomial pneumonia [6], length of stay, and wound healing time [19]. A dose finding study including 131 patients showed that the procedure is safe and can eventually be conducted without trace element monitoring [23], as proposed by the Lausanne authors. The proposed doses adapted to body surface are safe in children [35]. Brazilian data confirm the clinical benefit of such supplementation combining zinc with vitamins C and E in children [2].

19.2.2.4.2 Vitamins

Vitamin status is also seriously altered, and the requirements are increased due to the elevated metabolic rate required for healing. This is particularly true for the vitamin B and vitamin C. Low circulating concentrations of antioxidant vitamins, α-tocopherol and ascorbic acid, have repeatedly been shown.

Vitamin C has even been used at high pharmacological doses during the first 24 h after major burns to contain the capillary leak and stabilize endothelial function. Tanaka et al. have shown that 0.6 mg/kg body weight (110 g in a 70 kg patient) delivered for the first 24 h is associated with a 30% reduction of fluid requirements during the resuscitation phase [36].

Vitamin D deficiency develops in all burns, becoming clinically relevant from the second month after injury and contributes with the long bedridden periods to osteoporosis. It is caused by the reduced synthesis in the skin [18]. Administration of higher doses is required especially as the patients have increased calcium losses due to the bed rest. It has been shown that standard doses are not sufficient [28]. In a randomised trial using doses of 200,000 IU cholecalciferol, this dose was safe and efficient to correct hypovitaminosis D in burn adults [27]. In the latest ESPEN micronutrients recommendation, 4000–5000 IU/day should be administered to critically ill patients during the acute phase [3].

19.3 Feeding Route and Timing

Early enteral nutrition, i.e., within 6–12 h of injury, belongs to resuscitation, as providing a modest amount of feeds into the gut attracts blood flow in the mesenteric arteries [10], while the intestine is threatened by the early shock. Burns rarely cause direct injury to the gut. Further, its immediate use reduces the occurrence of ileus and gastrointestinal bleeding and reduces mortality [21]. As in all other acute conditions, no early full feeding should be attempted [32], but rather a progression over 3–4 days to the goal determined either by indirect calorimetry or with the Toronto equation.

The gastric route should be considered first. Nevertheless, in burns >40% TBSA, the frequent hydrotherapies and surgeries required for their treatment cause frequent fasting periods, which can be reduced if a postpyloric tube is used. In intubated patients, it enables stopping feeding just before the intervention and restarting it immediately at the end. In extubated patients, the agreement with the anaesthesiologists is a reduction of the fasting period to 3 h before the intervention.

The solutions should be high energy, high protein polymeric fibre containing solutions completed with glutamine supplements to reach the 2.0–2.5 g/kg/day protein targets [32]. Fibres should be integrated from the start. There is no hard evidence in this field, only clinical experience. Constipation can become a real problem in major burns due to the elevated doses of opioids required for pain control and the important fluid and electrolyte shifts. Early prevention is warranted from day 1, with fibres, in association with macrogol or similar osmotic agents. Oral opioid-antagonists is an option in the context of high opioid doses. In our hands, diarrhoea is rare. Rates up to 180 ml/h are well tolerated, optimal being around 150 ml/h. The fibre has the advantage of maintaining the microbiome [12].

Parenteral nutrition is required on occasions and may prove essential in case of gastro-intestinal complications. The same rules and indications prevail as in other critically ill patients.

19.4 Conclusion

In major burns, medical nutrition therapy is more than just providing energy and is essential for survival and recovery. As in other critical care conditions, overfeeding belongs to the past and should be prevented, even in this condition of higher energy requirements: monitoring of delivery is essential. Rather, the specific requirements of the burn healing process should be addressed. They start with the intense oxidative stress associated with burn injuries that can be significantly attenuated by the early intravenous repletion of endogenous antioxidants, particularly of trace elements Cu, Se, and Zn. Maintenance of the gut integrity is also an early priority, using enteral nutrition at low dose: the latter should be started immediately within hours after admission. Energy requirements should ideally be determined by repeated indirect calorimetry: alternatively, the Toronto equation provides a good guidance. Glucose and protein requirements are higher than in non-burn trauma patients, with a specific increased glutamine requirement.

References

1. Allard JP, Pichard C, Hoshino E, Stechison S, Fareholm L, Peters WJ, Jeejheebhoy KN. Validation of a new formula for calculating energy requirements of burn patients. JPEN. 1990;14:115–8.
2. Barbosa E, Faintuch J, Machado Moreira EA, Goncalves VR, da Silva MJ, Lopes Pereima RL, Fagundes M, Filho DW. Supplementation of vitamin E, vitamin C, and zinc attenuates oxidative stress in burned children: a randomized, double-blind, placebo-controlled pilot study. J Burn Care Res. 2009;30:859–66.
3. Berger MM, Shenkin A, Schweinlin A, Amrein K, Augsburger M, Biesalski HK, Bischoff SC, Casaer MP, Gundogan K, Lepp HL, de Man AME, Muscogiuri G, Pietka M, Pironi L, Rezzi S, Cuerda C. ESPEN micronutrient guideline. Clin Nutr. 2022b;41:1357–424.

4. Berger MM, Binnert C, Chiolero RL, Taylor W, Raffoul W, Cayeux MC, Benathan M, Shenkin A, Tappy L. Trace element supplements after major burns increase burned skin concentrations and modulate local protein metabolism, but not whole body substrate metabolism. Am J Clin Nutr. 2007;85:1301–6.
5. Berger MM, Binz PA, Roux C, Charrière M, Scaletta C, Raffoul W, Applegate LA, Pantet O. Exudative Glutamine losses contribute to the high needs after burn injury. JPEN. 2022a;46:782–8.
6. Berger MM, Eggimann P, Heyland DK, Chioléro RL, Revelly JP, Day A, Raffoul W, Shenkin A. Reduction of nosocomial pneumonia after major burns by trace element supplementation: aggregation of two randomised trials. Crit Care. 2006;10:R153.
7. Berger MM, Shenkin A. Trace element requirements in critically ill burned patients. J Trace Elem Med Biol. 2007;21(suppl 1):44–8.
8. Coudray-Lucas C, LeBever H, Cynober L, DeBandt JP, Carsin H. Ornithine α-ketoglutarate improves wound healing in severe burn patients: a prospective randomized double-blind trial versus isonitrogenous controls. Crit Care Med. 2000;28:1772–6.
9. Garrel DR, Razi M, Larivière F, Jobin N, Naman N, Emptoz-Bonneton A, Pugeat MM. Improved clinical status and length of care with low-fat nutrition support in burn patients. JPEN. 1995;19:482–91.
10. Gatt M, MacFie J, Anderson AD, Howell G, Reddy BS, Suppiah A, Renwick I, Mitchell CJ. Changes in superior mesenteric artery blood flow after oral, enteral, and parenteral feeding in humans. Crit Care Med. 2009;37:171–6.
11. Gore DC, Chinkes DL, Wolf SE, Sanford AP, Herndon DN, Wolfe RR. Quantification of protein metabolism in vivo for skin, wound, and muscle in severe burn patients. JPEN. 2006;30:331–8.
12. Green CH, Busch RA, Patel JJ. Fiber in the ICU: should it be a regular part of feeding? Curr Gastroenterol Rep. 2021;23:14.
13. Haines RW, Zolfaghari P, Wan Y, Pearse RM, Puthucheary Z, Prowle JR. Elevated urea-to-creatinine ratio provides a biochemical signature of muscle catabolism and persistent critical illness after major trauma. Intensive Care Med. 2019;45:1718–31.
14. Hart DW, Wolf SE, Herndon DN, Chinkes DL, Lal SO, Obeng MK, Beauford RB, Mlcak RP. Energy expenditure and caloric balance after burn: increased feeding leads to fat rather than lean sass accretion. Ann Surg. 2002;235:152–61.
15. Heyland DK, Wischmeyer P, Jeschke MG, Wibbenmeyer L, Turgeon AF, Stelfox HT, Day AG, Garrel D. A randomizEd trial of ENtERal Glutamine to minimIZE thermal injury (The RE-ENERGIZE Trial): a clinical trial protocol. Scars Burn Heal. 2017;3:2059513117745241.
16. Jeschke MG, Przkora R, Suman OE, Finnerty CC, Mlcak RP, Pereira CT, Sanford AP, Herndon DN. Sex differences in the long-term outcome after a severe thermal injury. Shock. 2007;27:461–5.
17. Kibor DK, Nyaim OE, Wanjeri K. Effects of enteral glutamine supplementation on reduction of infection in adult patients with severe burns. East Afr Med J. 2014;91:33–6.
18. Klein GL, Holick MF, Langman CB, Celis MM, Herndon DN. Synthesis of vitamin D in skin after burns. Lancet. 2004;363:291–2.
19. Kurmis R, Greenwood J, Aromataris E. Trace element supplementation following severe burn injury: a systematic review and meta-analysis. J Burn Care Res. 2016;37:143–59.
20. Kurmis R, Parker A, Greenwood J. The use of immunonutrition in burn injury care: where are we? J Burn Care Res. 2010;31:677–91.
21. Lam NN, Tien NG, Khoa CM. Early enteral feeding for burned patients: an effective method which should be encouraged in developing countries. Burns. 2008;34:192–6.
22. Lee JO, Gauglitz GG, Herndon DN, Hawkins HK, Halder SC, Jeschke MG. Association between dietary fat content and outcomes in pediatric burn patients. J Surg Res. 2011;166:e83–90.
23. Pantet O, Stoecklin P, Charriere M, Voirol P, Vernay A, Berger MM. Trace element repletion following severe burn injury: a dose-finding cohort study. Clin Nutr. 2019;38:246–51.
24. Patterson BW, Zhang XJ, Chen Y, Klein S, Wolfe RR. Measurement of very low stable isotope enrichments by gas chromatography/mass spectrometry: application to measurement of muscle protein synthesis. Metabolism. 1997;46:943–8.

25. Porter C, Hurren NM, Herndon DN, Borsheim E. Whole body and skeletal muscle protein turnover in recovery from burns. Int J Burns Trauma. 2013;3:9–17.
26. Rehou S, Shahrokhi S, Natanson R, Stanojcic M, Jeschke MG. Antioxidant and trace element supplementation reduce the inflammatory response in critically Ill burn patients. J Burn Care Res. 2018;39:1–9.
27. Rousseau AF, Foidart-Desalle M, Ledoux D, Remy C, Croisier JL, Damas P, Cavalier E. Effects of cholecalciferol supplementation and optimized calcium intakes on vitamin D status, muscle strength and bone health: a one-year pilot randomized controlled trial in adults with severe burns. Burns. 2015;41:317–25.
28. Rousseau AF, Damas P, Ledoux D, Cavalier E. Effect of cholecalciferol recommended daily allowances on vitamin D status and fibroblast growth factor-23: an observational study in acute burn patients. Burns. 2014;40:865–70.
29. Rousseau AF, Losser MR, Ichai C, Berger MM. ESPEN endorsed recommendations: nutritional therapy in major burns. Clin Nutr. 2013;32:497–502.
30. Rugg C, Strohle M, Schmid S, Kreutziger J. The link between hypermetabolism and hypernatremia in severely burned patients. Nutrients. 2020;12(3):774.
31. Ryan CM, Schoenfeld DA, Thorpe WP, Sheridan RL, Cassem EH, Tompkins RG. Objective estimates of the probability of death from burn injuries. New Engl J Med. 1998;338:362–6.
32. Singer P, Blaser AR, Berger MM, Calder PC, Casaer M, Hiesmayr M, Mayer K, Montejo-Gonzalez JC, Pichard C, Preiser JC, Szczeklik W, van Zanten ARH, Bischoff SC. ESPEN practical and partially revised guideline: Clinical nutrition in the intensive care unit. Clin Nutr. 2023;42:1671–89.
33. Stewart BT, Pham T, Cancio L, O'Keefe G, Nordlund MJ, Day AG, Heyland DK. Higher energy delivery is associated with improved long-term survival among adults with major burn injury: a multicenter, multinational, observational study. J Trauma Acute Care Surg. 2024;97:812–21.
34. Stoecklin P, Delodder F, Pantet O, Berger MM. Moderate glycemic control safe in critically ill adult burn patients – A 15 year cohort study. Burns. 2016;42:63–70.
35. Stucki P, Perez MH, Cotting J, Shenkin A, Berger MM. Substitution of exudative trace elements losses in burned children. Crit Care. 2010;14:439.
36. Tanaka H, Matsuda T, Miyagantani Y, Yukioka T, Matsuda H, Shimazaki S. Reduction of resuscitation fluid volumes in severely burned patients using ascorbic acid administration. Arch Surg. 2000;135:326–31.
37. Williams FN, Jeschke MG, Chinkes DL, Suman OE, Branski LK, Herndon DN. Modulation of the hypermetabolic response to trauma: temperature, nutrition, and drugs. J Am Coll Surg. 2009;208:489–502.
38. Wischmeyer PE. Glutamine: mode of action in critical illness. Crit Care Med. 2007;35(9 Suppl):S541–S44.
39. Wischmeyer PE. Glutamine in burn injury. Nutr Clin Pract. 2019;34:681–7.
40. Yang Y, Chen Q, Fan S, Lu Y, Huang Q, Liu X, Peng X. Glutamine sustains energy metabolism and alleviates liver injury in burn sepsis by promoting the assembly of mitochondrial HSP60-HSP10 complex via SIRT4 dependent protein deacetylation. Redox Rep. 2024;29:2312320.

Special Enteral Diets: Synbiotics

Arved Weimann and Geraldine de Heer

Focusing on the preservation of the gut microbiome, synbiotics reveal trophic effects in the colon promoting mucosal regeneration in balance with the microenvironment. Fiber has prebiotic effects and may be combined with probiotics. Synbiotics refer to the combination of both probiotics and prebiotics, containing *Lactobacillus* organisms alongside fiber. They have been also referred to as "ecoimmunonutrition" [3].

For formulae containing synbiotics with fiber and *Lactobacillus*, a significantly lower incidence of infections was shown in critically ill trauma patients [13], and after major abdominal surgery, involving pancreatic and hepatobiliary resections, as well as liver transplantation [10, 11, 22, 23, 26]. No difference was observed between the effects of living or heat-killed lactobacilli [21–23]. No influence was shown on the incidence of ventilator associated pneumonia (VAP) [12]. A study in brain injured patients [8] showed significant advantages of a formulae containing glutamine and probiotics with regard to infection rate and length of stay in the intensive care unit. In critically ill trauma patients, significantly lower intestinal permeability and infection rate were observed for synbiotics versus fermentable fiber alone, glutamine, or peptide diet [25].

A plenty of meta-analyses has been published. A meta-analysis of 34 randomized clinical trials with 2723 patients revealed for probiotic and symbiotic use in elective surgical patients a reduction of postoperative sepsis [5]. For trauma patients,

A. Weimann
Department of General, Visceral and Oncological Surgery, St. George Hospital,
Leipzig, Germany
e-mail: Arved.Weimann@sanktgeorg.de

G. de Heer (✉)
Department Intensive Care Medicine, University Hospital Hamburg Eppendorf (UKE),
Hamburg, Germany
e-mail: deheer@uke.de

a meta-analysis from 5 studies with 281 patients showed significant benefits with regard to a reduction of nosocomial infections, the rate of ventilator associated pneumonia, and the length of intensive care stay. No difference in mortality was observed [9]. The authors already pointed out the considerable heterogeneity of the included studies.

Concerns about giving synbiotics to patients with acute sepsis (APACHE II score > 15) have been drawn from a multicenter, randomized, double-blind, placebo-controlled study by [4]. 298 patients with predicted severe acute pancreatitis (APACHE II score > 8) were given probiotics via the enteral route. The results showed a significantly higher mortality rate in the probiotic group, in which nine of the patients also developed bowel ischaemia. The authors have suggested that the cause for the increased mortality could be due to an increased local oxygen demand caused by the enteral administration of probiotic bacteria. Together with an already reduced blood flow, this could have become a trigger for the bowel ischemia. A second explanation discusses the possibility of local inflammation of the mucosa caused by the probiotics, which has already been shown to be the case, in experimental studies with enterocytes [4]. It is also conceivable that the probiotics led to an increase in gas production in the intestine and that this distention caused reduced bowel perfusion. A combination of which may have led to detrimental bowel ischemia.

In another randomized controlled study from Spain in 89 patients with multiple organ failure (exclusion: neutropenia, acute pancreatitis), a synbiotic drink was enterally administered for 7 days. In the intervention group, lower serum lactate levels were found on the second day, higher fibrinogen levels on day 5 and 7, and lower dimer levels. While no difference in microbiological resistance was observed, the synbiotic group showed mucosa colonization by Candida which resolved after stopping symbiotic administration. The clinical course in the ICU was without difference [16].

In a systematic review including 23 randomized controlled trials about the use of probiotics in the critically ill, the rate of ventilator-associated pneumonia was significantly reduced with probiotics (risk ratio 0.75; 95% confidence interval 0.59–0.97; $p = 0.03$). There was a trend toward reduced intensive care unit mortality (risk ratio 0.75; 95% confidence interval 0.59–1.09; $p = 0.16$) without any effect on intensive care unit or hospital length of stay [20].

A meta-analysis of 30 studies including 2972 patients revealed a significantly decreased rate of infections (RR 0.80, 95% CI 0.68, 0.95, $p = 0.009$). Furthermore, a significant reduction of ventilator associated pneumonia was observed (RR 0.74, 95% CI 0.61, 0.90, $p = 0.002$). No impact was found on mortality, hospital length of stay, and rate of diarrhea. Regarding infection rate, the subgroup analysis showed that the administration of probiotics may be more beneficial than the combination with prebiotics [17]. A meta-analyses including 31 RCTs with 8339 patients confirmed the benefits of probiotics-supplemented enteral nutrition regarding the prevention and alleviation of ventilator associated pneumonia. Prebiotic supplementation was the most effective in preventing diarrhea [15]. In another recent meta-analysis including 14 studies, the incidence of diarrhea was just slightly reduced by probiotics and synbiotics [2]. A recent umbrella review of 30 meta-analyses showed [1] that probiotics significantly decreased

- Incidence of ventilator-associated pneumonia (VAP)
- Incidence of nosocomial infections
- Intensive care unit (ICU) length of stay
- Hospital length of stay
- ICU mortality
- Mechanical ventilation duration
- Duration of antibiotic use
- Diarrhea

Due to the heterogeneity of treatment regimen, no special species of probiotics can be recommended.

The German guidelines recommend probiotics (*Lactobacillus plantarum* and *Lactobacillus* CG) for patients with severe trauma and those undergoing liver transplantation [7].

The ASPEN guidelines (2016) suggest to consider a commercial mixed fiber formula if there is evidence for persistent diarrhea. Avoidance of both soluble and insoluble fiber is recommended in patients with severe dysmotility. A recommendation for the routine use of probiotics in ICU patients could not be given [19].

A recent meta-analysis of 71 studies with 8551 patients showed the benefits of probiotics and synbiotics only in lower quality studies [14].

In conclusion, there is limited safety of probiotics in the critically ill patient with typical side effects sepsis, fungemia, and even bowel ischemia [6].

Despite controversies and open questions, the administration of synbiotics for the maintenance of the microbiome is a challenging concept with possible impact on the incidence of ventilator-associated pneumonia infectious complications and diarrhea [1, 18]. The most appropriate species has not been elucidated yet. Therefore, more high powered clinical studies will be required.

References

1. Anvarifard P, Anbari M, Ghalichi F, Ghoreishi Z, Zarezadeh M. The effectiveness of probiotics as an adjunct therapy in patients under mechanical ventilation: an umbrella systematic review and meta-analysis. Food Funct. 2024;15:5737–51. https://doi.org/10.1039/d3fo04653b. PMID: 38771159.
2. Bagdadi B, Alqazlane A, Alotaibi M, Alamoudi A, Baghdadi L, MohammadMahmood A, Al-Neami I, Fageehi I, Salamah M, Majrabi S. The effectiveness of probiotics or synbiotics in the prevention and treatment of diarrhea among critically ill adults: a systematic review and meta-analysis. Clin Nutr ESPEN. 2025;65:218–26. https://doi.org/10.1016/j.clnesp.2024.11.025. Epub 2024 Dec 3. PMID: 39638033.
3. Bengmark S. Gut microbiota, immune development and function. Pharmacol Res. 2013;69:87–113.

4. Besselink MG, van Santvoort HC, Buskens E, Boermeester MA, van Goor H, Timmerman HM, Dutch Acute Pancreatitis Study Group, et al. Probiotic prophylaxis in predicted severe acute pancreatitis: a randomised, double- blind, placebo-controlled trial. Lancet. 2008;371:651–9.
5. Chowdhury AH, Adiamah A, Kushairi A, Varadhan KK, Krznaric Z, Kulkarni AD, Neal KR, Lobo DN. Perioperative probiotics or synbiotics in adults undergoing elective abdominal surgery: a systematic review and meta-analysis of randomized controlled trials. Ann Surg. 2020;271(6):1036–47. https://doi.org/10.1097/SLA.0000000000003581. PMID: 31469748.
6. Didari T, Solki S, Mozaffari S, Nikfar S, Abdollahi M. A systematic review of the safety of probiotics. Expert Opin Drug Saf. 2014;13:227–39.
7. Elke G, Hartl WH, Kreymann KG, Adolph M, Felbinger TW, Graf T, de Heer G, Heller AR, Kampa U, Mayer K, Muhl E, Niemann B, Rümelin A, Steiner S, Stoppe C, Weimann A, Bischoff SC. Clinical nutrition in critical care medicine – guideline of the German Society for Nutritional Medicine (DGEM). Clin Nutr ESPEN. 2019;33:220–75. https://doi.org/10.1016/j.clnesp.2019.05.002. Epub 2019 Jul 9. PMID: 31451265.
8. Falcao de Arruda IS, de Aguilar-Nascimento JE. Benefits of early enteral nutrition with glutamine and probiotics in brain injury patients. Clin Sci (Lond). 2004;106:287–92.
9. Gu WJ, Deng T, Gong YZ, Jing R, Liu JC. The effects of probiotics in early enteral nutrition on the outcomes of trauma: a meta-analysis of randomized controlled trials. JPEN J Parenter Enteral Nutr. 2013;37:310–7.
10. Kanazawa H, Nagino M, Kamiya S, Komatsu S, Mayumi T, Takagi K, Asahara T, Nomoto K, Tanaka R, Nimura Y. Synbiotics reduce postoperative infectious complications: a randomized controlled trial in biliary cancer patients undergoing hepatectomy. Langenbeck's Arch Surg. 2005;390:104–13.
11. Kinross JM, Markar S, Karthikesalingam A, Chow A, Penney N, Silk D, Darzi A. A meta-analysis of probiotic and synbiotic use in elective surgery: does nutrition modulation of the gut microbiome improve clinical outcome? JPEN J Parenter Enteral Nutr. 2013;37:243–53.
12. Knight D, Gardiner D, Banks A, Snape SE, Weston VC, Bengmark S, Girling KJ. Effect of synbiotic therapy on the incidence of ventialtor associated pneumonia in criically ill patients: randomised, double-blind, placebo-controlled trial. Intensive Care Med. 2009;35:854–61.
13. Kotzampassi K, Giamarellos-Bourboulis EJ, Voudouris A, Kazamias P, Eleftheriadis E. Benefits of a synbiotic formula (Synbiotic 2000Forte) in critically Ill trauma patients: early results of a randomized controlled trial. World J Surg. 2006;30(10):1848–55. https://doi.org/10.1007/s00268-005-0653-1. PMID: 16983476.
14. Lee ZY, Lew CCH, Ortiz-Reyes A, Patel JJ, Wong YJ, Loh CTI, Martindale RG, Heyland DK. Benefits and harm of probiotics and synbiotics in adult critically ill patients. A systematic review and meta-analysis of randomized controlled trials with trial sequential analysis. Clin Nutr. 2023;42(4):519–31. https://doi.org/10.1016/j.clnu.2023.01.019. Epub 2023 Feb 7. PMID: 36857961.
15. Li C, Lu F, Chen J, Ma J, Xu N. Probiotic supplementation prevents the development of ventilator-associated pneumonia for mechanically ventilated ICU patients: a systematic review and network meta-analysis of randomized controlled trials. Front Nutr. 2022;9:919156. https://doi.org/10.3389/fnut.2022.919156. PMID: 35879981; PMCID: PMC9307490.
16. López de Toro Martín-Consuegra I, Sanchez-Casado M, Pérez-Pedrero Sánchez-Belmonte MJ, López-Reina Torrijos P, Sánchez-Rodriguez P, Raigal-Caño A, Heredero-Galvez E, Zubigaray SB, Arrese-Cosculluela MÁ. The influence of symbiotics in multi-organ failure: randomised trial. Med Clin (Barc). 2014;143(4):143–9. https://doi.org/10.1016/j.medcli.2013.09.046. Epub 2014 Feb 21 (Spanish).
17. Manzanares W, Lemieux M, Langlois PL, Wischmeyer PE. Probiotic and synbiotic therapy in critical illness: a systematic review and meta-analysis. Crit Care. 2016;19:262–7.
18. Manzanares W, Langlois PL, Wischmeyer PE. Restoring the microbiome in critically ill patients: are probiotics our true friends when we are seriously ill? JPEN J Parenter Enteral Nutr. 2017;41(4):530–3. https://doi.org/10.1177/0148607117700572. Epub 2017 Mar 10.

19. McClave SA, Taylor BE, Martindale RG, Warren MM, Johnson DR, Braunschweig C, McCarthy MS, Davanos E, Rice TW, Cresci GA, Gervasio JM, Sacks GS, Roberts PR, Compher C; Society of Critical Care Medicine; American Society for Parenteral and Enteral Nutrition. Guidelines for the provision and assessment of nutrition support therapy in the adult critically ill patient: Society of Critical Care Medicine (SCCM) and American Society for Parenteral and Enteral Nutrition (A.S.P.E.N.). JPEN J Parenter Enteral Nutr. 2016;40(2):159–211. https://doi.org/10.1177/0148607115621863. Erratum in: JPEN J Parenter Enteral Nutr. 2016 Nov;40(8):1200. doi: 10.1177/0148607116670155. PMID: 26773077.
20. Petrof EO, Dhaliwal R, Manzanares W, Johnstone J, Cook D, Heyland DK. Probiotics in the critically ill: a systematic review of the randomized trial evidence. Crit Care Med. 2012;40:3290–2.
21. Rayes N, Hansen S, Seehofer D, Müller AR, Serke S, Bengmark S, et al. Early enteral supply of fiber and Lactobacilli versus conventional nutrition: a controlled trial in patients with major abdominal surgery. Nutrition. 2002;18:609–15.
22. Rayes N, Seehofer D, Theruvath T, Schiller RA, Langrehr JM, Jonas S, et al. Supply of pre- and probiotics reduces bacterial infection rates after liver transplantation- a randomized double-blind trial. Am J Transplant. 2005;5:125–30.
23. Rayes N, Pilarski T, Stockmann M, Bengmark S, Neuhaus P, Seehofer D. Effect of pre- and probiotics on liver regeneration after resection: a randomised, double-blind pilot study. Benef Microbes. 2012;3:237–44.
24. Rayes N, Seehofer D, Theruvath T, Mogl M, Langrehr JM, Nüssler NC, Bengmark S, Neuhaus P. Effect of enteral nutrition and synbiotics on bacterial infection rates after pylorus-preserving pancreatoduodenectomy: a randomized, double-blind trial. Ann Surg. 2007;246(1):36–41. https://doi.org/10.1097/01.sla.0000259442.78947.19. PMID: 17592288
25. Spindler-Vesel A, Benmerk S, Vovk I, Cerovic O, Kompan L. Synbiotics, prebiotics, glutamine, or peptide in early enteral nutrition: a randomized study in trauma patients. JPEN. 2007;31:119–26.
26. Sugawara G, Nagino M, Nishio H, Ebata T, Takagi K, Asahara T, Nomoto K, Nimura Y. Perioperative synbiotic treatment to prevent postoperative infectious complications in biliary cancer surgery: a randomized controlled trial. Ann Surg. 2006;244:706–14.

Part IV
Special Aspects

Early Mobilisation in ICU

Laura Homann and Stefan J. Schaller

21.1 Introduction

Modern intensive care has improved the survival rates of critically ill patients over the past decade and reduced mortality risk following discharge from the intensive care unit (ICU) [1–3].

However, patients continue to suffer from long-term decreased functional ability and a lower physical quality of life after ICU discharge [4]. This includes limitations in exercise ability, ICU-acquired muscle weakness (ICUAW), and physical and psychological sequelae [2, 5]. These limitations directly affect patients and have consequences for the socio-economic system, such as increased costs and greater utilisation of the social health system [2].

L. Homann
Charité – Universitätsmedizin Berlin, Corporate Member of Freie Universität Berlin and Humboldt Universität zu Berlin, Institute of Clinical Nursing Science, Berlin, Germany
e-mail: laura.homann@charite.de

S. J. Schaller (✉)
Medical University of Vienna, Department of Anaesthesia, Intensive Care Medicine and Pain Medicine, Clinical Division of General Anaesthesia and Intensive Care Medicine, Vienna, Austria

Charité – Universitätsmedizin Berlin, Corporate Member of Freie Universität Berlin and Humboldt Universität zu Berlin, Department of Anaesthesiology and Intensive Care Medicine (CCM/CVK), Berlin, Germany
e-mail: stefan.schaller@meduniwien.ac.at

To address these long-term challenges, clinical practice guidelines recommend the implementation of early mobilisation in the ICU [6, 7]. Early mobilisation is a crucial component of the rehabilitation process. It has been proven to be an effective and safe intervention for enhancing the long-term quality of life and functional outcomes of critically ill patients [8–10].

21.2 Definition of Early Mobilisation

Even though early mobilisation is used worldwide, there is still no universal agreement on the definition, the optimal time for initiation or form of mobilisation [8, 11]. This lack of consensus hinders a standardised and widespread clinical implementation [8]. Early mobilisation is an exercise intervention that initiates and supports passive or active movements in patients to promote and maintain their mobility. It is based on a reproducible and physiological approach [8, 12]. The goal is to initiate early mobilisation as soon as it is deemed safe, typically when patients are physiologically stable enough to be mobilised [11]. For example, the patient mobilised into the chair in Fig. 21.1. He had a temporary external ventricular drainage due to a ventricular shunt defect and was first passively and later actively mobilised to a chair as soon as it was deemed safe. Currently, the timing of early mobilisation

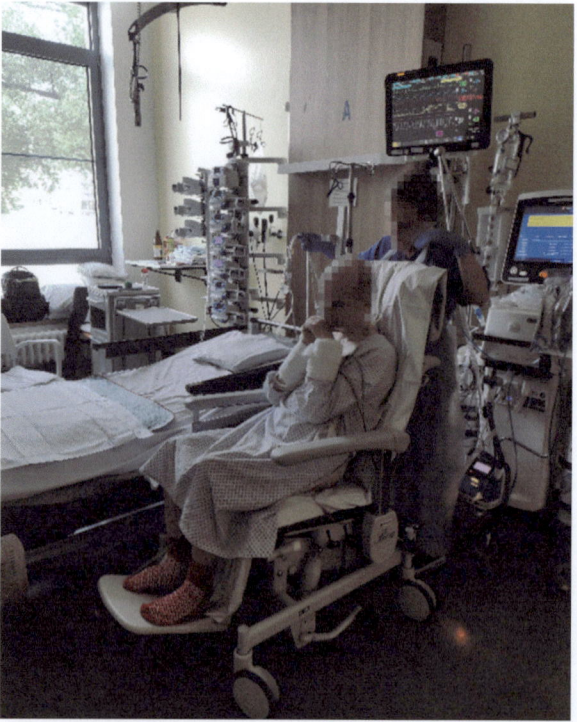

Fig. 21.1 Sitting of a patient with an external ventricular drainage

varies from less than 24 h after mechanical ventilation to more than 1 week after ICU admission. Researchers have concluded that intervening with early mobilisation within 48–72 h of mechanical ventilation is optimal for improving clinical outcomes [8]. The German guideline on "Positioning and Mobilisation of Critically Ill Patients in Intensive Care Units" defines early mobilisation as initiating mobilisation within 72 h after admission to the ICU [7].

21.3 Types of Mobilisations

Mobilisation can occur in three different ways, depending on the activity level: passive mobilisation, passive-active mobilisation, and active mobilisation. Existing mobilisation protocols usually contain passive and active elements in a graduated approach depending on the patient's condition [3]. The lowest level is passive mobilisation, and the highest is independent walking [3, 13]. Figure 21.2 shows an example of a passive transfer of an amputee patient into a chair, assisted by two physiotherapists and one nurse. Including passive forms of mobilisation has the advantage that patients can receive mobilisation in every phase of the disease [14]. Based on this, there are two known mobilisation concepts: (1) passive-active and (2) active concepts. Passive-active mobilisation concepts combine passive and active elements regarding mobilisation. One such concept is the "Surgical Optimal Mobilisation Score" (SOMS), shown in Fig. 21.3 [3, 14]. Every day, mobilisation goals will be defined by an interprofessional team based on the clinical condition of the patient and the mobility algorithm of the SOMS. The clinical team will then work together throughout the day to achieve the patient's daily goals [14, 15]. Active mobilisation concepts, such as the one used in the

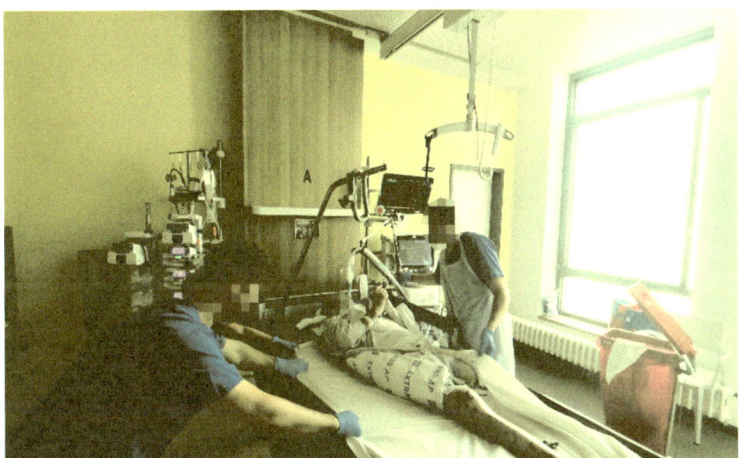

Fig. 21.2 Passive transfer of a patient into a chair

Fig. 21.3 SOMS (3, 13)

SOMS	Description
0	No activity
1	Passive range of motion
2	Sitting
3	Standing
4	Ambulation

ICU-MS	Definion
0	Passively rolled or passively exercised by staff
1	Sitting in bed, active bed exercises
2	Passively moved to chair (no standing)
3	Sitting over edge of bed
4	Standing with or without assistance
5	Transferring bed to chair
6	Marching on spot (at bedside)
7	Walking with assistance of two or more people
8	Walking with assistance of one person
9	Walking independently with a gait aid
10	Walking independently with out a gait aid

Fig. 21.4 ICU Mobility Scale (IMS) according to [17]

TEAM Trial, which is based on the ICU mobility scale (IMS), require muscle activity from the patient [16]. Patients will be assessed daily based on their clinical condition and the IMS level, for details, see Fig. 21.4. Unlike the SOMS, this approach aims to start with the highest possible mobilisation level, which can be reduced during the day if necessary. Additionally, only active mobilisations count to fulfil the protocol [16]. For instance, as shown in Fig. 21.5, passive sitting does not contribute to the fulfilment of active mobilisation concepts. This requires considerable time and personal effort [3].

In conclusion, early mobilisation should be goal-directed and protocol-based therapy, which includes passive and active components [12, 13].

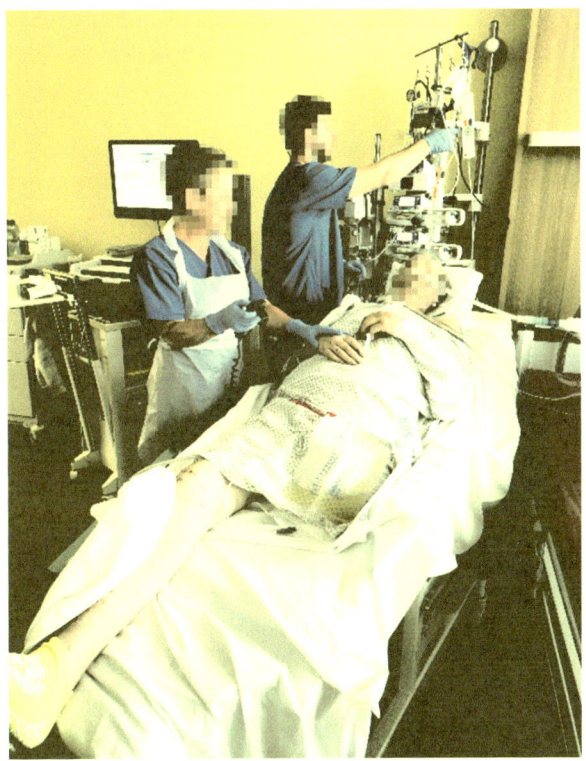

Fig. 21.5 Passive mobilisation into sitting position of an amputee patient

21.4 Effects of Early Mobilisation

Early mobilisation demonstrates positive effects that can be observed in the short and long term. These effects include changes in ventilation, functional ability, and quality of life. Concerning the short-term effects of respiration, early mobilisation has been shown to improve outcomes related to weaning and mechanical ventilation. In detail, early mobilisation compared to standard care positively influenced the duration of ventilation and ICU length of stay, the incidence of ICUAW and ICU-related complications such as ventilator-associated pneumonia, deep vein thrombosis and pressure sores, and physical function at hospital discharge, with conflicting results on hospital length of stay [18, 19]. Early mobilisation reduced the incidence but showed only minor differences in delirium-free days. However, early mobilisation does not affect ICU and hospital mortality [18, 19]. Regarding functional ability and muscle strength, potential effects of early mobilisation have been demonstrated in smaller studies, indicating to enhance patients' mobility throughout their ICU admission, improve functional mobility at hospital discharge, and present promising discharge disposition [10, 13]. Patients who underwent early mobilisation achieved higher levels of mobilisation during their ICU stay and left the ICU with a higher level of mobilisation compared to standard care [13].

Data about the long-term effects of early mobilisation is more challenging to interpret. On the one hand, it has been demonstrated that early mobilisation might be the first known intervention to improve long-term cognitive impairment in ICU survivors after mechanical ventilation. A long-term study comparing the effects of early mobilisation conducted by occupational therapy and physiotherapy with standard care revealed a reduction in rates of cognitive impairment after 1 year (24% vs. 43%). Furthermore, the early mobilisation group had fewer cases of ICUAW (0% vs. 14%) and higher physical health in terms of quality of life. However, there was no difference in functional independence between the two groups. It is essential to understand that in the study by Patel et al., the control group received nearly no mobilisation [20]. Controversially, an increase in early active mobilisation did not result in a more significant number of survival days or days spent outside the hospital setting, which was investigated in the TEAM trial, the largest long-term study in the field. The intervention of early active mobilisation did not significantly change the number of days alive and out of the hospital at 6 months. There was also no difference between the groups regarding mortality, number of ventilator-free days, health-related quality of life, and function. It is essential to understand that the standard care group received active and passive mobilisation of above-average quality in the TEAM Trial. The main differences to the intervention group were that active and passive components were used and some timing differences. Consequently, the TEAM trial shows a dose-ceiling effect of mobilisation but not the ineffectiveness of early mobilisation [4].

In summary, the positive effects of mobilisation are not limited to short-term benefits but also the long-term well-being of critically ill patients.

21.5 Safety, Dosage, and Individualisation

The question of whether early mobilisation can harm patients arises regularly. It can be asserted that, in general, mobilisation in the ICU is safe and feasible for every patient. However, rare unwanted effects may occur in isolated cases [21]. To counteract this, there should be clearly defined guidelines for each therapy. Protocol-based mobilisation enhances feasibility and improves the safety of the mobilisation treatment itself [22]. It has also been shown that implementing a safety protocol leads to more automatic initiation of (early) mobilisation, thereby avoiding detrimental delays for patients [23, 24]. For example, a traffic-light system has proven effective. It determines when mobilisation should be withheld (red), when individual consultation is necessary (yellow), or when it can proceed without consultation (green) [11]. Furthermore, it has been observed that internal contraindications and termination criteria within the ICU increase patients' safety [3]. Other principal factors for implementing early mobilisation and safety aspects include the expertise of the treating team. The availability and utilisation of specific mobilisation equipment might facilitate the mobilisation process. As demonstrated in Fig. 21.6, a specialised physiotherapist is using a walking frame to provide adequate support to the patient and to maintain safety. Daily assessment of the patient's physiological condition

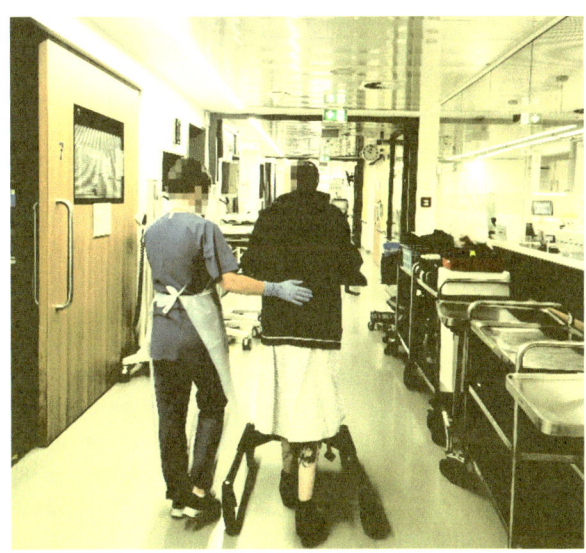

Fig. 21.6 Walking with a patient with ICUAW

regarding suitability for mobility activities and considerations for concluding a mobilisation session should be discussed [6, 11].

Literature has shown that when mobilising severely affected patients, the dosage of mobilisation is crucial to prevent potential unwanted effects. The mobility dosage comprises duration, intensity (especially level), and frequency of mobilisation. There is some evidence that increased mobilisation duration and higher mobilisation levels are associated with overall better treatment outcomes, as opposed to increasing the frequency of therapy sessions [25–27]. Since the TEAM trial, however, we must be aware that an upper limit of meaningful intensity must be considered. Furthermore, recent studies indicate that mobilisation duration lacks a modifying effect on diverse patients, which is essential for resource allocation [28]. The evidence concerning mobilisation in the context of neurointensive care with critically ill patients is still highly limited [3]. However, studies involving patients in stroke units have indicated that the dosage (duration, frequency, level of mobilisation) may impact the outcome. Evidence suggests that shorter units distributed throughout the day have a more positive effect on the outcome than a single prolonged unit [29]. If this can be extrapolated to neurocritical care patients in an ICU is unknown. An additional particular subgroup consists of patients with aneurysmal subarachnoid haemorrhage and older patients with functional limitations upon ICU admission. For this group of individuals, it is still being determined what extent of mobilisation is appropriate and which resources need to be allocated to achieve positive results [3]. But in general, all patients should be mobilised if there are no contraindications [12].

There should be an individualised approach for each patient, considering their current medical condition [28, 30]. This approach may enable the adjustment of the personalised mobilisation of critically ill patients, thereby improving outcomes [28]. Furthermore, it has been shown that a protocol-based approach with integrated safety criteria enhances the safety of mobilisation treatment. Daily re-evaluation and pre-defined individual daily therapy goals support successful and safe implementation [12].

21.6 What Else Needs to Be Considered

21.6.1 Barriers and Facilitators of Early Mobilisation

Barriers continue to exist in the early mobilisation of critically ill patients [3, 23]. These barriers can be categorised as patient-related barriers (e.g., physiological instability and medical devices), structural barriers (e.g., limited staff, financial resources, and equipment), procedural barriers (e.g., lack of coordination and delayed screening for eligibility), and cultural barriers (e.g., prior staff experience and ICU priorities for patient care) [23, 24]. Hospitals are generally encouraged to create the necessary personnel and material conditions to perform guideline-compliant early mobilisation [12]. Moreover, institutionalising early mobilisation can help reduce financial, personnel, and equipment-related barriers [23]. The active early mobilisation of ICU patients is a remarkably complex task, not only due to the severity of the patient's illness but also because these patients require numerous cables and tubes for monitoring and therapy, which translates into an increased amount of time for preparation and overall time spent with the patient (example in Fig. 21.7) [31]. Therefore, early mobilisation is not solely the responsibility of physiotherapists but the entire critical care team. Tasks should be adjusted and coordinated according to the expertise of each professional group, further highlighting the importance of optimal internal communication for effective collaboration within the interprofessional team [12]. It is advisable to use a structure or protocol adapted to the individual ICU that allows for algorithm-based mobilisation goals, including an opportunity for all team members to raise concerns and ensure the flow of information regarding mobility goals and achievements across staff and over time [13,

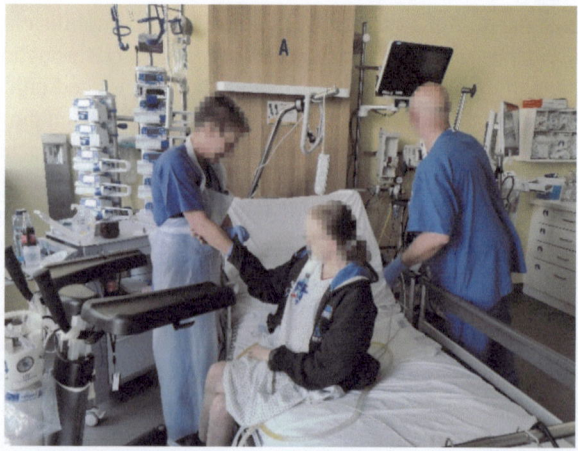

Fig. 21.7 Preparation of a Patient for Mobilisation

23]. It should be ensured that interprofessional team meetings (rounds) and interprofessional training occur regularly [24].

Other critical factors for successful implementation include the presence of experts or so-called "champions." Mobility champions can help develop a culture of prioritising mobilisation through leadership and communication skills to educate, train practical skills, coordinate, and promote patient mobilisation [24, 32]. They can support staff with an emphasis on safety and practical skills to improve the team's confidence and capabilities [32].

21.6.2 Additional Therapeutic Approaches in the Mobilisation and Treatment of Critically Ill Patients

The interventions to be considered include active functional mobilisation, in-bed cycle ergometry, electrical muscle stimulation (with or without passive/active exercises), tilt tables, and various rehabilitation equipment [33]. There is no benefit to adding in-bed cycling, electrical stimulation, or specific training formats in addition to a standardised early rehabilitation program [34, 35]. This highlights that functional exercises such as standing, sitting, or walking are the most effective exercises [6, 36]. However, technical aids such as in-bed cycle ergometry or muscle stimulation can provide alternatives when there are insufficient human resources [3].

21.7 Nutrition and Mobilisation

The combination of protein-rich nutritional therapy and exercise has become a recent focus in the critically ill, yet evidence remains limited [37]. Although it has often been studied separately in previous research, it is frequently performed combined in clinical practice. We still need to explore the mutual benefits of combined interventions of nutrition and exercise, which may augment gains in muscle mass, strength, and physical function in critical illness [37]. Caution is necessary, as the publication of the EFFORT trial revealed that providing protein to the acutely critically ill patient may have unintended negative consequences [38, 39]. The metabolic demands of exercise are poorly understood in the ICU setting. Recent research has highlighted significant heterogeneity in energy requirements between critically ill individuals undertaking the same functional activities [40]. Energy requirements are higher in the critically ill than healthy individuals [40]. Mobilisation and nutrition are interconnected, and the nutrient requirements depend on the activity's duration and intensity. It has been demonstrated that protein intake during or immediately after strength training increases muscle protein synthesis, but continuous protein intake can negate this physiological process due to the "muscle full effect" [41]. In this regard, intermittent nutrition in conjunction with resistance training can enhance protein turnover in critically ill patients [42]. The idea is that the combination of early mobilisation and early nutrition (within 72 h after ICU admission) may effectively increase muscle mass (or prevent its atrophy), enhance physical functioning and independence, and prevent ICUAW [43, 44]. The combined intervention might benefit nutritional status more than standard care and promote improvement in muscle strength [43]. In a similar approach, they found better muscle volume maintenance by combining high protein intake, early mobilisation, and electrical muscle stimulation. These findings only exist because a high protein delivery target provided greater benefits for muscle volume maintenance than medium protein delivery, but only when combined with active early rehabilitation and electrical muscle stimulation [45]. Further data from a single-centre study from Brazil compared high protein intake and resistance training using cycle ergometry. They suggested a positive impact on the physical quality of life and reduced mortality rates of critically ill patients [46]. These results will need further exploration in large multicentre trials.

The ICU population is highly heterogeneous in terms of admission diagnoses and comorbid health statuses, as well as pre-ICU health factors such as comorbidities, age, sex, and baseline nutritional status. These aspects impact the response to exercise and nutrition [47]. Therefore, an individualised approach considering different therapies and dosage levels of nutrition and mobilisation, as well as the overall condition of the patient, is sensible [37]. It is unlikely that one strategy alone will be successful in modifying this, but nutrition and exercise are likely to have an essential synergistic role [41].

In conclusion, procedural questions regarding the combination of training and nutrition still need to be answered in critically ill patients: What kind of protein (combination)? What dose of protein is optimal? Is the timing essential (continuous vs. bolus; before or after a training session)? What mobilisation and what mobilisation dose would show the best effectiveness in these combinations?

21.8 Summary

It can be concluded that performing mobilisation early after ICU admission is essential for successful treatment. Although firm conclusions cannot yet be drawn regarding the type, timing, or dose of early mobilisation, it is necessary to individualise the approach for each patient, considering their current medical condition and adjusting mobilisation therapy accordingly. Furthermore, goal-oriented and protocol-based therapy should be implemented, incorporating both passive and active elements. Including safety criteria for mobilisation in the protocol enhances the safety and feasibility of the treatment. Interprofessional collaboration is crucial to improve the implementation and safety of patient mobilisation. Therefore, regular meetings and interprofessional training should be emphasised. The use of technical aids, such as a bed bicycle or muscle stimulation, is not superior to functional training but might be helpful to alternatives if functional training is not possible.

Comment All patients provided written informed consent to use their pictures for this publication.

References

1. Rawal G, Yadav S, Kumar R. Post-intensive care syndrome: an overview. J Transl Int Med. 2017;5(2):90–2.
2. Herridge MS, Tansey CM, Matte A, Tomlinson G, Diaz-Granados N, Cooper A, et al. Functional disability 5 years after acute respiratory distress syndrome. N Engl J Med. 2011;364(14):1293–304.
3. Fuest K, Schaller SJ. Early mobilisation on the intensive care unit: what we know. Med Klin Intensivmed Notfmed. 2019;114(8):759–64.
4. Investigators TS, the ACTG, Hodgson CL, Bailey M, Bellomo R, Brickell K, et al. Early active mobilization during mechanical ventilation in the ICU. N Engl J Med. 2022;387(19):1747–58.
5. Fazzini B, Markl T, Costas C, Blobner M, Schaller SJ, Prowle J, et al. The rate and assessment of muscle wasting during critical illness: a systematic review and meta-analysis. Crit Care. 2023;27(1):2.
6. Lang JK, Paykel MS, Haines KJ, Hodgson CL. Clinical practice guidelines for early mobilization in the ICU: a systematic review. Crit Care Med. 2020;48(11):e1121–e8.
7. Schaller SJ, Scheffenbichler FT, Bein T, Blobner M, Grunow JJ, Hamsen U, et al. Guideline on positioning and early mobilisation in the critically ill by an expert panel. Intensive Care Med. 2024;50(8):1211–27.
8. Ding N, Zhang Z, Zhang C, Yao L, Yang L, Jiang B, et al. What is the optimum time for initiation of early mobilization in mechanically ventilated patients? A network meta-analysis. PLoS One. 2019;14(10):e0223151.
9. Tipping CJ, Harrold M, Holland A, Romero L, Nisbet T, Hodgson CL. The effects of active mobilisation and rehabilitation in ICU on mortality and function: a systematic review. Intensive Care Med. 2017;43(2):171–83.
10. Schweickert WD, Pohlman MC, Pohlman AS, Nigos C, Pawlik AJ, Esbrook CL, et al. Early physical and occupational therapy in mechanically ventilated, critically ill patients: a randomised controlled trial. Lancet. 2009;373(9678):1874–82.
11. Hodgson CL, Stiller K, Needham DM, Tipping CJ, Harrold M, Baldwin CE, et al. Expert consensus and recommendations on safety criteria for active mobilization of mechanically ventilated critically ill adults. Crit Care. 2014;18(6):658.
12. Schaller SJCSM. Lagerungstherapie und Mobilisation von kritisch Erkrankten auf Intensivstationen. In: (DGAI) DGfAuIeV, editor. S3-Leitlinie AWMF; 2023.
13. Schaller SJ, Anstey M, Blobner M, Edrich T, Grabitz SD, Gradwohl-Matis I, et al. Early, goal-directed mobilisation in the surgical intensive care unit: a randomised controlled trial. Lancet. 2016;388(10052):1377–88.
14. Schaller SJ, Stauble CG, Suemasa M, Heim M, Duarte IM, Mensch O, et al. The German validation study of the surgical intensive care unit optimal mobility score. J Crit Care. 2016;32:201–6.
15. Schaller SJ, Scheffenbichler FT, Bose S, Mazwi N, Deng H, Krebs F, et al. Influence of the initial level of consciousness on early, goal-directed mobilization: a post hoc analysis. Intensive Care Med. 2019;45(2):201–10.
16. Presneill JJ, Bellomo R, Brickell K, Buhr H, Gabbe BJ, Gould DW, Harrold M, Higgins AM, Hurford S, Iwashyna T, Neto AS, Nichol A, Schaller SJ, Sivasuthan J, Tipping C, Webb S, Young P, Hodgson CL. Protocol and statistical analysis plan for the phase 3 randomised controlled Treatment of Invasively Ventilated Adults with Early Activity and Mobilisation (TEAM III) trial. Crit Care Resusc. 2021;23(3):262–72. https://search.informit.org/doi/10.3316/informit.148294150680332.
17. Hodgson CL, Bailey M, Bellomo R, Berney S, Buhr H, Denehy L, Gabbe B, Harrold M, Higgins A, Iwashyna TJ, Papworth R, Parke R, Patman S, Presneill J, Saxena M, Skinner E, Tipping C, Young P, Webb S; Trial of Early Activity and Mobilization Study Investigators. A Binational Multicenter Pilot Feasibility Randomized Controlled Trial of Early Goal-Directed Mobilization in the ICU. Crit Care Med. 2016;44(6):1145–52. https://doi.org/10.1097/CCM.0000000000001643. PMID: 26968024.

18. Klem HE, Tveiten TS, Beitland S, Malerod S, Kristoffersen DT, Dalsnes T, et al. Early activity in mechanically ventilated patients – a meta-analysis. Tidsskr Nor Laegeforen. 2021;141(8). https://doi.org/10.4045/tidsskr.20.0351.
19. Worraphan S, Thammata A, Chittawatanarat K, Saokaew S, Kengkla K, Prasannarong M. Effects of inspiratory muscle training and early mobilization on weaning of mechanical ventilation: a systematic review and network meta-analysis. Arch Phys Med Rehabil. 2020;101(11):2002–14.
20. Patel BK, Wolfe KS, Patel SB, Dugan KC, Esbrook CL, Pawlik AJ, et al. Effect of early mobilisation on long-term cognitive impairment in critical illness in the USA: a randomised controlled trial. Lancet. Respir Med. 2023;11:563.
21. Nydahl P, Sricharoenchai T, Chandra S, Kundt FS, Huang M, Fischill M, et al. Safety of patient mobilization and rehabilitation in the intensive care unit. Systematic review with meta-analysis. Ann Am Thorac Soc. 2017;14(5):766–77.
22. Morris PE, Goad A, Thompson C, Taylor K, Harry B, Passmore L, et al. Early intensive care unit mobility therapy in the treatment of acute respiratory failure. Crit Care Med. 2008;36(8):2238–43.
23. Bakhru RN, McWilliams DJ, Wiebe DJ, Spuhler VJ, Schweickert WD. Intensive care unit structure variation and implications for early mobilization practices. An international survey. Ann Am Thorac Soc. 2016;13(9):1527–37.
24. Dubb R, Nydahl P, Hermes C, Schwabbauer N, Toonstra A, Parker AM, et al. Barriers and strategies for early mobilization of patients in intensive care units. Ann Am Thorac Soc. 2016;13(5):724–30.
25. Paton M, Lane R, Paul E, Cuthbertson GA, Hodgson CL. Mobilization during critical illness: a higher level of mobilization improves health status at 6 months, a secondary analysis of a prospective cohort study. Crit Care Med. 2021;49(9):e860–e9.
26. Winkelman C, Sattar A, Momotaz H, Johnson KD, Morris P, Rowbottom JR, et al. Dose of early therapeutic mobility: does frequency or intensity matter? Biol Res Nurs. 2018;20(5):522–30.
27. Scheffenbichler FT, Teja B, Wongtangman K, Mazwi N, Waak K, Schaller SJ, et al. Effects of the level and duration of mobilization therapy in the surgical ICU on the loss of the ability to live independently: an international prospective cohort study. Crit Care Med. 2021;49(3):e247–e57.
28. Fuest KE, Ulm B, Daum N, Lindholz M, Lorenz M, Blobner K, et al. Clustering of critically ill patients using an individualized learning approach enables dose optimization of mobilization in the ICU. Crit Care. 2023;27(1):1.
29. Bernhardt J, Churilov L, Ellery F, Collier J, Chamberlain J, Langhorne P, et al. Prespecified dose-response analysis for A Very Early Rehabilitation Trial (AVERT). Neurology. 2016;86(23):2138–45.
30. Hodgson CL, Kho ME, da Silva VM. To mobilise or not to mobilise: is that the right question? Intensive Care Med. 2023;49:1000.
31. Benjamin E, Roddy L, Giuliano KK. Management of patient tubes and lines during early mobility in the intensive care unit. Hum Factors Healthc. 2022;2:2.
32. Parry SM, Remedios L, Denehy L, Knight LD, Beach L, Rollinson TC, et al. What factors affect implementation of early rehabilitation into intensive care unit practice? A qualitative study with clinicians. J Crit Care. 2017;38:137–43.
33. Hodgson CL, Schaller SJ, Nydahl P, Timenetsky KT, Needham DM. Ten strategies to optimize early mobilization and rehabilitation in intensive care. Crit Care. 2021;25(1):324.
34. Fossat G, Baudin F, Courtes L, Bobet S, Dupont A, Bretagnol A, et al. Effect of in-bed leg cycling and electrical stimulation of the quadriceps on global muscle strength in critically ill adults: a randomized clinical trial. JAMA. 2018;320(4):368–78.
35. Eggmann S, Verra ML, Luder G, Takala J, Jakob SM. Effects of early, combined endurance and resistance training in mechanically ventilated, critically ill patients: a randomised controlled trial. PLoS One. 2018;13(11):e0207428.

36. Waldauf P, Jiroutkova K, Krajcova A, Puthucheary Z, Duska F. Effects of rehabilitation interventions on clinical outcomes in critically ill patients: systematic review and meta-analysis of randomized controlled trials. Crit Care Med. 2020;48(7):1055–65.
37. Chapple LS, Parry SM, Schaller SJ. Attenuating muscle mass loss in critical illness: the role of nutrition and exercise. Curr Osteoporos Rep. 2022;20(5):290–308.
38. Haines RW, Granholm A, Puthucheary Z, Day AG, Bear DE, Prowle JR, et al. The effect of high protein dosing in critically ill patients: an exploratory, secondary Bayesian analyses of the EFFORT Protein trial. Br J Anaesth. 2024;133:1192.
39. Heyland DK, Patel J, Compher C, Rice TW, Bear DE, Lee ZY, et al. The effect of higher protein dosing in critically ill patients with high nutritional risk (EFFORT Protein): an international, multicentre, pragmatic, registry-based randomised trial. Lancet. 2023;401(10376):568–76.
40. Black C, Grocott M, Singer M. The oxygen cost of rehabilitation interventions in mechanically ventilated patients: an observational study. Physiotherapy. 2020;107:169–75. https://doi.org/10.1016/j.physio.2019.06.008. Epub 2019 Jul 2. PMID: 32026817.
41. Bear DE, Parry SM, Puthucheary ZA. Can the critically ill patient generate sufficient energy to facilitate exercise in the ICU? Curr Opin Clin Nutr Metab Care. 2018;21(2):110–5.
42. Arabi YM, Casaer MP, Chapman M, Heyland DK, Ichai C, Marik PE, et al. The intensive care medicine research agenda in nutrition and metabolism. Intensive Care Med. 2017;43(9):1239–56.
43. Zhou W, Yu L, Fan Y, Shi B, Wang X, Chen T, et al. Effect of early mobilization combined with early nutrition on acquired weakness in critically ill patients (EMAS): a dual-center, randomized controlled trial. PLoS One. 2022;17(5):e0268599.
44. Heyland DK, Day A, Clarke GJ, Hough CT, Files DC, Mourtzakis M, et al. Nutrition and Exercise in Critical Illness Trial (NEXIS Trial): a protocol of a multicentred, randomised controlled trial of combined cycle ergometry and amino acid supplementation commenced early during critical illness. BMJ Open. 2019;9(7):e027893.
45. Nakamura K, Nakano H, Naraba H, Mochizuki M, Takahashi Y, Sonoo T, et al. High protein versus medium protein delivery under equal total energy delivery in critical care: a randomized controlled trial. Clin Nutr. 2021;40(3):796–803.
46. de Azevedo JRA, Lima HCM, Frota P, Nogueira I, de Souza SC, Fernandes EAA, et al. High-protein intake and early exercise in adult intensive care patients: a prospective, randomized controlled trial to evaluate the impact on functional outcomes. BMC Anesthesiol. 2021;21(1):283.
47. Amundadottir OR, Jonasdottir RJ, Sigvaldason K, Jonsdottir H, Moller AD, Dean E, et al. Predictive variables for poor long-term physical recovery after intensive care unit stay: an exploratory study. Acta Anaesthesiol Scand. 2020;64(10):1477–90.

Ethical Challenges of Artificial Nutrition in Intensive Care: Navigating the Borders Between Self-Determination, Authenticity, and Best Interest

Norbert W. Paul

22.1 Introduction

Quite some time ago and almost forgotten, the internationally discussed case of Terri Schiavo triggered a remarkable amount of medical attention [1, 2] on the issue of total parenteral nutrition, which is still widely discussed in public—often emotionally and controversially [9]. When it comes to the pros and cons of total parenteral nutrition, especially in intensive care, physicians and nurses tend to have strong opinions that are rooted in moral concepts that reflect on how to deal with the issue based on everyday morality. The same holds true, however, for other forms of (artificial) nutrition in intensive care settings.[1] Nasogastric tubes are often discussed in the context of discomfort while tubes applied by percutaneous endoscopic gastrostomy (PEG-tubes) often trigger debates on the prolongation of life at the actual end of life or—more general—against the background of medical futility. Neither recent case law nor legislative acts did so far ameliorate the situation mainly because they do not help to (and do not intend to) evaluate ongoing individual cases and acute situated decision-making. The third amendment to the German *Betreuungsrecht* (Care Act) from 2009 [5] specifies the decisive role of the will of the patient, which may also be expressed by an authorized representative, an agent, or a legal proxy as the linchpin of decisions on therapeutic aims. In this context, the supreme court of Germany (Bundesgerichtshof, in short BGH) issued several verdicts regarding the termination of artificial nutrition of a highly dependent and demented patients,

---

[1] Artificial or clinical nutrition often also called nutritional therapy includes oral, enteral and parenteral ways of artificial feeding.

N. W. Paul (✉)
Universitätsmedizin Mainz, Institute for the History, Theory and Ethics of Medicine, Mainz, Germany
e-mail: norbert.paul@uni-mainz.de

starting with a highly controversial case of the transection of the PEG-tube of a demented mother by her daughter on 25 June 2010 (2 StR 454/09, Karlsruhe). The legislation of the German Federal Court of Justice (BGH) and subsequent amendments place the weighting of prolonging life and prolonging suffering exclusively in the hands of patients, their representatives, or their legal proxies. However, the definition of the medically indicated options for diagnosis and treatment remains the task of the physician. The question of whether medical expertise or a close personal relationship is the decisive factor for the prolongation of nutrition is thus complicated. A ruling by the German Federal Supreme Court (Bundesgerichtshof, BGH) underlined the fact that medical professions and their indications can play the leading role in deciding whether or not to prolong the life of a (suffering) patient by means of artificial nutrition, even for several years. In this case, a son sued his father's doctor because his father, who was suffering from dementia, was kept alive for several years by means of artificial nutrition in a subjectively distressing state. The Federal Court of Justice (BGH) ruled that the doctor could not be held responsible for the continuation of artificial nutrition, even though the legal representative had not been involved in the decision-making process. The Federal Court of Justice stated that the prolongation of life could not be understood as harm to the patient or to others, such as the patient's family (Federal Court of Justice judgement of 2 April 2019, VI ZR 13/18). This verdict created an uncertainty among medical professionals. As a consequence, medical practice has become more "defensive," neglecting or hesitating to withdraw life-prolonging measures and particularly forms of nutrition which are often understood to be "only" caring for the fundamental physical needs, even in the case of futility. It is precisely at this point that ethical reflection is on demand.

In light of the legal uncertainty, it is important to emphasize that in situations in which the patient's long-term survival can only be ensured through the long-term use of artificial nutrition, decisions about therapeutic goals are not only based on the medical indication, but also have to take into account specific ethical dimensions. These dimensions must be addressed in a participatory process [20] which acknowledges the decisive role of a patient's will, often communicated by legal proxies, relatives or in advanced directives. In contrast to questions of everyday morality, a theoretically and methodologically well-founded clinical ethics must examine legitimacy and justifiability because of universal ethical principles and norms [13] against the background of possible courses of action and taking into account evaluative [19] and normative aspects of each case.

In post-war Anglo-Saxon medical ethics, the principle of patient self-determination and autonomy became the linchpin of decision-making, overcoming the now outdated paternalistic doctor-patient relationship [10] in favor of a cooperative doctor-patient relationship, in which the doctor as medical expert is in a symmetrical relationship with the patient as expert in life-world goals and values, guided by a self-determined will. This is now the gold standard in most Western health care systems. In addition, several constructs of the presumed will of incapacitated patients have been given considerable scope for interpretation, both ethically and legally. Of relevance to issues of nutrition in intensive care settings particularly in the light of futility are the current expressed will of the patient who has sufficient capacity, the previously expressed will of incapacitated patients, often recorded in the patient's will, the expressed will of an authorized representative or agent, and the presumed will, often derived from earlier life decisions. In the following, we will discuss where, from an ethical point of view, the boundaries between different concepts of the patient's will in relation to artificial nutrition for intensive care patients play a significant role. This includes practices of assessing the personal value systems of a patient and his or her significant others in ensuring the patient's best interests. Finally, it needs to be discussed how the physician's role can be reconciled with the patient's self-determination in which form ever.

22.2 Forms of Self-Determination and Some Critical Remarks on the Concept of Autonomy

22.2.1 Definitions

Autonomous will of a patient is ideally based on information and individual (rational) deliberation, is related to personal value systems, and is freely formed and expressed in the context of medical decision-making. It can take many forms (e.g., gestural, verbal, or written). In the clinical context, it must always be ensured that the patient, who is sufficiently capable of reasoning, is able to form his convictions based on comprehensive and extensive information. This requirement already raises questions about the concept of autonomy: How autonomous are children and adolescents? Where are the limits of psycho-cognitive competence that are essential for self-determination (for example, in the case of dementia or intellectual limitations) [18]? What personal burdens experienced in the course of the illness (fear, despair, anger) do influence or hamper our free will? What are the intellectual capacities needed to build an adequate "breadth and depth" of knowledge, medical indications, and their consequences?

In the context of advance care planning and advance directives, a previously *expressed will* formulated in anticipation of a situation that has not yet occurred is also considered autonomous, if it meets the above criteria. It is often not clear whether the writer has made the expressed will after rational reflection and in an informed and independent manner, given the form and content of the patient's instructions. Ultimately, an incapacitated patient's agent or guardian (since the patient's incapacity is the precondition for applying the patient's advance decision in the first place) decides whether the document is applicable to individual living and treatment conditions.

The *presumed will* is an expression of the patient's beliefs if he or she were able to do so and is therefore a matter of best judgement. So, the presumed will does not exist "naturally" but must be investigated. Usually, this exploration is done by reference to narratives. Narrative accounts of the patient's life, his or her value system, previous life decisions (especially regarding health and illness), and reports and assessments from loved ones form the basis for establishing presumed will. As with any interpretation, even a thorough one, there is an inherent danger that the presumed will projects one's own or others' assumptions and beliefs onto the presumed wishes of the patient.

Especially authorized representatives or agents, who are simultaneously advocating the patient's wishes and are close to him, frequently face the problem of overlaying the patient's presumed will with personal emotions or interests. Oftentimes it is unascertainable in how far volitions claimed by representatives correspond to the patient's desires or whether they are biased by the representative's value-systems, convictions, emotions, and interests. Therefore, the avoidance of misuse of warrants plays a decisive ethical and legal role in clinical contexts.

22.2.2 Critical Remarks on the Concept of Autonomy

Aside from these rather structural limitations of the concept of patient autonomy, some conceptual borders, which are of particular interest in case of questions of life support and nutrition, need to be discussed. The first difficulty results from the requirement of knowledgeability when forming a self-determined will. Particularly those patient's provisions which have been composed without lived experience regarding end-of-life situations oftentimes waive unwanted treatments (97.8%) and explicitly waive parenteral nutrition (98.9%), as studies have shown [16]. Sometimes, however, this decision is triggered by experiences or on reports of hearsay from the patient's personal environment. Comprehensive clarification of the indication of parenteral or otherwise supported nutrition, its different procedures (including the combination of procedures of parenteral nutrition and enteral nutrition), indication of the adjustment of supported nutrition and so on, does usually not form the basis of this decision. In contrary, to be nourished is understood as one of the most natural and often delightful processes in human life and artificial nutrition is often understood as a significant loss of autonomy and quality of life. This impact of lay perceptions is not surprising, since according to [16], only 7.3% in a sample of respondents stated that they had support of a physician in their composition of a patient's provision. Thus, after the commencement of the third amendment to the German National Care Act (Betreuungsrecht) statements such as "I don't want to be attached to any tubes at any point" or "I want every available medical treatment (except parenteral nutrition) as long as there is still hope for me, otherwise I request to die in a humane and dignified manner" are fully valid in Germany, despite the fact that they leave much room for interpretation. Therefore, it needs to be resumed that in dealing with patient's provisions, legal certainty, which helps the patient's will to fully develop, has apparently been established but the applicability is limited by (a) a lack of knowledge and personal experience with end-of-life situations, (b) abstinence from professional medical support in formulation advance directives, and (c) relatively reduced statements with regard to values and beliefs being the driving forces behind the directives. How far this declared will is attuned to the scope of the decision and based on information and reflection can still only be assumed. Thus, preference needs to be given to patients' current and informed decisions for or against treatments including nutrition in each individual case. Even though in some cases these decisions may not comply with the ideal of informed, rational decision-making rooted in the concept of autonomy, the decision's authenticity can often be established in direct conversations. As has already been outlined, this may also be one of the central issues in the case of volition by authorized representatives and/or agents. For this reason, the additional reconstruction of the patient's presumed will should always be brought into consideration alongside the representatives' reports.

A more subtle problem is rooted in the apparent disembodiment of the concept of autonomy. Particularly, the notion that nutrition is a natural, joyful, and very individual act of a person does challenge (rationally justified) concepts of autonomy [6]. Ingestion not only serves to cover our daily physiological need, but is also related to lust or disgust, pleasure or aversion, and always refers to (possibly new) experiences pertaining to the life-world and to social participation. Decisions by patients and/or of authorized representatives and agents are thus always placed within the context of a subjective corporal-bodily world of experience, which is rarely explicitly included into clinical-ethical considerations. The reason for this neglect may lie within the methodological uncertainty of dealing with a phenomenon, which can only be accessed via narratives—if narratibility is established. This interpretative access is thus always context-bound and can only be situatively developed. Nevertheless, especially the thematization of the subjective, bodily dimension, which for the patient is related to different ways of ingestion, may contribute to protecting the decisions' authenticity (see below).

22.3 Authenticity, Best Interest, and Healthcare

As the previous discussion shows, the patient's expressed will, sometimes through a proxy, must be accompanied by further ethical considerations to ensure that the decision for or against parenteral nutrition represents the patient's best interest, both in terms of treatment and therapeutic goals. However, medical care should not define the best interest of the patient in terms of a professional and generalizable judgement alone. Particularly, weighting the opportunity costs [7] of supported or parenteral nutrition and the achievable "quality-adjusted life years" (QUALYS) would inevitably lead to neo-paternalism and an unacceptable asymmetry in the doctor-patient relationship, resulting in a clear shift within the power of interpretation to the detriment of the patient. The main reason is a silent shift from an individualized approach in appreciation of the person the patient is to a more utilitarian approach. This has been demonstrated in a case of the Federal Court of Justice (BHG judgement of 2 April 2019, VI ZR 13/18). From an ethical standpoint, the process of defining therapeutic aims is adequate, when it is situated, individually adjusted, based within the patient's value-system and when patient or representative adopt the expert role in what pertains to the life world and thus assess the life- and treatment situation. This position poses the difficulty that accepting the role in the decision-making process (role-making) is accompanied by basic requirements directed at the holder of this position (role-taking). Artificial nutrition and hydration in clinical settings thus need guidelines. Druml et al. [8] provided a valuable guideline for shared decision-making beyond existing consensus papers. Right at the beginning the authors state that "This guideline provides a critical summary for caregivers in regard to the ethics of artificial nutrition and hydration therapy" ([8]:546). While this is tremendously helpful, the ethical argumentation hinges (only) on the four principles of biomedical ethics as championed by Beauchamp and Childress [3]. From a clinical ethics perspective, therefore, the paper does not address the limits of autonomy beyond the specific conditions required for informed decision-making.

This is where the concept of authenticity comes into play. Authenticity has unfortunately long since been neglected in most approaches to clinical ethics, partly because decision-making beyond informed consent is often equaled with medico-legal or forensic risk. From an ethical perspective, though, the authenticity of a decision can be used as a criterion in an individual case if it is understood normatively and not perceived according to a model of personal conformity, i.e., if a person's actions or statements are in accordance with his or her intentions. Rather, authenticity needs to be understood as an epistemological term in this context. Perceived in such an evaluative manner, authenticity means that a person's decisions or intentional actions provide information about the person's stances and attitudes toward the overall goal of the decision and/or the therapy—if one will in a hermeneutical manner. The difficulty lies in the distinction between intentional and unintentional actions. This problem is reflected in the debate about whether the repeated refusal of food by people with dementia is to be understood as an intentional act, and thus as a form of natural volition, or as an under reflected, situated aversion. The problem is exacerbated in the case of patients whose individual intentions are unknown and whose interests are expressed exclusively by authorized representatives or agents. Typically, this problem arises in the case of neonates and infants and regularly results in an almost indistinguishable overlap between the intentions of the parents and the (presumed) best interests of the child. Similarly, decisions supported by legal proxies of dementia patients may be biased on the one hand by the interests or emotions of those who are supposed to speak for the patient, or simply by a lack of knowledge of the patient's life story in those frequent cases where elderly people without family or friends become incapacitated and are supported—in most Western countries—by a professional legal proxy. From the perspective of clinical ethics, however, the best evaluative approach to this issue is to develop the differences and similarities between the personal best interest and the best interest of the patient, a process often based on narrative methods and evaluations. Reconstructive clinical ethics is based on this kind of "contextual reconstruction" and has been quite successful in distinguishing the best interests and presumed will of patients from the assumptions, interests, and emotions of their (legal) representatives.

22.4 Nutrition, Prolongation of Life, and Prolongation of Suffering

One of the most difficult areas of ethics is the moral intuition that often arises in the context of assisted or artificial nutrition. Not infrequently, relatives or caregivers express the opinion that the patient would not live a "worthwhile" or "dignified" life. This position aims to balance the protection of life against the protection of dignity, which also seems problematic given history of abusive euthanasia during the Nazi regime in Germany [4]. The extent to which a patient is merely alive but not a participant in life is often almost impossible to judge from the outside and should therefore not be the subject of medical or nursing considerations. The assessment of an individual's quality of life is a highly personal consideration, or at least an individual's perception, and can only exceptionally be transferred to a person familiar with the individual's values and life choices.

Nevertheless, the extent to which prolonging life primarily means prolonging suffering, or merely prolonging suffering [12], can and should be critically examined from the perspective of a physician and/or nurse. It must also be considered whether the measures taken (e.g., parenteral nutrition) are suitable to make a preventive, curative, or palliative contribution to the therapeutic goal and the treatment goal, whether curative or palliative [11]. There are usually three options for such an indication for artificial nutrition based on the overall therapeutic goal:

1. When artificial nutrition is essential to maintain life in the context of an overriding curative or palliative therapeutic goal, it is medically indicated and its desirability and applicability assessed in collaboration with the patient or their representative.
2. The desirability and applicability of artificial nutrition should be assessed in cooperation with the patient or his representative, weighing the prolongation of life against the prolongation of suffering, if nutrition is provided solely for the purpose of maintaining life without any other reason for treatment [17].
3. If measures of artificial nutrition serve to maintain life without achieving additional curative or palliative therapeutic goals, they can only be justified from a palliative perspective and should be evaluated for their ability to alleviate suffering in cooperation with the patient or his representative according to their desirability and applicability.

It would be going too far at this point to explore the concept of dignity in depth. Suffice to say, though, that in addition to the dignity that is intrinsic to each human being and is based on their existence and being (ontic dignity), there is also a phenomenological source of dignity that takes the subject and their sense of self, which even may rest on a minimal cognitive state, as the starting point for ethical reflection, and a dignity that takes as a reflexive source the continuous "updating" of the subject on the basis of their values. Therefore, taking into account actualized value systems and choices, as well as the indication of parenteral nutrition, which, in the case of cognitive limitations, is linked to a minimal sense of self and capacity to suffer, always contributes to the recognition and development of the patient's dignity. It is the reciprocal, valid realization of the human encounter at the bedside that ultimately feeds the relational source of dignity in medical and nursing practice.

22.5 Conclusions for Clinical Practice

With regard to the indication of artificial nutrition, medical problem-solving is faced with the challenge of reflexively incorporating into the decision-making process the ethical dimensions of physicians' actions, which are publicly discussed and charged with personal value systems.

The same applies in the context of the seeming supremacy of the personal or representative will of the person concerned and the reconstructive, presumptive will of the person concerned. A constant contextualization and possible re-evaluation of the patient's will against the background of the given life and treatment situation is required due to the pragmatic and systematic limitations of the concept of autonomy. The methods of clinical ethics that have now been established for this purpose have only recently become part of the training of doctors and nurses, and this is not the case everywhere. Where there is no clear authority for clinical ethics and no specific authority—such as a theoretically and methodologically well-founded ethics committee—is available, a systematic examination of the following aspects can be a helpful guide for the layperson in clinical ethics:

1. Reconstruction: The reconstruction of the treatment situation should, in addition to medical facts, always include the social background and the culturally influenced value-system of a contextualized evaluation.
2. Analysis: The analysis of all treatment options (including those which are immediately declined) should, in addition to the critical assessment of individual competence in the treatment application, also comprise principles and norms to evaluate courses of action. The following questions are of major interest: Does the treatment result in additional suffering, which could have been avoided or is the treatment and its additional strain inevitable in order to prevent greater suffering and harm? Which volition expresses the patient, or by their authorized representative or agent, with reference to the viable options? Can the procedures be executed according to need and performance?
3. Critical evaluation: Ultimately, the normative evaluation of treatments of parenteral nutrition needs to assess the treatment's applicability, desirability, and justifiability against the backdrop of the information gathered in step 1 and 2.
4. Application: Finally, a concept of implementation needs to be developed which, whether parenteral nutrition is executed or not, includes the patient's preferences, the aims and limits of medical care and especially the subjective, culturally and socially influenced perception of suffering and alleviation, which is also tied to the body, into the situative evaluation and implementation of the therapeutic strategy.

In conclusion, parenteral nutrition poses specific ethical challenges to medical and nursing decision-making and performance. Expertise in clinical ethics is therefore particularly desirable but is currently not available in all places. This is most notably true for the availability of clinical ethics services in institutions for the elderly or in the context of outpatient and ambulatory care. The heuristic developed from the broad theoretical debate on reconstructive ethics and integrative particularism can help to make a medically reasonable, ethically justifiable, and socially desirable decision for or against parenteral nutrition in each individual case, with regard to the ethical dimensions outlined here, namely, the ethical dimensions of autonomy, authenticity of decisions, best interests of the patient, and medical and nursing care, which can make a decisive contribution to the endowment of dignity.

References

1. Ankermann E. Verlängerung sinnlos gewordenen Lebens? Zur rechtlichen Situation von Koma-Patienten. Medizinrecht. 1999;17:387–92.
2. Annas GJ. 'Culture of life' politics at the bedside: the case of Terri Schiavo. NEJM. 2005;352:1710–5.
3. Beauchamp TL, Childress JF. Principles of biomedical ethics. Oxford: Oxford University Press; 1989 and following editions.
4. Binding K, Hoche A. Die Freigabe der Vernichtung lebensunwerten Lebens. Leipzig: Ihr Maß und ihre Form; 1920.
5. Borasio GD, Heßler H-J, Wiesing U. Patientenverfügungsgesetz: Umsetzung in der klinischen Praxis. Dtsch Arztebl. 2009;106/40:A1952/B1675/C1643.
6. Böttcher B, Paul NW. Personale Autonomie: Diskussion eines zentralen ethischen Konzepts am Beispiel von fertilitätsprotektiven Maßnahmen bei Krebspatientinnen. Ethik in der Medizin. 2012. https://doi.org/10.1007/s00481-012-0186-8. Published online on 12 February 2012.
7. Callahan CM, Buchanan NN, Stump TE. Healthcare costs associated with percutaneous endoscopic gastrostomy among older adults in a defindes community. Am Geraitr Soc. 2001;49:1525–9.
8. Druml C, Ballmer PE, Druml W, Oehmichen F, Shenkin A, Singer P, Soeters P, Weimann A, Bischoff SC. ESPEN guideline on ethical aspects of artificial nutrition and hydration. Clin Nutr. 2016;35(3):545–56.
9. Gjerdingen DK, Neff JA, Wang M, Chaloner K. Older persons' opinions about life-sustaining procedures in the face of dementia. Arch Fam Med. 1999;8:421–5.
10. Krones T, Richter G. Die Arzt-Patient-Beziehung. In: Schulz S, Steigleder K, Fangerau H, Paul NW, editors. Geschichte, Theorie und Ethik der Medizin: Eine Einführung. Frankfurt/M: Suhrkamp; 2006. p. 94–116.
11. Lorenzl S. Flüssigkeit und Ernährung am Lebensende. Entscheidungsfindung und medizinisch-ethische Problembereiche. Z Med Ethik. 2010;56:121–30.
12. Oehmichen F. Künstliche Ernährung bis zum Lebensende? Berl Ärzte. 2001;6:21–3.
13. Paul NW. Klinische Ethikberatung: Therapieziele, Patientenwille und Entscheidungsprobleme in der modernen Medizin. In: Junginger T, Perneczky A, Vahl CF, Werner C, editors. Grenzsituationen der Intensivmedizin: Entscheidungsgrundlagen. Heidelberg: Springer; 2008. p. 207–17.
14. Paul NW. A closer look at health and disease as prerequisites for diagnosis and prognosis. Med Stud: Int J Hist Philos Ethics Med Allied Sci. 2010;2(2):95–100.
15. Paul NW. Clinical ethics counseling: therapeutic goals, the patient's will and decision-making problems in modern medicine. Formos J Med Humanit. 2010;11(1&2):19–36.

16. Paul NW, Fischer A. Patientenverfügung: Wahrnehmung und Wirklichkeit. Ergebnisse einer Befragung. Dtsch Med Wochenschr. 2008;133:175–9.
17. Schweidtmann W. Ethische Begründung und Grenzen der Ernährungstherapie bei onkologischen Patienten. Akt Ernähr Med. 2001;26:170–3.
18. Simon A. Ethische Aspekte der künstlichen Ernährung bei nichteinwilligungsfähigen Patienten. Ethik Med. 2004;16:211–6.
19. Synofzik M, Marckmann G. Sondenernährung. Die Bedeutung evaluativer Vorstellungen eines guten Lebens für die Entscheidungsfindung. Zeitschrift für medizinische Ethik. 2010;56:143–58.
20. Tolmein O. Die rechtlichen Rahmenbedingungen der sogenannten künstlichen Ernährung. Z Für Med Ethik. 2010;56(2):159–67.
21. Walensi M, Inthorn J, Paul NW. Willensfreiheit, Determinismus und die Abwägung eines vorab erklärten autonomen Willens im Falle einer natürlichen Willensäußerung. Int Z Philos Psychosom. 2016;1:1–16.

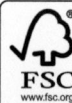

MIX
Papier aus verantwortungsvollen Quellen
Paper from responsible sources
FSC® C105338

If you have any concerns about our products,
you can contact us on
ProductSafety@springernature.com

In case Publisher is established outside the EU,
the EU authorized representative is:
Springer Nature Customer Service Center GmbH
Europaplatz 3, 69115 Heidelberg, Germany

Printed by Libri Plureos GmbH
in Hamburg, Germany